Hidden Terrors

HIDDEN TERRORS

The Scourge of Cholera in Jackson's America

by

PAUL KELTON

OXFORD
UNIVERSITY PRESS

OXFORD
UNIVERSITY PRESS

Oxford University Press is a department of the University of Oxford.
It furthers the University's objective of excellence in research, scholarship,
and education by publishing worldwide. Oxford is a registered trade mark of
Oxford University Press in the UK and in certain other countries.

Published in the United States of America by Oxford University Press
546 Fifth Avenue, New York, NY 10036, United States of America.

Library of Congress Cataloging-in-Publication Data
Names: Kelton, Paul author
Title: Hidden terrors : the scourge of cholera in Jackson's America / by Paul Kelton.
Description: [New York] : [Oxford University Press], [2026] | Includes
bibliographical references and index.
Identifiers: LCCN 2026007348 | ISBN 9780197772089 hardback |
ISBN 9780197772102 epub
Subjects: LCSH: Cholera—United States—History—19th century |
Cholera—Social aspects—United States—19th century
Classification: LCC RC131.A2 K45 2026
LC record available at https://lccn.loc.gov/2026007348

DOI: 10.1093/oso/9780197772089.001.0001

Printed by Sheridan Books, Inc., United States of America

The manufacturer's authorized representative in the EU for product safety is
Oxford University Press España S.A. of Parque Empresarial San Fernando de Henares,
Avenida de Castilla, 2 – 28830 Madrid (www.oup.es/en or product.safety@oup.com).
OUP España S.A. also acts as importer into Spain of products made by the manufacturer.

MIX
Paper | Supporting
responsible forestry
FSC® C008955
FSC
www.fsc.org

For Caroline, Bradley, and Katherine

Contents

Acknowledgments

SINCE 2017, I have been incredibly fortunate and grateful to have the support of the Robert David Lion Gardiner Foundation and Stony Brook University. I began this book during my first year at Stony Brook and could not have known at the time that I would be writing about a pandemic during a pandemic. The experience has been surreal, to say the least, and one that increased the necessity that all scholars typically face of relying on the help of others to complete our projects.

Librarians and archivists at the repositories where I conducted research deserve more appreciation than I can give. Special thanks go to the staff at the following: Western History Collection at the University of Oklahoma, Helmerich Center for American Research at the University of Tulsa, Kansas State Historical Society, Houghton Library at Harvard University, Huntington Library, the Historical Society of Pennsylvania, Albert and Shirley Small Special Collections at the University of Virginia, Virginia Historical Society, the Library of Virginia, Southern History Collection at the University of North Carolina at Chapel Hill, Rubenstein Library at Duke University, Yale University libraries (Cushing/Whitney Medical, Sterling Memorial, and the Beinecke), Maryland Center for History and Culture, National Archives and Records Administration at College Park, Maryland, Filson Historical Society, William L. Clements Library at the University of Michigan, New Jersey State Archives, New Jersey Historical Society, Historical Society of Princeton, Firestone Library at Princeton University, Wright Library at Princeton Theological Seminary, Alexander Library at Rutgers University, the Historic New Orleans Collection, Hill Memorial Library at Louisiana State University, Howard-Tilton Memorial Library at Tulane University, Wilson Library at Millsaps College, Pennsylvania State Archives, Swem Library at the College of William and Mary, South Carolina Historical Society at the College of Charleston, General Theological Seminary, New York Historical Society,

New York Public Library, New York Society Library, Fales Library at New York University, Carl A. Kroch Library at Cornell University, Columbia University libraries (Campbell and Butler), Oneida County (NY) Historical Society, Fenimore Art Museum, and Bird Library at Syracuse University.

The staff at several archives I could not visit graciously responded to queries, tracked down sources, and promptly fulfilled duplication requests. Special thanks go to Conner Prairie, Metropolitan Government Archives of Nashville and Davidson County, Hodges Library at the University of Tennessee, Chester County (PA) History Center, Cincinnati Museum, Dolph Briscoe Center for American History at the University of Texas at Austin, Somerville (MA) Museum, Archdiocese of Boston, South Caroliniana Library at the University of South Carolina, Colonial Williamsburg Foundation, Rauner Library at Dartmouth College, Mississippi Department of Archives and History, New Orleans Public Library, Missouri Historical Society, and Miner Medical Library at Rochester University. Stony Brook University's Interlibrary Loan Department proved to be indispensable, and I thank them for going above and beyond in trying to get hard-to-obtain materials. I know that I am overlooking some and regret that the above list is not exhaustive of the dedicated professionals who have helped me and so many of my peers do the job we love to do.

As I worked to piece this book together, I consulted with several experts in subjects that have been relatively new to me. David Sack and John Booss tutored me on cholera's etiology and pathology; Joshua Rothman, Robert Gudmestad, and Calvin Schermerhorn explained the complexities of the domestic slave trade, as did Kari Winter, who generously shared photocopies of important letters; Kerby Miller, William Watson, and April Masten pointed me to source materials and insights on Irish immigration and labor history; Kristin O'Brassill-Kulfan and Donna Rilling helped me understand Philadelphia's urban environment. Claudio Saunt and Cristina Snyder graciously shared their knowledge of Choctaw removal and primary documents that were immensely helpful. David S. Jones, Paul Gilje, Gary Anderson, Jon Earle, Leslie Tuttle, Virgil Dean, Gregory Evans Dowd, Tai Edwards, Sarah Ahmedani, Sarah Jourdain, Paul Gootenberg, Sara Lipton, and David Wrobel have all steered me in constructive directions, and I appreciate their support and encouragement through the years.

Opportunities to present portions of my work at academic conferences and seminars have been crucial, and I appreciate comments, questions, and encouragement that I received from my fellow panelists and audience members. I benefited from the exchange of ideas with Angela Pulley Hudson,

Mikaëla Adams, Jacob Lee, and Sari Altschuler during a panel at the 2018 Organization of American Historians annual conference. I presented a long and clunky draft of what became several chapters at a session of the New York Academy of Medicine's History of Medicine and Health Working Group in March of 2020. There, I met Charles Rosenberg, whose classic work *The Cholera Years* had inspired me many years before to think about microbes as important historical actors. His response to my project proved invaluable, as did the comments of Nancy Tomes (who also arranged for me to present to the working group), David Barnes, Alix Cooper, and other participants. It was an honor to present at the NYU Atlantic History Workshop and obtain feedback from Nichole Eustace, Elizabeth Ellis, Elise Mitchell, Kevin Kenny, and others. Nick Wilson and Mohammad Ballan invited me to present portions of the work during the Initiative for Historical Social Science at Stony Brook University, where my generous colleagues in the history and sociology departments gave my scholarship critical attention in its final stages.

The production of this book would not have been possible without many people. Several research assistants not only accelerated the acquisition of sources but also helped me conceptualize the story I wanted to tell. Thank you, Alec Lurie, Nathan Greenhaw, Lance Boos, Kevin Murphy, Andrew Ehrinpreis, Kayla Huaranga, Bradley Kelton, and Katherine Kelton for all your invaluable aid. Erin Giuliano, Roxanne Fernandez, and Ming Huang, with unsurpassed professionalism and efficiency, managed the "paperwork" involved in making assistantships happen and getting research expenses paid.

I was fortunate to be introduced to Franchesca Rodriguez through Gil Jang of Stony Brook's Geospatial Center. Franchesca is an amazing mapmaker, and I appreciate her creativity and hard work. Kristy Adams proved not only to be an accomplished photographer but also did some skilled sleuthing to track down historical markers and monuments in New Jersey. Selina Bartlett (Allen Memorial Art Museum, Oberlin College), Laura Keim (Stenton Museum), Danielle Ullrich (Belmont Mansion), and Jack Green (Cocks Art Museum, Miami University of Ohio) provided timely assistance in obtaining reproductions of several portraits that are found in this book. Rada Radojicic of Oxford University Press and Ethiraju Saraswathi of Straive have been a joy to work with and have made this book much better.

The entire manuscript would not be what it has become without the careful attention of several people. Susan Ferber, my editor at Oxford University Press, provided encouragement from the beginning and focused her sharp editorial vision on each chapter, and for that I am grateful. Kyle Harper pushed me to amplify connections that I had not developed as well as they could have been. Vaughn Scribner identified many places of redundancy and verbosity, and I cannot thank him enough for his generous attention to the manuscript. Cynthia Yaudes produced an excellent index, and Cindy Angelini has skillfully edited the entire work. Susan, Kyle, Vaughn, Cynthia, and Cindy indeed made this book better, but any mistakes, omissions, or lack of clarity in my prose are entirely my own.

This book has been an eight-year project, and my family is probably happier than I am in its completion. When friends and visitors asked me what I was working on, my wife, Stephanie, son, Bradley, and daughters, Caroline and Katherine, often cringed as I launched into a discussion about cholera, a disease that few people want to hear details about, particularly at the dinner table. Thank you for your patience and understanding of how important it has been for me to tell a story that needs to be told. Stephanie, an accomplished author and scholar, always championed my work, provided her own critical read of key portions, and pushed me to be a better writer. But, most importantly, she encouraged me to join her on a fishing excursion or a walk around our neighborhood when I most needed a break. Caroline, Bradley, and Katherine all finished high school and began college as I worked on this book. The greatest joys of my life have been being a father to them and watching them mature into the remarkable young adults they have become. To them I dedicate this book.

Note on Sources

NINETEENTH-CENTURY MANUSCRIPT sources often do not follow modern conventions. Writers may have inconsistent spelling, grammar, and punctuation. Faded ink, torn pages, and difficult-to-read penmanship compound the problems. When quoting from these sources, I have made corrections to accord to modern usages for the ease of readers and to avoid the excessive and invasive insertion of "*sic*" into the text. Minor corrections to quotes from newspapers and other printed sources have been made in cases of spelling mistakes due to typesetting errors and in some cases in which the published words do not conform to modern conventions and contemporary American instead of English spelling, for example, "every one" instead of "everyone," "christian" instead of "Christian," and "labour" instead of "labor."

Introduction

"Great Heaven! how awful do I feel in contemplating the approach of cholera," Sarah Haynsworth Gayle confided in her diary. Gayle, Alabama's First Lady, made the entry on July 6, 1832, just two days after Tuscaloosa's *Spirit of the Age* announced that the "Asiatic Spasmodic Cholera" was raging in Canada. "In some places it has been more fatal than in England, nearly all dying who were attacked," the paper declared. The disease had arrived in Quebec in early June, quickly spread to Montreal, and appeared to be on its way to New York City. Forty people were dying daily in Quebec, where "this terrible malady progressed so rapidly, that death ensued from four to twelve hours." Gayle despaired at the terrible news. She called the disease "the Destroying Angel" and remarked, "my fears could not be more harrowing." While she took solace that her life was "in the hands of a good God," she ended her entry with foreboding. "There is no possibility that Alabama will escape the general scourge."[1]

Many other Americans revealed similar anxieties in their private journals and letters. Thomas Knight, a resident of a small New York town on Lake Ontario, described cholera in his diary as a "dreadful scourge" that "made its horrific appearance" in Canada. He added, "Its terror seems not to have diminished in its journey."[2] Elam Tilden of New Lebanon, New York, called cholera "a pestilence walking in darkness" and warned his son Samuel, the future governor of their state, that "there seems to be no safety anywhere."[3] Alfred Robinson of Williamsburg, Virginia, emphatically termed the disease a "*monster*" and told his brother in Richmond to expect an outbreak near him in the coming months.[4] Delila Hurd of New Bern, North Carolina, admitted that she "cannot reasonably hope to ever see all my friends again" and prepared "for the worst."[5]

Americans had good reason to be afraid as a global pandemic came their way. Throughout 1831 and the first half of 1832, US newspapers published international reports of cholera breaking out of South Asia, ravaging Eastern

Europe, spreading westward across the continent, and arriving on the British Isles. Descriptions of its victims experiencing ghastly symptoms—vomiting, explosive diarrhea, and painful spasms—filled these reports. The illness distorted the body, with victims turning blue, collapsing into an unresponsive state, and often perishing within twelve hours of first becoming sick. Victims might wake up healthy, eat a hearty breakfast, and go about their day, only to begin to feel ill by nightfall and not awaken the next morning. Theories circulated about the cause of the disease as well as why some people survived and others did not, but mystery and exoticism surrounded it.

Western Europeans and Americans had long called ordinary diarrhea "cholera," but the disease that had been devastating a vast swath of people was something different, a much more severe illness that required a distinguishing descriptor. Some called it "spasmodic" for its violent symptoms; some called it "Asiatic" or "Indian" for its supposed geographic origins; some called it "malignant" to indicate it was more severe than the usual diarrhea; others, such as the editors of *Spirit of the Age*, used a combination of descriptors. Whatever people called it, countless Asians and Europeans had succumbed to the disease before it arrived in Canada.

Many Americans, though, mocked those who let themselves become afraid of what was at best seen as exaggerated information and at worst fabricated accounts. One Yale student, Alexander Smith Johnson, informed his mother that he and his classmates were "not much alarmed" about the news from Canada. But some of their classmates were exceptions and deserved derision. These students, according to Johnson, came down with "newspaper symptoms of the disease," and one who went to the doctor with an ailment he thought was cholera "has been laughed at very much."[6] James Savage of Boston echoed Johnson. "All New York and New England is going mad," he wrote to a friend in Vermont. "But the first burst of terror to the ignorant," he claimed, would quickly disappear when the truth of the disease became more widely known. "The great nuisance of our country, the million and one newspapers, propagate lies in all directions," Savage declared, adding that only a few editors do not follow "the usual style of spreading false news."[7]

Other Americans tempered whatever fear they had with a belief in cholera's discriminating nature. The disease might be real, they assured each other, but it would spare native-born white Protestants. Jabez Colt of New York City admitted to his brother that "accounts from Canada are truly frightful" but pointed to the supposed fact that cholera found "fit subjects" only among Catholics—Irish immigrants and "filthy" French Canadians.[8]

Martha Randolph, daughter of the late Thomas Jefferson, read the "frightful accounts of the cholera at Quebec and Montreal" and became anxious about her daughter, Ellen Wayles Coolidge, and her son-in-law, Joseph Coolidge, Jr. Their New England residence, she thought, was too close to the growing calamity, and she wanted them to join her in Washington, DC.[9] "Believe me, and not for worlds would I deceive you," her son-in-law wrote back to her, "there is no more fear of the cholera in Boston than there is in Heaven, to those whose situation and character is such as yours and ours."[10]

Discussion over the coming storm played out in Congress as well. On June 6, before Americans even knew cholera had arrived in Quebec, the General Synod of the Reformed Dutch Church in North America met in New York City and called for the nation to observe "a day of Fasting and Humiliation." The Synod, whose members had certainly read dire accounts of the disease's spread across Europe, believed that "our beloved country is at this time threatened with an awful pestilence."[11] To make the formal appeal to Andrew Jackson, the body appointed Reverend John Schermerhorn, a man particularly suited to influence the president. Schermerhorn was one of the rare religious leaders in the nation to publicly support the administration's Indian Removal Act of 1830, a controversial policy that was then deporting thousands of Indigenous peoples from their homes east of the Mississippi to lands set aside for them in the West.

Jackson rebuked his ally's request, however. "I concur with the Synod in the efficacy of prayer and in the hope that our country may be preserved from the attacks of pestilence," the president replied, but the Constitution's separation of church and state could not be violated. Amid "the *apprehensions* that the Cholera may visit our land," Jackson concluded, congregations, local governments, and even states might choose collective appeals to the Almighty, but the federal government should not interfere in religion.[12]

After news circulated in US newspapers of cholera's arrival in Canada, the president's political opponents tried to use his opposition to a national prayer to embarrass him. On June 27, Henry Clay—a senator from Kentucky, the leading candidate to oppose Jackson in the coming presidential election, and not a particularly devout Christian himself—introduced a resolution to ask the president to set aside a solemn day for Americans to make a collective appeal to God. Americans, Clay's resolution proclaimed, should ask the Almighty to bestow "blessings upon our country, and . . . avert from it the Asiatic scourge which has reached our borders." The senator did not mince words about the potential storm. "Asiatic cholera," he declared, "now hangs on our borders in its most frightful form." "Hitherto, the skill of medical science, liberal and enlightened as it now is, has been altogether incompetent to provide a sure and effective remedy."[13]

Jackson's ally Senator Littleton Tazewell of Virginia spoke against the resolution on constitutional grounds as well as by minimizing the threat. The United States, the senator argued, was in for a light blow if any: "It would probably rage, and prove extensively fatal among emigrants, being a disease which was engendered by the filth which attends squalid poverty; and, until our situation shall be so changed as to reduce us to similar poverty, there was no reason to fear it." A national day of prayer would only make things worse by adding "to the existing excitement on the subject, interrupting the ordinary course of business, and throwing everything into a state of confusion."[14]

In the end, there would be no national day of prayer. The resolution passed in the Senate, gaining thirty ayes and thirteen nays, but a majority in the House of Representatives remained loyal to the president's position. Jackson's allies managed to send the measure to committee, where it would die.[15]

The prayer debate ground to a halt just as the nation's experience with the deadly bacteria *Vibrio cholerae* took off. Coming in waves and striking in each year from 1832 to 1836, cholera caused episodes of mass mortality in nearly every state and territory of the United States. Outbreaks erupted not only in the nation's cities but also in small towns, rural farms, prisons, and plantations. It popped up in places as unlike and distant from each other as the thriving urban seaports of the East Coast and Indigenous villages on the Great Plains, and it affected people as different from one another as middle-class Protestants and Irish Catholic laborers as well as white enslavers and the people of color they exploited. Those who succumbed included great numbers of unnamed poor and ordinary people as well as business owners, judges, ministers, legislators, military officers, physicians, editors, and many other individuals from middle-class and affluent American families. For four years, the pathogen had taken victims from all ranks and devastated communities across the nation of some 13.7 million people, and then it disappeared for over a decade.[16]

Surprisingly, historians have left cholera's sweep through the entire US during the 1830s unexamined.[17] Countless volumes on the Jacksonian years exist, which collectively show how heated and divided the American public became over internal improvements, tariffs, the National Bank, Indian Removal, slavery, and other controversies. Scholars, however, have barely acknowledged that the pandemic occupied the attention of Americans as intensely as, if not more so than, other issues.[18]

Cholera ignited a contest that engulfed the nation. It was not just a life-and-death struggle between humans and deadly bacteria but also a contest over the meaning of the pandemic. On one side, people with powerful public voices demonstrated a degree of unity that has largely gone unnoticed in Jackson's America. Except for the proposed prayer resolution, cholera did not become a partisan issue and did not affect national politics in significant ways. Instead, newspaper editors, ministers, social reformers, municipal officials, medical writers, and other persuasive people coalesced around a set of beliefs that minimized cholera's lethal power. They imagined the disease as only capable of exploding among the impoverished, dependent, and degraded subjects of monarchical and authoritarian regimes of Asia and Europe. Its visit to the democratic and prosperous US, they believed, would be limited to relatively few people whose individual failings—eating rotten foods, drinking alcohol, neglecting to seek medical treatment, and maintaining otherwise filthy lifestyles—made them vulnerable.

On the other side was *Vibrio cholerae*. The germ, of course, could not literally speak for itself; scientific breakthroughs that have allowed us to understand microbes were decades away. But its actions demonstrated abundant evidence to counter those who minimized its power. It stayed longer than anticipated, went places it was not supposed to go, and killed people thought to be safe. Even some Americans with wealth and influence expressed fears, privately and sometimes publicly, of their own susceptibility. Cholera, moreover, made this universal vulnerability increasingly apparent as deaths of supposedly respectable people became shockingly numerous and undeniable. Some Americans became true believers that cholera was a deadly, indiscriminate, and pervasive disease.

Vibrio also made a strong case that prosperity, equality, and justice did not reign in the United States as extensively as people with powerful public voices imagined. The pandemic exposed xenophobia, exploitation, ethnic cleansing, and enslavement that pervaded the nation. The disease exploded in the cramped dwellings, work camps, poorhouses, hospitals, and prisons that many recently arrived Irish immigrants found themselves in. It circulated along the western waterways and trails on which deported Indigenous peoples were forced to travel. It erupted among enslaved workers in Southern cities and plantations and decimated African Americans trafficked as part of the booming interstate slave trade. The bodies of the exploited, deported, and commodified were no match for cholera. The disease's supposedly debauched victims, whose bad choices caused their own suffering and death, in reality included a disproportionate number of Irish immigrants, Indigenous peoples, and people of color thrust into deadly circumstances not of their own making.

Still, the silent bacteria could not win the contest over meaning. Voices that dominated the public sphere rang loudly throughout the pandemic, shouting that their nation's experience conformed to expectations. A coterie of people amplified and perpetuated a delusive narrative that individuals who lacked self-discipline and morality made themselves vulnerable to infection and death. In the process, the powerful hid cholera's diverse impacts and dimmed the light that a deadly disease shone on the dark side of their democratic experiment.[19]

That cholera's first sweep through the United States is a sad story goes without saying—thousands of people lost their lives to a gruesome disease that physicians did not understand. Not until the 1860s would scientists develop germ theory—the idea that a microscopic organism invaded a human body, reproduced in it, caused illness, and then passed on to another body wherein it caused the same disease. Medical authorities also were decades away from comprehending the pathogen's fecal–oral route of transmission and connecting outbreaks to sewage-inundated drinking water. Cholera's symptoms could be identified, but the mechanisms involved in making people sick were not. Doctors were unaware that *Vibrio* released toxins that paralyzed the lower digestive system, prevented water absorption, and induced voluminous stool filled with white flakes of intestinal tissue and blood plasma. Physicians observed that some people had mild cases and others more severe, but they could not have known that the number of bacteria ingested (dosage) and stomach acid levels of its victims affected the outcomes. Small doses could lead to mild, even imperceptible cases, while large doses into less acidic stomachs led to rapid dehydration, organ failures, and death within hours of infection. Whether mild or severe, the disease triggered an immune response that left survivors with lifelong protection.[20]

Medical scientists were aware that the disease originated in South Asia, but the ecological processes involved in its emergence as a human infection would not be pieced together until the twentieth century. Throughout most of its history, *Vibrio* remained restricted to the Sundarbans—an extensive wetland area of the Ganges Delta along the Bay of Bengal. There, the bacteria thrived in warm waters and were particularly adapted to copepods—small aquatic crustaceans (2 mm to 17 mm), which can be found in all types of water. *Vibrio* stuck to egg sacs and interior linings of their hosts, which then infested a variety of sea life, including barnacles, mollusks, and algae. Occasionally, the bacteria spilled over to humans when they used the

Sundarbans wetlands for hunting, fishing, and gathering, and ingested copepods that had infested drinking water or shellfish.

Imperialism provided the means for *Vibrio* to break out of its original habitat. Around 1760, the British East India Company began cutting down the Sundarbans forests, constructing rice plantations, bringing in labor to work in the aqueous environment, commanding their own army to maintain control, and accelerating ship traffic to and from the region. Amid the disruptions, *Vibrio* may have broken out and caused epidemics in some parts of India as early as the 1780s, but it was not until 1817 that a pandemic began. It started in the Ganges Valley, where the bacteria infected Hindus on their religious pilgrimage, accompanied them back home, and ignited outbreaks throughout India. Cholera followed Muslims from South Asia making their pilgrimage to Mecca, hitched rides with caravans destined for Baghdad and other Middle Eastern trading centers, and penetrated southern Russia.

The pathogen spread to the Far East as well. Ships sailing from South Asian ports carried *Vibrio* across the Indian Ocean and into the Pacific by way of infected passengers, contaminated water casks, and marine creatures attached to their hulls.[21] Crews of cholera-ridden vessels also likely expelled the deadly germ into new environments through bilge water—the foul brew that collected at the bottom of the boat that consisted of sea spray that splashed upon the deck, rain that periodically doused ships as they cross the Atlantic, and the vomit and excreta of passengers who could not make it to toilets that drained directly into the sea. After being pumped from arriving ships, the bacteria then colonized local sea life, particularly during warm weather, and became a hazard for peoples who fished, swam, bathed, or, more dangerously, drank the water.[22] Europe escaped this first pandemic, but before outbreaks ceased in 1824, millions had become infected, from Jordan to Japan, and untold numbers perished.

Western medical writers observed cholera's destructive power in South Asia and initiated a debate that would carry into the 1830s. Some writers advocated the contagion theory of disease, which envisioned some illnesses stemming from a chemical poison emitted from an ill individual that another person contracted directly or indirectly by handling contaminated clothing or other objects. Smallpox was an analog. Not only did people understand the contagious nature of this disease, but they also knew that once one got it, one would not get it again. Deliberate infection with cowpox, moreover, had been successfully demonstrated to give one lifelong immunity to smallpox as well. This process, which became called vaccination, gave medical science a boost of confidence in the early nineteenth century. Cholera deflated that confidence, but at least to some theorists, it seemed to behave like smallpox and could be controlled like a contagious disease. Since this new disease traveled along transportation routes, exploded in previously unexposed communities, and frequently ran through entire households, health authorities could best respond with quarantines, travel restrictions, and other containment measures.

Most medical writers, however, believed cholera to be atmospheric in nature. Contagion theory could not account for the fact that many doctors and attendants did not become sick, even though they had close contact with patients. The disease also skipped over some communities that lay on the same communication routes as afflicted places and left some neighborhoods unscathed while inflicting serious damage on adjacent ones. Cholera also exhibited a seasonal nature. Although infections during the cold seasons were observed, the disease spiked as the weather warmed. Cholera, the medical writers believed, then resembled yellow fever, a disease theorized at the time to be associated with changes in the weather, chemical compounds that flowed with the winds, electrical energy, or other phenomena. Locally produced miasma, according to most medical writers, played a role as well. Bad air arising from carcasses, manure, cesspools, stagnant water, rotting foods, unventilated dwellings, and crowds, according to this theory, either by itself or in combination with atmospheric influences, caused disease. Restricting the flow of people and commerce, thus, were not necessary; instead, sanitation efforts were. Keeping streets, alleys, yards, docks, and homes clean and dry offered protection. Moving to higher locations was thought to be the surest route to avoid the pestilential air.

While disagreeing about the origins of cholera, members of the medical establishment shared the same basic understanding of the human body and what was needed to restore health when the malady seemed to be at work. Western physicians like those educated in the premier US medical school at the time—the University of Pennsylvania—still adhered, in the 1830s, to humoral theory, an idea that went back to the ancient Greeks. People maintained proper health, they believed, when their bodily fluids—blood, yellow bile, black bile, and phlegm—stayed in balance. Doctors thus resorted to individualized interventions to bring about equilibrium, often employing bold, or "heroic," therapies to produce the desired result: bleeding to relieve the body of excess blood; emetics to induce vomiting and expel excess yellow bile; purgatives such as calomel (a mercury-based compound) to promote elimination of black bile; and sedatives such as laudanum (an opium-based drug) to reduce irritability. Faced with actual and suspected cases of cholera, professionally trained physicians turned to their tool kit of heroic medicines and therapies.

In doing so, scientifically minded physicians joined ranks with religiously minded social reformers to promote morality as the key to surviving cholera. First, abstinence from alcohol was essential. Liquor and other intoxicating beverages disrupted the constitutional balance of humors and put a drinker's body beyond the reach of heroic medicine's efficacy. Second, cleanliness of bodies, homes, and neighborhoods inhibited miasmatic influences, which, if they did not cause the illness, at least made one predisposed to it. Third, individuals had to exercise vigilance and responsibility in policing their own bodies, or the bodies that they claimed responsibility for. The slightest digestive unease or diarrhea, or so-called premonitory symptoms, necessitated immediate medical intervention. Prudent people often agreed to be bled and dosed with calomel and laudanum when they thought the disease was coming on; impoverished, incarcerated, and enslaved people were often involuntarily subjected to the same heroic interventions. Because many of their patients never had active *Vibrio* infections, doctors consequently claimed much success in their response. They reflexively described patients whom they lost as intemperate, filthy, or derelict in calling for medical assistance in time. Conversely, morality, especially in the forms of temperance, cleanliness, and prudence, generally kept one healthy, and in cases of illness, these behaviors allowed medicine to work, whether a contagion or atmospheric influence had precipitated sickness.[23]

Physicians and moral reformers were not necessarily wrong to associate poor health outcomes with poverty, squalor, and inebriation. People chronically malnourished, infected with multiple diseases, and suffering from alcoholism certainly had weakened immune systems in which a deadly disease like cholera could quickly end fatally. Drunkenness was also a social problem in the nineteenth century that reformers genuinely wanted to solve. Per capita liquor consumption was astounding before 1840. A lack of clean water led people to drink hard cider, beer, rum, whiskey, and other intoxicating beverages in amounts unsurpassed in any subsequent period of American history. Alcohol abuse led to lost jobs, broken homes, disabilities, and incarceration. Reformers took action to protect not only the addicted but also family and community members who suffered significant harm.[24]

To lump all drinkers into the intemperate masses that cholera deliberately targeted has no basis in science, however. Modern studies suggest that moderate ethanol intake generally increases stomach acid. Gut acidity, to be sure, depends on a variety of other factors, especially diet. Ethanol may have had little prophylactic benefit for those who had relatively low acid levels to begin with, especially when they ingested large doses of *Vibrio*. Still, it is plausible that people who habitually drank enhanced their body's efforts to kill the invading microbes and thus staved off *Vibrio*'s most severe impact.[25]

The biological need to quench thirst, rather than moral choices, led to cholera outbreaks. That *Vibrio* found its way disproportionately into the bodies of the poor and powerless had everything to do with the unequal access people had to safe and clean ways to hydrate themselves. The wealthy could import spring water from distant sources to avoid drinking notoriously foul local supplies and could afford to flee outbreaks, while the impoverished could afford neither of these privileges. Grossly overgeneralizing disease victims as intemperate thus obscured the social determinants of health that played such a crucial role in shaping the pandemic.

Historians cannot fault people of the past for failing to have a modern understanding of epidemiology, microbiology, and medicine. The lack of knowledge about cholera in the 1830s understandably elicits our empathy for earlier generations. They went through a tragic experience that future generations eventually learned from. Scientists have developed knowledge and technologies to protect people from deadly pathogens. In developed countries, modern sewage and water filtration systems had eliminated cholera's menace, as well as that of a number of other waterborne germs, by the early twentieth century. Modern medical practitioners, furthermore, can save lives by administering intravenous injections of rehydrating fluids, antibiotics that can kill bacteria, and even a vaccine that can provide long-term immunity against *Vibrio*.

Cholera, to be sure, has not disappeared. Deadly outbreaks have recently occurred in the wake of natural disasters and civil wars in impoverished places such as Yemen and Haiti. Climate change has further increased the danger and, along with war, led to record number of cases in Syria and Lebanon in November of 2022.[26] In a sense, though, these modern tragedies confirm how transformative modern sanitation and medical technologies have been to a large portion of the global population. Recent outbreaks serve, much as the 1830s pandemic should, as object lessons in the importance of clean water, robust public health systems, and access to medical care.

The purpose of this book is not to repeat the well-known story of scientific progress. Americans were no closer to understanding cholera in 1836 than they were in 1832. Four years of struggle with the disease only reinforced flawed medical notions and perpetuated social injustices. Americans emerged by 1836 even more convinced that cholera was a disease that could be easily cured with proper medical treatment and that those who died did so because of their own bad choices.

Research for this book began before 2020, but the story of a nation's experience with a global pandemic during its early history has become even more imperative to tell with the arrival of COVID in our own time. Our struggle with a novel disease has made me even more determined to recover the experiences of people who lived and died during a previous pandemic.[27] I hope that we do not allow the experiences of the afflicted to become hidden behind a veil of elite perspectives that minimizes the suffering of others and ignores the social injustices that have produced vulnerabilities. Cholera in Jacksonian America can warn us about the perils of clinging to convictions based on flawed assumptions during times of uncertainty and the dangers of purposely forgetting about calamities that have exposed ugly realities of the world in which we live.

This book traces cholera's sweep through the United States in the 1830s chronologically, showing how during five annual waves of outbreaks, powerful people used their public voices to hide the pandemic's terrors. This process began even before *Vibrio* started to replicate in New York City's water supply in June of 1832. As chapter 1 shows, American newspapers were filled with accounts of a strange, new scourge spreading in Asia and Europe. These stories illustrate that preconceived notions about cholera's selective predation on the poor, filthy, and debauched had already been firmly established before it actually arrived. Chapters 2 through 8 follow *Vibrio* as it crossed the Atlantic and jumped from place to place on the Eastern Seaboard during the summer and fall of 1832. Chapter 9 switches focus to the Trans-Appalachian West, showing how the pathogen spread into the interior and then down the Mississippi from October to December. Cincinnati and New Orleans experienced devastating blows from the pandemic's first wave that confounded all expectations. Chapters 10 and 11 take deep dives into the disease's intersection with the ongoing deportation of Indigenous Choctaws and trafficking of enslaved African Americans into the lower Mississippi Valley. Chapter 12 illustrates how temperance advocates in early 1833 employed the nation's previous experience with cholera to bolster their drive to stamp out inebriation in the country and, in doing so, solidified a false narrative about cholera's choice to discriminately prey on drunks. Chapter 13 focuses on the second wave during 1833, with a particular focus on one of the hardest-hit cities in the United States: Lexington, Kentucky. Chapter 14 finishes the pandemic with the outbreaks that occurred in 1834, 1835, and 1836. While weakening in intensity in these latter years of the pandemic, *Vibrio* still laid bare the contradictions to the story that powerful public voices continued to tell about the disease.

The moralizing narrative that elites tried to create about the pandemic did not match the horrible reality that many Americans experienced during the deadly pandemic. By bringing this discrepancy to light, *Hidden Terrors* aims to treat the people who lost their lives during this American tragedy with the empathy they deserve.

1

Entertaining Fear

A DISTANT PANDEMIC STOKES AMERICAN IMAGINATIONS

ON CHRISTMAS DAY in 1830, the ship *Czarina*, which left from the Baltic in the middle of the fall, arrived in Boston with news that cholera had infected some eight thousand people in Moscow, four thousand of whom had died.[1] "Accounts from Russia continue to be afflicting," a New York newspaper reported on December 30. "The cholera has spread to the new provinces of South Russia; it has hitherto defied medical treatment." The epidemic produced an appalling and extremely rapid mortality. "Out of 200 who are attacked daily with this complaint," the article stated, "100 die in the course of 24 hours."[2]

The distant tragedy conjured up images of a biblical plague or the infamous Black Death of fourteenth-century Europe. "This fatal epidemic, having ravaged a large portion of Asia, is fast spreading in Europe," the *New England Palladium* reported. "Fears are entertained, and not without reason, that it may extend to America. Providence seems to have directed that the human race, at stated periods, should be visited with pestilence."[3]

Would the mysterious and fatal disease cross the Atlantic? Americans increasingly thought so as more and more bad news arrived from Europe. A mass print-media environment existed in Jackson's America that kept people informed of a deadly scourge ravaging Poland, Hungary, Austria, Prussia, England, Scotland, Ireland, and France. A system of roads, rivers, and canals along with advancements in steamboat technology linked Americans together into a network in which information flowed at a rapidly escalating volume and pace. Editors exchanged newspapers with each other through the US postal system, published information lifted from other sources (often without attribution), and informed readers of happenings in places they probably had never been to and maybe never would.[4] Throughout 1831 and the first half of 1832, readers from Maine to Missouri learned that a deadly disease appeared to be unstoppable in Europe, and they could not help but entertain fears of a scourge of their own country.

People with powerful public voices told them not to. They intervened, telling them time and again that these fears had no place in a nation of liberty, prosperity, and self-discipline.

In the spring of 1831, cholera marched alongside Czar Nicholas I's soldiers as they traveled across Russia and into Poland to crush a rebellion of independence-minded subjects. *Vibrio* took lives on both sides, most notably that of the Russian Army's commander, Field Marshal Karl von Diebitsch. Diebitsch went to bed on June 9, 1831, feeling ill and awoke at two in the morning "indisposed."[5] One hour later, a doctor observed the telltale signs of the dreaded disease. The field marshal suffered severe cramping, labored breathing, delirium, and then coma. By noon he had become a corpse.[6]

Diebitsch's death could not hinder Russian progress. The czar's forces crushed the Poles, and the rebels finally surrendered in October, but deadly bacteria had inflicted greater damage than the troops. The pandemic ravaged the Polish army and infiltrated the cities of Pułtusk, Warsaw, Kraków, and Poznań.[7]

The pathogen, meanwhile, advanced through other parts of Eastern and Central Europe. Outbreaks erupted in the principalities of Moldavia and Wallachia, then part of the Russian Empire.[8] There, six thousand people in present-day Romania reportedly perished "in a short time."[9] *Vibrio* penetrated the Galicia region of the Austrian Empire and continued "spreading frightfully."[10] The Austrian government, convinced of cholera's contagiousness, enacted martial law in the affected area and established a *cordon sanitaire* along the Galician and Hungarian border. "Every transgressor is immediately tried and shot," readers learned from one commonly circulated story.[11] Such authoritarian measures did not work. The pandemic continued to spread and had encompassed a broad swath of the Austrian Empire by that fall.[12]

Social unrest added to the chaos. Hungarian peasants believed that people were dying because aristocrats had poisoned wells across the land. As rumors spread, castles were sacked, lords chased off, and property destroyed. Soldiers came in to quell the unrest, but peasants fought back. One military officer, according to a widely circulated account, was "bound, tortured with scissors and knives, then beheaded, and his head fixed on a pike as a trophy." Peasants also drowned an official who accompanied the military, broke his carriage into pieces, and discovered chloride of lime inside. They forced one of the official's servants to eat the cleaning product until "he vomited blood, which again confirmed the notion of poison." "So the bands went from village to village," the account read, "wherever a nobleman or physician was found, death was his lot." The Hungarian peasantry's identification of well water as the source of cholera was not the lesson of this widely circulated story. Instead, the account emphasized how the aristocracy kept the lower classes in a state of "ignorance and brutality," consequently leading them to act on their unenlightened beliefs in a violent manner.[13]

Czar Nicholas I also grappled with cholera-induced social unrest. Residents of St. Petersburg began to fall to the disease in increasing numbers throughout June 1831.[14] The royal family and affluent residents fled, while imperial officials took infected people to hospitals and kept them there surrounded by armed guards. The poor thought such measures amounted to murder. Attendants at the hospitals, they believed, served up poison and even buried patients alive. Rioters attacked the hospitals, dragged out their friends, and in some cases killed medical personnel.[15] St. Petersburg remained unsafe from disease into the fall. As of November 3, an official total of 9,228 cases and 4,745 deaths had been recorded.[16]

By then, cholera had spread throughout the Baltic and into the German lands. Statistics indicated a case fatality rate that reached nearly 50 percent in Riga, Latvia, during the spring.[17] Outbreaks followed in the port cities of Libau (Latvia), Palanga (Lithuania), and Gdańsk (Poland). By August 1, a reported 1,500 residents fled Berlin before any infections had been officially reported.[18] Cases began to pop up there by early September, leading to further flight from the Prussian capital.[19] John A. Cuthbert, a US consul in Germany, informed Americans that cholera in Berlin "loses nothing of its virulence" and that individuals stricken with the pestilence "have died in less than six hours."[20] Next was Hamburg, a sovereign city-state on the Elbe River that bustled with commerce. "This is a new instance of the very capricious march of this pestilence," American editors repeated from English papers, "for, without touching at any intermediate spot, it appears to have leaped at once from Berlin to the mouth of the Elbe."[21]

In the United States, calls to quarantine incoming ship traffic from Europe became more pronounced. Medical policing of incoming ship traffic had been common at US ports, although it had remained under the control of local rather than federal authorities. Health officers could use their discretion in determining whether passengers carried smallpox or other diseases thought to be contagious and could direct ships to anchor at the quarantine grounds. There, passengers were isolated at a lazaretto—a building often found at ports to house infected people until their symptoms cleared. Merchandise also came under scrutiny. Crew members of ships had to unpack their cargo, air it out, and douse items with chloride of lime, vinegar, or other disinfecting agents. Passengers also had to wash their clothes and, in some cases, burn or sink them. Finally, the ships themselves were entirely cleaned.

Ships also came under suspicion of introducing diseases considered noncontagious. Miasmatic influences that caused disorders at the point of departure could invade a ship's hold, remain on items, and jeopardize people who entered the ships or handled the cargo at the destination port. For this reason, ships sailing from the Caribbean and arriving in the United States during the warm season were automatically anchored at the quarantine ground for more extensive inspections and cleaning.[22]

Uncertainty about cholera's nature led to debate about restrictive measures. On August 6, 1831, Walter Bowne, mayor of New York City, issued one of the first of many proclamations that American municipalities would make to deal with the threat. Bowne ordered that any ship coming from an infected place automatically had to anchor at the quarantine ground and undergo rigorous inspection before any crew or cargo could leave it.[23] The mayor's proclamation did not mandate that all cargo be taken off a suspect vessel, which worried some New Yorkers.[24] A rural resident, for example, warned that infected goods unloaded in New York City would bring "the new and dreadful scourge of the human family" inland, where it would kill country as well as urban dwellers.[25] Bowne responded to these general fears by ordering port authorities to mandate that crews of ships arriving from the Baltic unload and disinfect their goods before delivering them to merchants.[26]

Other US cities followed New York's lead but not without controversy. Ports from Maine to Georgia stepped up policing of vessels from Europe through the remainder of the summer of 1831.[27] Editors of a Providence, Rhode Island, newspaper lauded its city's enactment of quarantines as necessary to keep out a disease that carried "with it terror and dismay wherever it makes its appearance."[28]

Business interests found the public health measures disruptive and found allies in the medical establishment. Dr. Joseph Mather Smith, a professor at the New York College of Physicians and Surgeons, lectured the public that cholera was not contagious and "all quarantine regulations and public enactments are in fact nullities." His reading of the evidence from Asia and Europe led him to conclude that "the electrical state of the atmosphere" gave rise to the pandemic and that human attempts to turn it away were futile. He stopped short of concluding that cholera would or would not arrive in America, but he gave a vague hope that if "the destroying angel light upon our shore," prudent behavior might spare his countrymen from high levels of mortality.[29]

Philadelphia's *Journal of Health*, representing the views of the city's medical elite, gave a sterner warning about the dangers of policing and explained that old-world tyranny contributed to cholera's virulence. Quarantines were ridiculous for an atmospheric disease, they explained. The editors counseled their readers that "the only effectual means of escaping" was to maintain a "good wholesome diet, regular exercise, temperance in all things, a cheerful temper and undaunted spirit."[30] The Austrian emperor's restrictive public health measures, they added, were designed to stop Polish liberalism from spreading and best understood as "an engine in the hands of despotism, for the suppression of liberty." The editors gave no credence to the Hungarian peasants' beliefs that poisoned water led to cholera deaths but did sympathize with them for being confined in a "sickly district" where they remained "breathing an impure air" and "kept in perpetual agitation and terror." The *Journal* concluded that policies based on outdated contagion theory were "old women's tales and vulgar prejudice."[31]

Ominous news of cholera's passage across the English Channel, though, kept the debate over quarantines alive. The news started trickling in at the beginning of 1832, and by February it had become quite clear to Americans that port cities in Northern England and Scotland had fallen into the pandemic's grip.[32] An article from the London *Sun*, reprinted in multiple US newspapers, declared the disease a "plague" that traveled "with a giant's speed, and more than a giant's energy," striking the "Young and old—the feeble and the strong—the dissolute and the abstemious." It had caused "terrific" mortality, and panic ensued. The scourge, the article declared, "rages like a devouring flame, with a suddenness and phrenzy almost without parallel in the annals of infectious visitations."[33]

News from the United Kingdom led to calls for the US federal government to enact a national quarantine law. On January 5, the New York Board of Health met, considered the new information from Britain, and formulated a short memorial to Congress.[34] The pandemic, according to the memorial, had taken "not less than fifty millions of the human family" since breaking out of South Asia in 1817. The United States would "not be exempt from . . . this frightful malady," and the federal government should consider restrictive measures on incoming ship traffic and send a sanitary commission to Europe and Asia "to collect all the facts relating to the means of preventing, and remedies to be applied to, this fatal disease."[35] Legislation enacting a national quarantine law and a sanitary commission, though, never came out of a Congress dominated by states' rights Jacksonian Democrats.[36]

Meanwhile, a piece from the London *Quarterly Review* enthralled the American reading public. The essay promoted contagion theory and appeared in excerpted form in the New York *Daily Advertiser* and other papers under the title "Horrors of the Cholera Morbus." The piece proclaimed "the birth of new pestilence" that had "swept off at least *fifty millions*" of the human race. "It has mastered every variety of climate, surmounted every natural barrier, conquered every people." Grown men could collapse within fifteen minutes of becoming sick and death could ensue within an hour. Symptoms included "exhausting evacuations of a peculiar character, intense thirst, cold blue clammy skin, suffused filmy half-closed eyes, cramps of the limbs, extending to the muscles of respirations, and . . . an unimpaired intellect." "If the detail we have given be pursued with common attention," the piece concluded, "the reader cannot but be impressed with a conviction as deep as that felt by ourselves that *the disease has been propagated by contagion*."[37]

Excerpts of the London *Quarterly Review* essay circulated widely in a variety of forms. The Boston *Courier*'s editors prefaced their summary of the piece with a comparison to the Black Death, when people left others to die, civil rule collapsed, and robbers and murderers ran rampant. The "poor and the destitute are hardly more liable than the rich" to suffer, the *Courier* concluded, while calling for stricter quarantine measures throughout the nation.[38] A letter from "Cassandria," which cited the *Quarterly Review* piece and called for more vigilance, appeared in the New York *Evening Post*. "Every instance of . . . negligence on the part of our city authorities should be marked and reprobated," Cassandria declared, "and the public journalist who would counsel a relaxation of our quarantine laws, in order to give facilities to commerce at the hazard of our very existence, should be condemned as the enemy of this country."[39]

Renewed calls for stepping up quarantines received support at the local level. In February and March, New York City, Philadelphia, Portsmouth, Boston, and other ports all added ships from the United Kingdom to the list of those to undergo rigorous inspection.[40]

Despite resurging anxiety, most of the medical establishment remained staunchly opposed to quarantines. The wide circulation of the London *Quarterly Review* piece drew the ire of Dr. Paul F. Eve of Savannah, Georgia. Having graduated at the University of Pennsylvania, Eve went to Paris in 1829 for surgical lessons but abandoned those to join the Polish rebels fighting against the czar.[41] After returning to the United States, he wrote a letter shaming the editor of the Charleston, South Carolina, *Courier* for publishing contagionist views. Contagion, Eve argued, was a superstition of aristocrats, "who have never seen a case of Cholera, nor have ever visited a place where it is has existed." To support his charge, he cited his service in Poland, where he treated numerous cholera victims and had a case of the disease himself. He also detailed the activities of his colleague, Parisian physician François Foy, who "inhaled the breath of the dying sufferer, he put on the shirt and got into the bed of the dead patient, he drank the matter ejected from his stomach, he even infused into his own veins the blood drawn from the Choleric—and all this with only a slight nausea and head-ache." Eve added more reassurance by pointing out that "Errors in diet" and exposure to the elements served as exciting causes that took predisposed victims, including "the glutton" Russian Field Marshal Diebitsch, "the impoverished Pole," and "the drunken Englishman."[42]

Other noncontagionists fired back as well. Philadelphia's *Journal of Health* described the pandemic's victims so far as "miserable, servile, and ignorant." Resigning themselves to "slavish fears, to a death which they conceived inevitable, the peasants of the Old World neither asked nor allowed of the administration of means of relief." Alcohol and bad food added to their predisposition.[43] Philadelphia's *National Gazette* echoed such views. "The imaginations of some good American folks are already cholera-stricken," the editors decried. Americans, they claimed, need not worry: "The cholera finds aliment in the squalid wretchedness and brutal habits of the European populace;—its natural prey is not abundant in our country. Its haunts are, very narrow, dirty streets and lanes, filthy hovels, and generally those scenes where indigence and vice wallow in their extreme misery, grossness and turpitude."[44]

More reassurance came from Dr. Charles Mifflin. Another University of Pennsylvania–trained physician, Mifflin served as a surgeon aboard a St. Petersburg–bound ship. He ended up treating patients in Russia's capital in September and October of 1831 and then returned to the United States in January of 1832.[45] New York City's *Daily Advertiser* subsequently published Mifflin's observations, which then circulated in multiple newspapers.[46] The doctor maintained that local factors energized the atmospheric influences that caused cholera, with the most glaring of these factors being poverty. "I never saw at home," he stated, "such evidence of degradation and misery, as attach to the lower classes that fell under my observation in Russia." Cholera did take the lives of some middle- and upper-class people, but these deaths stemmed from alcohol consumption, "irregularities in living," "high excitement," and other issues. He concluded with confident words, stating, "should it please an all wise Providence to send this Epidemic to our Shores, the general *improved* habits of our people... will so far arrest its fatality, as to leave it among the ordinary diseases to which we are more or less exposed."[47] Mifflin thus added his voice to the choir expressing confidence that America's prosperous and self-disciplined population had nothing to fear.

More news kept coming during the spring as ships arrived with the latest ominous accounts from Europe. Seventy-three new cases and forty-one deaths occurred in London on the single day of March 18. The epidemic continued to grow in the capital, with deaths surpassing the thousand mark by April 5, 1832.[48]

Next came Paris. "The ravages of the disease are not confined, as in England, to the lower classes," a translated and reprinted letter from a French newspaper proclaimed. The dead included a baron, a baroness, a count, the chief of division in the Department of War, a former dean of the Faculty of Medicine, and many doctors. "The terror is... extreme in the finest parts of Paris," the letter added.[49] Social upheaval added to the frightful situation. Mobs burst into the hospitals where impoverished people were taken against their will, "saying that the cholera is a mere invention of the Government, who has poisoned both the casks of the water-carriers, and the tanks of the wine merchants." Ragpickers, who scavenged the city's rubbish for cloth and other items to resell, chafed at extra rounds of trash collection, attacked garbage collectors, and threw up barricades in various parts of the city. On the roads leading out of the city, angry mobs attacked the vehicles of the wealthy, who had loaded what they could and attempted to flee the violence and cholera.[50] One account claimed cholera had caused "the death of TWENTY THOUSAND persons," which turned out to be rather close to the total fatalities of 18,000 people during that tragic spring in a city of 785,000.[51]

Then Le Havre, France, and Dublin, Ireland, succumbed to the pandemic. Both seaports sent multitudes of ships and people to North America, and both began to see cases at nearly the same time. By April 18, the disease began to erupt among German and Swiss immigrants within four miles of Le Havre. Cholera, it was reported, "triumphed over every individual who has been attacked."[52] By early May, the disease began to take the lives of Dubliners and spread to other locations in Ireland.[53]

Amid the gloomy news coming from Western Europe, the Philadelphia Board of Health attempted to calm anxieties while at the same preparing people for what, by that time, many Americans thought to be the inevitable

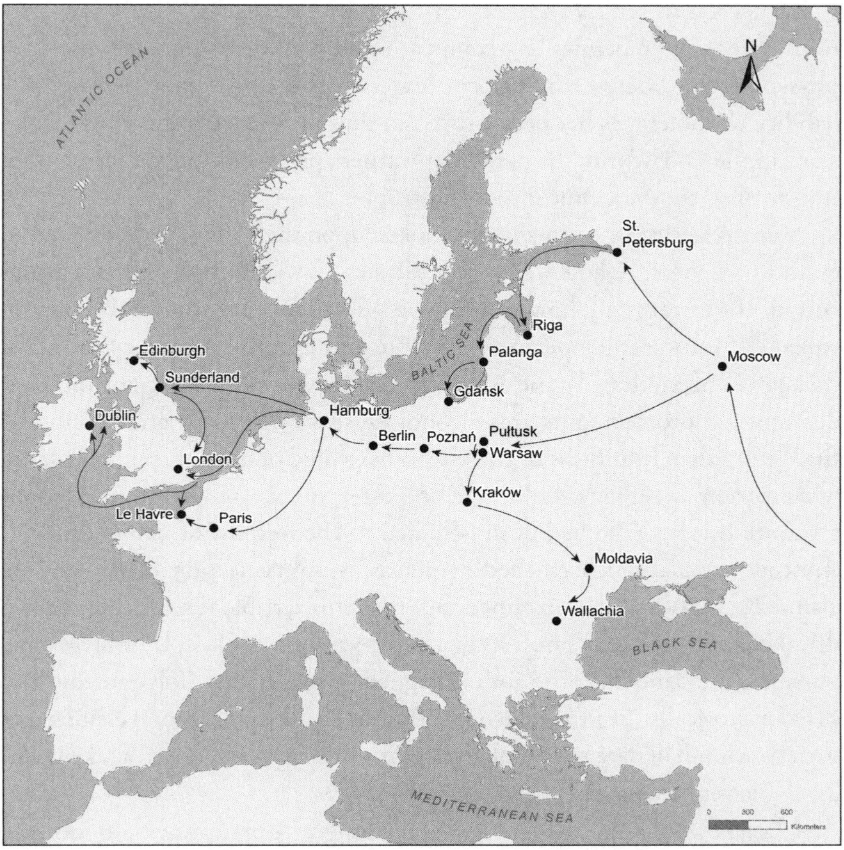

Spread of Cholera, 1830–May 1832. Map by Franchesca Rodriguez, Geospatial Center, Stony Brook University.

arrival of the disease.[54] The board circulated a pamphlet, "Nature of Cholera—Quarantine—Health Police," authored by Drs. John T. Sharpless, George F. Lehman, and Jesse Reading Burden. These professionally trained physicians had just returned from a conference with their New York City peers and, not surprisingly, derided quarantines and travel restrictions as ineffective against atmospheric diseases. The best prevention, the pamphlet advocated, involved the individual prudence of their fellow Americans. "Personal cleanliness, regular habits, and temperance should be recommended to all," the physicians declared, "as it has been observed, whenever and wherever the cholera has prevailed, it has seized upon, as its first and easiest victims, the dirty, debauched, and intemperate classes of society." The United States thus stood a good chance to get off lightly, as the disease's "fatality will be lessened still more, by the improved habits of our people, and their intelligence."

Danger, however, lay ahead if Americans gave in to fear. "The best protection against all epidemics is a composed and confident state of mind," the physicians emphasized, adding that "excessive fear has always increased the liability to cholera, as has been proven in Europe." Strict and useless regulations in the Old World, the pamphlet warned, provoked "public terror" that transformed the pandemic into a catastrophe.[55]

Some Americans, astonishingly, looked upon the coming pandemic as an event to welcome. "Cholera May Be a Blessing," a widely reprinted article suggested. The disease had shown itself to be "a scourge of Providence, brought in to aid the cause of Temperance." The "vicious and the irregular are almost exclusively its victims."[56] The American Temperance Society cited the pandemic when promoting its anti-alcohol cause, stating in a national circular that "more than four fifths of those who have died of cholera, that pestilence which is now sweeping over Europe, and threatens also to visit our own country, were persons who had been addicted to the free use of strong drink."[57] Another article, which reached audiences in every section of the nation, claimed it was "a well ascertained fact that this terrible disease traces out a drunkard with about as sure a scent as a blood-hound [finds] the object of its pursuit." The pandemic, the author feigned, was "a melancholy remedy," but asked rhetorically, "if Providence sees fit thus to purify the moral elements of society, who shall dare to complain? Let rum-drinkers in America take warning while yet the curse is a stranger to our shores."[58]

Cholera would not be a stranger much longer. Americans would soon see if they were in for the light blow from a selective predator that temperance advocates, medical authorities, and editors would have them believe.

2

"An Irish Emigrant Died at Montpelier"

CHOLERA ARRIVES IN NORTH AMERICA

ON JUNE 19, 1832, a resident of Concord, New Hampshire, penned a letter "in haste." "The cholera has arrived at Montpelier, Vt.," he wrote to an acquaintance in Boston. "One case occurred there yesterday—an Irish Emigrant."[1] The Boston *Post* published the letter, many newspapers reprinted it verbatim, and others summarized its contents: "An Irish emigrant died at Montpelier."[2] Alarm reverberated across the country.

Further details circulated in later editions. The deceased was a woman who had stayed in Burlington in the same "poor Irish hovel" where "a child died suddenly of some disease of the bowels," where a man died "in a fit of intemperance," and where a female succumbed to an "undoubted case of the cholera."[3] The immigrant left Burlington before the latter two deaths occurred, and after traveling on foot for two days, she stopped near Montpelier for the night. She had become desperately ill on arrival, leading residents to call Dr. Dewey to attend her. Dewey described her, her husband, and their five children as "wretched emigrants, directly from Ireland, through Quebec and Montreal." The doctor could do nothing for her. She perished the following morning at five o'clock.[4]

This Irish mother, whose name remains absent from the historical record, was among the first people on US soil who succumbed to the global pandemic. Cholera erupted in Quebec during the first week of June and reached Montreal on the ninth. Soon thereafter, suspected cases began to pop up not only in Burlington and Montpelier but also in towns in New York along the Lake Champlain–Hudson corridor, which had recently been connected by a canal. Something ominous was happening on the country's northern border, but native-born Americans would hardly know the half of it.

The unnamed Irish woman who perished was part of a larger exodus from her homeland that had accelerated after 1815. Ireland's population had steadily increased during the first three decades of the nineteenth century, but under British imperial rule, very few Catholics owned land. British landlords rented plots to tenants, who then sublet smaller portions to poorer families. With the end of the Napoleonic Wars, crop prices collapsed, and landowners raised rents and increased evictions to turn land into pasturage.[5] Crop failures exacerbated the situation. Even before the more infamous famine of the 1840s, agricultural crises led to localized starvation in 1822, 1825–1829, and 1831–1832.[6]

Impoverished Irish had few options in their homeland. The UK Parliament removed a tariff that protected Irish producers, leading English manufacturers to dump vast quantities of inexpensive cloth in the Irish markets.[7] The mechanization of spinning after 1828 worsened the problem. Textile industries in Ireland never recovered.[8] Economic deprivation led tens of thousands of Irish to migrate annually to North America by the 1830s. Most disembarked at Quebec as fares to British Canada were cheaper, but many subsequently crossed the border into the United States, where wages were higher.

US immigration policies made it relatively easy for the Irish to become citizens. The US Naturalization Act of 1795 allowed "any alien, being a free white person" to gain citizenship after five years of residency, with one full year of residency in a single state. The individual also had to demonstrate proof of good moral character, swear an oath to the Constitution, and renounce allegiance to any foreign government. States could restrict immigration if they chose to do so, but none did prior to 1832. There would be no national restriction until the Chinese Exclusion Act of 1882. Until millions arrived with the onset of the potato famine of the 1840s, no serious effort was made to define the Irish—or, for that matter, any other national or ethnic groups coming from Europe—as a race apart from people of English descent; being of European descent and white were, at the time, synonymous.[9]

Coming to America was a grueling process even without the threat of cholera. Many gathered at Irish ports—Dublin, Belfast, or Cork—but the bulk of North America–bound ships anchored in Liverpool. Steamboats had decreased the time and costs required to get from Ireland to Liverpool. Many Irish had been in Great Britain for some time, looking for work, before heading to America. Finding a vessel to take them was fraught with obstacles. Housing in Liverpool and other port cities was notoriously squalid, so migrants sought to get on a ship as soon as possible. Multiple hucksters worked port cities and preyed on emigrants, selling tickets for ships that would never arrive or did not even exist.[10]

Once aboard ships, emigrants faced an arduous multiweek journey. Profit-minded owners emptied their holds of American products—cotton, grain, timber, and potash—and sought to pack their filthy vessels with iron, chemicals, manufactured goods, and people for their return voyages. Ship proprietors allotted their emigrant passengers only a few square feet each below decks, where they ate, slept, and toileted in cramped and poorly ventilated quarters.[11] Affluent travelers, paying for more spacious and airy cabins, brought aboard wine, coffee, tea, and soda water, while steerage passengers relied upon daily rations of notoriously foul and stagnant water from the casks that the crew had filled before departing. A cut in rations or even running out of water was not uncommon as journeys took longer than planned when calm winds slowed progress or storms blew ships off course.[12] Along with dehydration and exhaustion, diseases found opportune conditions to spread aboard transatlantic ships. In normal years, about 2 percent of passengers did not complete the crossing alive, due to smallpox, typhus, dysentery, and other illnesses.[13]

Cholera substantially increased the risks of transatlantic travel. Dublin, Liverpool, and other ports that emigrants typically traveled from began to have cases in April 1832 just as the spring shipping season began to pick up after its regular winter lull. Then crews packed hundreds of emigrants between decks of several ships setting out for North America. Many of these voyages ended in tragedy.

The proprietors of the *Brutus* crammed 330 emigrants, described as "destitute poor," into every space that did not carry cargo and, on May 18, set sail for Quebec.[14] On the twenty-seventh, a man became ill but recovered. After a stormy night on June 2, the cases of cholera jumped from three to twenty-one, and the situation worsened over the next three days. One passenger reported, "it is impossible to describe the scene of misery . . . people dying in every direction, the greater number of them destitute of the common articles of bed covering." Burials at sea became frequent. The splashing of the corpses into the Atlantic so frightened healthy passengers that they made every effort to sequester themselves from the ill. With many of the ship's crew dead or incapacitated, the captain had little choice but to return to Liverpool. The *Brutus* arrived back at port on June 13 having lost seventy-nine passengers. Healthy passengers disembarked and remained in quarantine, while the noticeably ill remained aboard.[15] Six more of the emigrants died in the ensuing days, bringing the death toll to eighty-six.[16]

Accusations immediately began after the *Brutus* came back to England. The Liverpool *Mercury* received letters that questioned whether the ship's proprietors took on more passengers than the law allowed and whether they supplied the emigrants with foul water.[17] Editors of the Liverpool *Courier* did not object to emigration, believing that England needed to relieve itself of "redundant population," but they decried the business aspect of it as inhumane. "It is horrible to hear of wretched emigrants contracted for at so much per head and for a certain limited space, as we bargain for the calves or pigs."[18] London's *Medico-Chirurgical Review* gave such accusations medical backing. "The state of crowding, the condensation of human effluvia, the scanty food, and the great deficiency of clothing, account, in a great measure, for the fatality of the attack," the editors charged. "Those only who have seen ships with emigrants for America, can form an idea of the misery and crowding, and bad air... in the 'tween decks."[19]

Bad water, not foul air, made the passengers sick. Before setting sail from Liverpool, the ship's crew did what they always did to prepare for the month-long journey across the Atlantic: they filled casks with drinking water from local supplies.[20] With an outbreak ongoing in Liverpool since April, some of these casks undoubtedly teemed with *Vibrio*. Perhaps the first one was uncontaminated and then, a week into the journey, people began to sicken after drinking water from a newly opened and contaminated one. The first passenger became ill nine days post departure, after all. Affluent passengers fared better since they consumed brewed tea or coffee, in which the boiling process killed bacteria, and could rely upon personal stores of wine or soda water. Impoverished emigrants, meanwhile, "chose" between tainted water or abject thirst.

Several other ships sailed into the Atlantic that terrible spring with cholera infesting either the bodies of passengers or the water put aboard. Thirty-two men, women, and children perished aboard the *Hebron*, which had come out of Dublin, before it arrived in Quebec on May 25. British officials examined the vessel as it anchored at quarantine, concluded that no one had arrived ill, and made the dubious determination that cholera had not been the culprit.[21] A later examination of Quebec's quarantine records revealed that cholera struck passengers of at least three other ships: the *Constantia* arrived from Limerick on April 28 after burying twenty-nine at sea, the *Robert* from Cork on May 14 after burying ten, and the *Elizabeth* from Dublin on May 28 after burying twenty-nine.[22] It was just a matter of time before a *Vibrio*-laden ship crossed the Atlantic and ignited an outbreak at its North American location.

Troubling signs became clear during the first week of June as the volume of ship traffic reached its annual peak. Some sea captains defied health orders at the crowded port of Quebec. They sailed past the quarantine station at Grosse Isle, went directly to the city's wharves, and disembarked passengers eager to end their miserable experiences on the unsanitary vessels.[23] Haggard medical officers at Grosse Isle often took a captain's word about sickness and directed passengers to Quebec or upriver to Montreal with only minimal screening.[24] The inflow was immense. Some four thousand immigrants reportedly arrived on just the two days of June 7 and 8.[25] A more specific count indicated that 10,599 immigrants arrived between the second and ninth—only 4,502 fewer than had arrived over the previous five months combined.[26]

Concern about cholera understandably grew. On June 3, the *Carricks* from Dublin arrived at Grosse Isle after reportedly losing forty-two passengers to "an unknown disease." Three days later, the Quebec Board of Health sent Dr. Morrin to investigate the strange sickness. Morrin learned from the captain that none of the deaths had occurred within three weeks of the ship's arrival. The captain, his crew, and some passengers left quarantine the following day, even though Morrin, upon his return to Grosse Isle, found some of the immigrants sick with an illness "resembling cholera." The doctor, however, either could not convince or did not try to convince city authorities that the feared scourge had arrived. On June 8, the board of health formally denied the existence of cholera.

The following day, cases of the disease became too obvious to ignore. The Quebec *Mercury* reported that between the morning of the eighth and afternoon of the ninth, fifteen cases and seven deaths occurred from what some doctors believed to be "Spasmodic Cholera." Six of the seven dead were immigrants who might have arrived sick, but one was a Canadian who worked on the transit boats between Grosse Isle and the city. Mortality continued to increase both at the quarantine station and within the city itself. By June 15, the daily death toll had reached one hundred.[27] North America's experience with the global cholera pandemic had begun.

This critical moment occurred when *Vibrio* started to replicate in Quebec's water supply. The bacteria likely traveled in the guts of multiple transatlantic passengers who found their way into the city during the first week of June. Immigrants and sailors stayed in boarding houses and used outhouses and other receptacles that drained waste into the groundwater. The pathogen then infiltrated local wells, particularly those that served as a source of water for the city's poor. People also relied on the St. Lawrence itself, which almost certainly teemed with *Vibrio* as European vessels pumped out their contaminated bilge water and introduced bacteria-carrying marine life. The summer temperatures accelerated the multiplication of the bacteria, which would only be checked by a dearth of non-immune victims or the return of cold weather, several months away.

Within a few days, cholera infested Montreal's water supply too. On June 9, the steamboat *Voyageur* brought the corpse of an Irish immigrant, "who had been suddenly attacked with every symptom of cholera," into Montreal's port. Another passenger became ill with unmistakable signs of cholera and died within twenty-four hours of arrival.[28] Cases soon began to erupt among French and English Canadian residents. The city's medical board was not convinced that the disease had actually arrived and kept news of the deaths quiet for about a week.[29] On June 17, however, the daily death toll surpassed one hundred, forcing an official acknowledgment of the outbreak.[30]

In both Montreal and Quebec, newcomers were subjected to a terrifying situation. Sick upon arrival, they were sent directly to inadequate hospitals. These filled beyond capacity. Doctors had to wear clogs because of the buildup of filth on the floors, staff abandoned their posts, and officials could not find enough people to provide care. Officials rounded up people who had become ill and had no one to care for them or whose impoverished conditions made them appear to be a threat to public health. Against their will, these people found themselves in places where, if they did not have cholera yet, they now stood a good chance of soon contracting it.[31]

Mary McLean Walsh understood these horrors all too well. Mary, her seven siblings, and their parents left Leitrim, Ireland, on May 10, 1832. They all survived the voyage, but Walsh, who described herself as "a perfectly healthy Irish girl of sixteen" at the outset of the journey, suffered an unidentifiable illness during the monthlong voyage. The family faced the specter of a deadly outbreak on arrival. Walsh described Quebec as "a plague-stricken city; where men, women and children, smitten by cholera, dropped in the streets to die in agony, where business was paralyzed, and naught prevailed but sorrow mingled with dead and gloom."[32]

While walking along the wharf, Walsh collapsed. When she awoke, she found herself in one of the makeshift hospitals. "I was now in a veritable house of torture, where the most appalling shrieks, groans, prayers and curses filled the air," she recounted. The constant hammering of workmen outside the hospital making one casket after another haunted her for the rest of her life. She convalesced for six weeks, aided in part by a nurse who disobeyed the doctors' orders and allowed her to drink water and warm broth, unknowingly providing the most important thing to aid recuperation—rehydration. When Walsh left the hospital, she saw the flames of bonfires consuming the apparel of cholera's victims. She was unaware that three of her siblings' clothes "were in that burning pile" until she met her "Mother, dressed in deep mourning, her pretty face sad and care-worn when she told me I was the only one of her four sick children who had survived."[33]

Mary McLean Walsh's siblings were just a few of the thousands swept away by cholera. Health officials reported that 3,451 people, or 12 percent, of Quebec's total population of 28,000 perished, while 4,000, or 15 percent, of Montreal's population of 27,000 died before the outbreaks burned out late in the summer.[34] Newcomers accounted for about one-third of the deaths. Five percent of all immigrants who came in 1832, according to the British agent in charge of migration, fell to the fatal disease.[35]

Survivors understandably tried to get out of Quebec and Montreal as fast as they could. Some escaped into Upper Canada, where jobs working on farms or constructing, operating, and maintaining Ontario's developing canal system awaited them but where cholera would continue its destruction into the fall. Many others thought better opportunities lay to the south. Immigrants crossed the US-Canadian border in June 1832 in search of desperately needed wages. Cholera, though, continued to present troubles, as did the resistance of native-born Americans seeking to keep them out.

In Plattsburgh, New York, a town on Lake Champlain sixty miles south of Montreal, an immigrant man perished on June 9.[36] Four more fatal cases occurred over the course of a week. "Our village is in great alarm," one resident wrote in a public letter, while reassuring readers that cases "have been confined to Canadians, and Irish of the very lowest order as to filth and intemperate excess."[37] City officials expected steamboats to continue service but to refuse passage for "Vagrants, Paupers or diseased persons."[38] By June 21, three more fatal cases occurred, all described by the town's board of health as "persons who lived in intemperance and in filthy places."[39]

Across Lake Champlain, immigrants faced severe opposition from Vermonters. Towns near the Canadian border mobilized militias, policed boat traffic on Lake Champlain, and stopped travelers on the paths and roads that cut across the border.[40] Steamboat companies reassured the public that, while they would still run, they would no longer transport foreigners.[41] Such efforts, according to one account, kept three thousand immigrants stuck on the Canadian side of the border.[42]

Halting the influx of newcomers delighted Dr. Benjamin Lincoln, secretary of the Burlington Board of Health. He disdained the Irish, not because he suspected them of spreading contagion, a theory he did not believe in, but because he viewed them as morally inferior. Lincoln publicly disparaged one of the pandemic's victims in his town as "an Irishman by the name of Barlow, a noted drunkard, who had been drunk all the week" and another as "Mrs. McFarlane, an Irish woman, of very intemperate habits."[43] His disdain was more obvious in his private correspondence. "I think it ridiculous to try to keep out cholera by Sentinels," Dr. Lincoln confided to his father, "but if we can frighten Paddies off we shall keep off a much greater evil than Cholera."[44]

By the time Lincoln penned his xenophobic comment, steamboats with numerous immigrants had reached Whitehall, a town at the junction of Lake Champlain and the canal. One vessel tried to land on June 14 with the corpse of a man who had recently been in Montreal.[45] Whitehall authorities met the suspected vessel as well as others with an armed force and prevented their landing.[46] Incoming boats had to either turn around with their passengers or deposit them at "obscure" places away from the town.[47]

Albany's city officials enacted measures immediately upon hearing news of cholera's arrival in Canada. On the evening of the fourteenth, the marshal stopped three boats and prevented passengers from disembarking until the health officers could inspect them. Some of the travelers did not want to take their chances, "jumped on shore, and came to the city on foot." The marshal subsequently stopped any more boats from approaching by removing the cranks from the canal locks. The editors of the Albany *Argus* published an extra edition on the evening of the fifteenth that declared, "The first step [to stop cholera] is to check the tide of emigration from the infected places in Canada, to this city."[48] Despite the prevalence of noncontagion doctrine in public discourse, contagion theory seemed to rule amid the immediate panic of civic leaders and native-born residents.

Immigrants arriving over the next several days found substantial obstacles. Guards stood at ferry crossings, turnpike gates, and other entry points into the city. Those who made it past the guards with "certificates of good health" found no boats willing to transport them farther down the Hudson and discovered the doors of Albany's lodging houses closed to them. The board of health authorized the stay of these stranded immigrants in temporary hospitals until they could be sent upriver to Troy, where they would quarantine on Green Island.[49] There, they were "hutted and kept under strict surveillance" by an "armed force."[50]

Immigrants experienced a tense and unwelcoming situation in Troy. On June 16, the chairman of the health committee tried to reassure residents. "For ourselves, we can see no reason for alarm or panic," D. Gardner proclaimed. "Let temperance in regimen, a good courage, and due caution be preserved, and there will be little cause for the apprehension of danger."[51]

Residents wanted more protection than temperance sermons. On June 17, city officials called out the militia to stop what Pastor Almon Underwood described as an expected "Irish insurrection." Underwood estimated that two to three hundred Irish immigrants who belonged "to the company that introduced the cholera into Canada" were being prevented from landing in the town. To Underwood's relief, they were forced into quarantine.[52] Troy residents remained on edge the following day. "There is a great excitement & agitation in the public mind respecting the cholera," Underwood recorded. "Probably there has never been more."[53] No reported violence occurred, however.

That the Irish were particularly singled out as a dangerous group can be seen by the treatment of one group of Welsh travelers. Around June 15, a boat with thirty to forty Welsh tried to land at Fort Miller, a way station halfway between Whitehall and Albany. The immigrants had originally arrived in Quebec in early June and departed there on the eighth, making their way down the St. Lawrence and then south into New York. By the time they reached Fort Miller, some had become ill and three had died.[54] Town authorities stopped the boat from unloading its passengers at the public landing and instead forced the immigrants into "shanties, surrounded by a guard."[55] An alderman of Albany's city council went to investigate the situation and sent back what he hoped to be reassuring news that the Welsh suffered from only ordinary diarrhea.[56] Another account repeated that the people seemed to be "generally neat and healthy."[57] Dr. Asa Fitch, who treated them, decried their detention as "highly injurious" and stated that locals need not fear giving them aid because their sicknesses stemmed from "exposure and hardships" rather than contagion.[58]

Irish-born newcomers would constitute the majority of the more than seven hundred immigrants held at Green Island. Dr. C. S. J. Goodrich of Troy attempted to justify the use of the quarantine when questioned by the noncontagionist medical establishment. "The object was not to prevent the introduction into the city of contagious disease," he claimed, "but to prohibit a mass of ill-clothed and unclean foreigners from entering and mingling with a dense foreign population already among us, and thereby exciting disease." The immigrants, Goodrich claimed, were better off at Green Island because there they could receive food and rest. The potential for panic among the native-born scared Goodrich the most. Without the detention of immigrants, he stated, "there would have resulted a total stagnation of business, and possibly many valuable lives lost through the excitement of fear."[59]

Even the Democratic state governor, Enos Thompson Throop, was not sympathetic toward immigrants. Throop and his fellow Jacksonians had courted the Irish vote and depended on their turnout for local, state, and federal elections. Cholera fears moved Throop to be more circumspect. In an address to the state legislature on June 21, he declared it "certain" that a "malignant disease . . . resembling the much dreaded Cholera is ravaging the hordes of squalid emigrants" in Quebec and Montreal and that many of these people "direct their course to the United States."

The governor hedged on contagion. On one hand, he voiced the possibility that cholera sprang up because of "very unfavorable circumstances under which an unusual number of the most destitute class of emigrants have been landed during the severe weather in a strange climate." On the other hand, he suggested that "inattention to cleanliness" as well as "enfeebling dissipations and excesses" would produce toxic conditions that could "expose our fellow citizens to the contagion of disease." He thus called for a rigid quarantine on newcomers immediately after they crossed the border from Canada.[60] So far the pathogen appeared to behave just as medical authorities had predicted, but travel restrictions, Throop seemed to be saying, were necessary in case the malady did not conform to expectations.

Just four days before New York's governor tied cholera to immigrants and their behavior, the unnamed Irish woman had perished in Montpelier. She should not be remembered as the caricatured figure who could be blamed for her own suffering, however. She arrived at her final destination burdened by *Vibrio* and grief. The eight-year-old girl who "died suddenly of some disease of the bowels" in Burlington was her daughter, a fact that did not appear in newspaper accounts.[61] Castigations of her as a "wretched" person of "the very lowest order" may have helped native-born residents feel more confident in their own safety, but they invited Americans to dehumanize her and to ignore the horrific demise experienced by those most exposed to the deadly disease.

Her life and death were part of a larger story in which massive numbers of Irish people undertook journeys of hope, hardship, and danger. Pushed by desperate economic circumstances and lured by cheap fares to board overcrowded and ill-supplied ships, impoverished Irish left for North America by the tens of thousands during the cholera year of 1832. *Vibrio* hitched a ride aboard many of their ships, forcing several vessels to turn back before getting far beyond the United Kingdom. Some immigrants witnessed the scourge killing dozens of their fellow passengers, debilitating many others, and then running its course before arriving at Quebec. Some immigrants arrived with cholera still raging on the ships that transported them, leading to days of confinement in unhealthy quarantine stations in Canada. Tired, hungry, dehydrated, and anxious to begin their new lives, many crossed the border seeking employment in the booming US economy. There, they met a largely unwelcoming, hostile, and fearful native population.

At every stage of their journey, immigrants were confronted with awful scenes of sick and dying fellow travelers. *Vibrio*, the invisible and yet to be known culprit, had transformed an already grueling process into one of real terror.

Its work in North America had just begun.

3

"It Is All a Humbug"

MORTALITY PEAKS IN NEW YORK CITY

JUDITH AND PETER Roosevelt's residency in New York City during the summer of 1832 worried their adopted son, Samuel Johnson, and his wife, Elizabeth. "I suppose you must partake of the general alarm which if I may judge from the papers is very great," Elizabeth wrote to her in-laws. She had just learned of cholera's presence in Quebec and admitted, "there is great cause for anxiety." Elizabeth told the Roosevelts that she and Samuel, an Episcopal minister, could host their New York City friends and relatives who might need a refuge from the coming scourge in their Hyde Park home. Come "without delay at the appearance of danger," she urged her in-laws. Still, she let the Roosevelts know that she expected the United States to experience a light touch. "I have no great fears for our country," she wrote. The nation lacked the crowding that existed in Europe, and Americans were not like "the poor houseless miserable emigrants" flocking into Canada. Samuel added to his wife's letter, claiming "there will be no extensive danger" and "that the cases will be *few*, and that all alarm will soon pass away."[1]

Anicartha Miller, daughter of Judge Sylvanus Miller, expressed a similar confidence. Soon after news broke of cholera's presence in Canada, Miller saw her neighbors preparing for the worst by hoarding chloride of lime as a disinfectant, purchasing the opium-based drug laudanum as a treatment, and packing up to leave on a moment's notice. "The first report of a case of Cholera in this city would I think set half of our citizens who could get away in motion," Anicartha wrote on June 20 to her older sister Margaret, who was then away from the city. She advised Margaret to postpone her planned visit to see the family but downplayed the potential threat. "I hope if the disease makes its appearance and the real extent of the danger becomes known, people will become more rational," she concluded. Anicartha added that she and the rest of the family were not alarmed. "Father still continues quite incredulous on the subject," she informed Margaret. "He says he believes that an ugly disease, probably cholera morbus is raging among the emigrants in Canada but as to Asiatic Cholera in this country, it is all a humbug."[2]

Other New Yorkers were less assured. "We in New York seem solemnly composed," Mary Suckley informed her father, a businessman who was visiting Washington, DC, at the time. "All Christians are engaged in prayer—it will be a merciful interposition of providence if we all are preserved."[3] Philip Hone wrote in his diary that cholera appeared "more mortal" in Canada than in Europe. "There can be little reasonable ground to hope for our exemption in New York from this dreadful scourge," Hone, a wealthy merchant and former mayor, declared. He decried the filthy state of his city, recording, "It must come, and we are in a dreadful state to receive it."[4]

For the weeks to come, New Yorkers remained on edge. Civic leaders and newspaper editors tried to downplay the threat and keep anxieties at bay in their city of some 225,000 residents, even as the pandemic gradually gained ground in the city.[5] As July's days passed, cholera increasingly showed itself to be anything but the "humbug" that some imagined it to be.

New York's editors delivered the frightful news of the novel disease's North American arrival while simultaneously echoing preconceived beliefs that their readers had little to fear. "In this city," the *Evening Post* asserted, "where the streets are wider and better ventilated, where the climate is as salubrious, the habits of the people as temperate, and the condition of the poorest classes far superior to that of those in London—we have no reasonable ground to fear a more sweeping mortality."[6] The *Morning Courier and New York Enquirer* informed its readers that "Much depends upon the state of the mind during the existence of Cholera" and assured them that "the habits of our people, their diet, and naturally cheerful dispositions, are considered certain evidences that when it does come among us, it will be in a mitigated form."[7]

The New York Board of Health—a political body composed of Mayor Bowne, City Recorder Richard Riker, and elected aldermen—did not ignore the potential threat. Municipal authorities increased policing of boats coming down the Hudson and enforced quarantines on those suspected of transporting ill passengers; levied fines on overland travelers who did not stop for inspection within a mile and a half of city hall; cancelled the city's Fourth of July celebration over a week in advance; ordered cleaning crews to give more attention to the city's filth; selected facilities to serve as temporary hospitals to receive an expected influx of cholera-infected patients; appointed a panel of physicians to serve as a Special Medical Council to advise them on the anticipated emergency; and posted placards around the city counseling people about cleanliness, temperance, prudence, and seeking prompt medical care should they experience symptoms. The board, in other words, tried to assuage the anxieties of people who held various beliefs about cholera's transmission—that it was contagious and incoming travelers would be screened, that it was a disease dependent on miasmatic conditions, and that behavioral choices would determine an individual's fate. Many nonetheless feared that they had not done enough, especially clearing the streets, alleys, gutters, and yards of standing water, manure, animal carcasses, and other miasmatic-causing wastes that accumulated.[8]

Cholera, as expected, found its way into New York, but officials proved reluctant to sound an immediate alarm. On Monday, June 25, a tailor named Fitzgerald became ill but began to feel better by the next morning. However, his two children suddenly sickened and died on Wednesday. Their mother succumbed next, developing symptoms on Thursday and dying on Friday. Physicians agreed that the Fitzgeralds, who had been living in Manhattan since May, had "Asiatic cholera," but they could not find any of the suspected predisposing causes. Doctors described the father as "a steady and temperate man" and the mother as "a neat housekeeper."[9] When Dr. James Manley reported the suspected cases to the board of health on June 30, he could not convince them that something unusual was beginning.[10] The next day's discovery of a corpse, identified as "an Irishman named O'Neil" whom a physician diagnosed as having been "seized with malignant cholera," did not move them either. Nor did reports of cases and a death in a boarding house.[11] When Dr. John Stearns pled with the mayor to publicly acknowledge that cholera had arrived, Bowne refused, claiming that the cases and deaths were nothing atypical.[12]

The Medical Society of New York, an independent association of respected physicians, pressed the emergency. On July 1, the doctors informed news editors that since June 27 a total of seven to ten cases had appeared. The *Standard* asserted in its July 2 issue, "CHOLERA IN NEW-YORK." The cases, the newspaper reported, were "so marked as to have no room for doubt," and the editors noted "that it has proved fatal to almost every individual attacked."[13] The *Journal of Commerce* similarly announced, "SPASMODIC CHOLERA IN NEW-YORK" and reported that several cases of "a very alarming character" had occurred with death following "after a short interval."[14] The *Morning Courier and Enquirer* acknowledged that "Asiatic Cholera has made its appearance in this city" and encouraged proper behavior to meet the moment: "With firmness, prudence, attention to cleanliness, temperance, and above all, a determined tranquility, we have not the slightest doubt, but it will prove mild and moderate."[15]

Other newspapers disparaged the Medical Society and denied the prevalence of the deadly malady. The *Evening Post*, which would prove to be the most skeptical of all outlets, claimed that one of the alleged cholera victims was a "filthy drunken wretch" who died "of his beastly excesses." To the idea that "Asiatic Cholera" was in the city, the editors declared, "Fudge!" The paper further condemned the physicians as overeager to render suspicious diagnoses without thinking about the panic that would ensue. "Have they considered what blow they are striking against the business of the city," the editors asked rhetorically, claiming that millions of dollars would be "prevented from flowing into New York."[16] The *American* lambasted the physicians' "alarm" as "mischievous."[17]

As the news broke, the board of health obfuscated. On July 2, it issued a report at 1:00 p.m., declaring that of the eleven deaths reported to them, five had "the appearance of Canadian Cholera" and one was "a case of decided Spasmodic Cholera." The board promised a more detailed report the next day. Municipal authorities, meanwhile, started to police the affected areas and interfered with Catholic wakes of suspected victims. Decaying corpses were thought to produce cholera-causing miasma, so health officials sought to bury bodies as quickly as possible. Grieving loved ones jumped on top of coffins to prevent them from being taken, and a melee broke out, with "black eyes and bloody noses" sustained on both sides.[18]

On the morning of the third, the board, in consultation with the Special Medical Council, backtracked from its statement of the previous day. Most of the eleven previously reported deaths plus an additional one that had occurred overnight, the board claimed, were "the ordinary cholera to which we are subjected at this season of the year." They included a shot against the Medical Society, instructing residents to reject any findings that did not come from the municipal government, and proclaimed that "in no former years has the number of deaths, in proportion to the population, been less than at present."[19]

Dr. Manley and other members of the Medical Society were appalled. Manley would later excoriate the Bowne administration, which he claimed had suppressed the truth "to deceive the public" into a false sense of security.[20]

The board of health, however, had significant support. "It may be doubted whether a single case of Asiatic Cholera . . . has yet occurred in this city," the *American* claimed. The *Morning Courier and Enquirer*, despite being one of the first newspapers to announce the novel disease's presence, backpedaled. Its editors claimed that "it is at least questionable if the Asiatic Pestilence exists at all in New-York." They warned that false reports could transform ordinary sickness into deadly maladies by the "terror" that they generated. The *Evening Post* declared that during the previous year, deaths from the usual illnesses had similarly increased as the summer heat intensified. John Pintard, a retired insurance executive, founding member of the New-York Historical Society, wealthy bank trustee, and *Evening Post* subscriber, privately agreed. In one of a series of letters he wrote to his daughter in New Orleans, he asserted that "nothing more than aggravated cases of cholera morbus, operative in intemperate subjects," had occurred. "At best we are likely to have a sickly season," he wrote, "but we are not timid & shall stand our ground."[21]

Thousands of New Yorkers disagreed. Immediately after papers reported the disease's presence on the second, city residents fled by the multitudes, just as Anicartha Miller predicted they would. It was not just a reflexive decision stemming from irrational panic. New Yorkers had known for some time that the disease could cause a horrible and quick death, and those who had the means to escape understandably did so. E. E. Briggs, for example, had his own doubts about the board of health's dismissive stance and called upon his family physician, who confirmed that "the real Asiatic" cholera had begun to spread. Briggs, a ship captain, decided to take his family to Sag Harbor on Long Island.[22] Several other newspapers, while not necessarily encouraging their readers to flee, did express their views that a novel malady had, in fact, taken root in the city.[23] "There is . . . no longer any question as to the existence of the dreaded Cholera, in its highest form of malignity," the *Commercial Advertiser* asserted on July 5. "There have been several cases to-day, some of which have already terminated fatally."[24]

The board of health came to accept reality as the number of sudden deaths spiked. On the fifth it announced that eleven people had died during the preceding twenty-four-hour period. Municipal authorities thus began the morbid daily reporting that cholera had forced European and Canadian cities to undertake as the pandemic swept westward. The death toll reached nineteen on the sixth. Mortality fell to twelve on July 7's report, but the board of health made a startling admission. The scourge had been spreading within the Bellevue complex over the previous ten days.[25]

Bellevue at the time served multiple functions and included a population of 1,650 inmates within an almshouse, a women's penitentiary, a jail for inmates convicted of state crimes, and a hospital for noncontagious yet gravely ill people who had no one to provide home care. Between June 24 and July 1, the city rounded up fifty-four vagrants and other impoverished people from various parts of the city and sent them into the complex. Some almost certainly carried *Vibrio*. Cases began in the almshouse, spread into the hospital as staff carried the sick there, and then broke out in the women's penitentiary. Thirty cholera cases and thirteen deaths occurred at Bellevue between June 27 and July 6.[26] City officials tried to alleviate crowding by releasing all healthy inmates convicted of no more than misdemeanors on their own recognizance and sending more serious offenders to penal facilities on Blackwell's Island (today's Roosevelt Island). The city could not find places to relocate most almshouse residents, however, and the disease continued to take a heavy toll among them.

Unlike the incarcerated, affluent people could remove themselves farther away from Manhattan. "A deep gloom has overspread our City," William Price wrote to an associate, claiming that seventy thousand residents left before July 8. "The panic far exceeds any thing of the kind you ever witnessed in the worst yellow fever visitations."[27] New Yorkers flocked to the homes of friends and relatives, rural resorts, and boarding houses throughout the mid-Atlantic and New England. "Two or three hundred passengers from N[ew] York arrive here every boat," a New London, Connecticut, resident observed on July 10.[28] According to some estimates, nearly half of the city's residents, or more than 112,000 people, left in July.[29]

Peter and Judith Roosevelt decided to stay. Their son Samuel, who read the *Evening Post*, was not entirely convinced that cholera had actually arrived in New York City, but the conflicting accounts made him "very anxious." "Do my dear parents shut up the house & come & spend the time with us, till the danger is overpast," he urged.[30] Judith Roosevelt responded to her son that she thought the alarm was "needless" as "the cases that have been reported have been brought on by imprudence." She added that no one would have paid attention to the cases had "Asiatic cholera" not been at the Canadian border. She still expressed a degree of Christian fatalism that was common for the time. "Why can we expect to be exempt when so great a part of the world has been scourged by it," she asked rhetorically. "We must look upon it as a peculiar visitation of the Almighty for the sins of the world." She appeased her son by telling him she and his father would leave for Hyde Park "should it become necessary and proper" to do so.[31]

The Roosevelts had some valid reasons to believe that it might not become necessary to evacuate their residence. Quebec, a city of twenty-eight thousand, saw one hundred daily fatalities in the ten days after cholera's arrival. During the entire ten-day period after the first reported cases in New York, the board of health counted only twenty-three total deaths, which skeptics questioned being the result of cholera. "When it touched... Quebec and Montreal," the *American* opined, "it blazed forth at once, and in few days swept away its hundreds of victims. Nothing of that sort has appeared here." Mortality increased in the city after the *American*'s dismissive statement, but rates still paled in comparison to European and Canadian cities. "Alarmists are... converting every bowel complaint into symptoms of Asiatic Cholera & every death into decided cases," Pintard informed his daughter. "Were it the true Asiatic it [would] have spread like wild fire."[32] The next day Pintard called those who fled "Cowards."[33]

Even editors who had been more circumspect early on started to question the severity of the situation. Mortality only increased to twenty-one on the eighth and then twenty-four on the ninth, prompting the *Commercial Advertiser* to conclude that the "number of deaths in proportion to the population, has been really comparatively trifling, the alarm which has prevailed may be considered unfounded."[34]

There were reasons, unbeknownst to New Yorkers, for cholera's slow start in their city. Everywhere *Vibrio* went, its assault followed unique patterns dictated by the ways people obtained their drinking water, where sewage drained, and the weather. New Yorkers relied on diverse and multiple sources for their water. Decades before the pandemic, Aaron Burr's Manhattan Company had received a charter to pipe water into businesses and residencies, but instead of expending its capital on running a pipeline from the relatively clean Bronx River as it was supposed to do, the institution functioned as a bank. It drew investors, lent money, collected interest, and grew into the behemoth that ultimately became today's JPMorgan Chase.

Its efforts to supply the metropolis's thirsty multitudes, meanwhile, floundered. Burr's company pumped foul liquid from the Collect Pond, an underground pool that filled with sewage-laden runoff from the surface of what is today Lower Manhattan. By 1832, Burr's company had managed to serve only one-third of the city with water delivered through a series of rotting wooden pipes. The remaining two-thirds relied on several local pumps that drew water from wells, which varied in depth, proximity to cesspools and outhouses, and vulnerability to infiltration from seawater. Wealthy New Yorkers could escape reliance on either the Manhattan Company or local wells by purchasing their water from vendors who trucked it into the city from cleaner sources in the countryside.[35]

The first neighborhoods that *Vibrio* infiltrated were those on reclaimed land along the east and west sides of Manhattan. There, shallow wells were most vulnerable to inundations from the twice daily high tides. These tides brought saltwater teeming with copepods and the contaminated bilge water from newly arrived ships. People traveling down the Champlain–Hudson corridor may have brought *Vibrio* into the city, but the concentration of initial cases near the wharves of the East and Hudson rivers suggests that ships arriving directly from Europe introduced the deadly pathogen.[36]

A drought that extended into the second week of July, furthermore, kept cholera restricted to a limited number of water sources, at least until July 9. Then rain broke the dry spell and carried *Vibrio*-loaded sewage to a wider range and variety of wells, causing a spike in mortality to forty-four on Tuesday, July 10.[37] Deaths remained near that level on Wednesday at fifty, Thursday at fifty-one, and Friday at forty-nine.

The skeptical press, however, continued to find reasons to declare that nothing unusual was happening. The *Evening Post* pointed to the board of health's report of the tenth as evidence of a false alarm. Physicians reported forty-four "malignant" cholera infections in private residences but only six of those cases terminating in death, leading the editors to suggest that disreputable doctors reported the slightest cases of diarrhea as a novel disease. Of the "alleged visitation of the Asiatic Cholera," the *Evening Post* exclaimed, "our opinion on this engrossing subject may be summed up in a very few words:—We have some Cholera in the city, and a great deal of Humbug."[38]

Affluent New Yorkers who stayed put adhered generally to the preconceived idea that cholera carefully chose its victims from the impoverished and imprudent. "We have *all* been under great alarm from this cholera," merchant James Lee wrote to an upstate doctor on July 9. The scourge, however, had "only visited the dissipated and filthy" and one person who had improperly taken medicine. Lee would stay in the city to receive merchandise from incoming ships until he found "matters worse than they are now."[39] Dr. Christopher Yates claimed to a colleague in Albany that New York had "an abundance of imaginary" cases and that the only severe illnesses occurred "among the poorer class of foreigners, and the poor filthy, and drunken."[40]

Pintard had the harshest judgment. "At present [cholera] is almost exclusively confined to the lower classes of intemperate dissolute & filthy people huddled together like swine in their polluted habitations," he wrote to his daughter on July 13. "A visitation like the present may work beneficially to promote Temperance, proving a blessing instead of a curse."[41]

Voices for temperance indeed rang loudly. The New York–based American Tract Society published Presbyterian minister Lyman Beecher's *An Appeal on the Subject of Cholera*, and city newspapers began to advertise it for sale on July 14. Already an internationally renowned advocate for moral reform, the American pastor preached abstinence, not merely from hard liquor but also from beer, wine, hard cider, and other intoxicating beverages, as the sure route to well-being.[42] "The dark wing of the destroying angel, whose sword has smitten the nations of Asia and Europe, now shadows our own threshold," he exclaimed in his *Appeal.* He charged that "America too needs the scourge" because of failure to observe the Sabbath as well as "Obscene impurities, drunkenness, profaneness, and infidelity." He cautioned that danger lay in store for everyone if they did not "bow in submission to the chastisements of the Almighty, repent and seek pardon and salvation whilst they may be found." If not, sinners would be subject to "the unspeakable terrors of the vengeance of an insulted God!" Repentant Christians might die, but it was their duty "to set an example of calm courage, of mild resignation, of active self-denying benevolence" so that others might ask for forgiveness and also find reward in heaven.[43]

The Episcopal minister Samuel Johnson almost certainly believed that his parents were pious Christians, but he worried. He had received his mother's letter telling him that, for the time being, she and his father would stay in the city. Samuel urged her to reconsider. He had come around to believing a "fierce epidemic" reigned in the city and noticed that cases had been occurring closer and closer to his parents' home on Desbrosses Street. "It is true, the *Evening Post* keeps up its courage & so do you, as your letter shows, and the poor who have few comforts & the dirty & vicious are the main sufferers," Samuel prefaced his appeal, "but yet would it not be the safer, to shut up house till the danger is over & come up & remain with us till then[?]"[44] Judith and Peter Roosevelt did not find the situation bad enough to flee, however.

On July 14 a critical transition occurred. The death toll reached sixty-six, dashing hopes that the outbreak had climaxed. It was not only the growing numbers of New Yorkers succumbing to the scourge but also the identities of some who died that increased the alarm. In the early morning hours of the thirteenth, General Alexander P. Muir, the commissary general of the New York State National Guard and president of Aetna Insurance Company, began vomiting, purging, and cramping. By noon he was a corpse.

The following day, the press reported his death. The *Morning Courier and Enquirer* announced Muir's demise along with that of Mr. S. J. Tobias, "a highly respected importer," and appeared to make an about-face on views it had earlier expressed. "The pestilence does not confine itself to the poor and destitute, but attacks indiscriminately all who come within its range," the editors remarked, seeming to be persuaded by cholera's real power. The editors declared that "it becomes our duty to say frankly to our fellow citizens, that the disease is on the increase and in no way mitigated in its violence." They furthermore cast doubt about the city's official numbers for the week that had just ended. The *Morning Courier and Enquirer* estimated that the real toll was not the forty-three to forty-four average daily deaths that the board of health reported but more than seventy per day.[45]

Others did not budge from their preconceived notions. The *Evening Post* explained that the forty-year-old Muir had suffered from a previous illness, and on the day before his death, he overexerted himself by walking an entire mile home from work. When he became ill, he delayed calling on a physician until it was too late. The *Evening Post* also doubted Muir's diagnosis. One of the attending doctors supposedly told the paper's editors that "the disease was decidedly *common cholera*" rather than the more deadly novel variety.[46] All the details proved that nothing "unusually alarming" was occurring and that the *Morning Courier and Enquirer* deserved chastisement for declaring otherwise.[47]

While editors argued about a dead insurance executive, *Vibrio* escalated its assault on the city's population. The board of health reported seventy-four fatalities in its report on July 15.

That day stood out vividly for a young city resident. James Riker, Jr., who was ten years old at the time, recounted four years later that "a gloomy solitude pervaded every thing" as cholera came to the city. The family closed its store for lack of business and "scarcely ventured farther than the apothecary's opposite to obtain drugs." He did, however, make a daily trip to the office of Dr. White, who posted the board of health's reports on his door. "We watched this bulletin with a good deal of interest," he recalled. On the morning of the fifteenth, the experience became even more real for him. His grandmother Mary Van Arsdale developed symptoms that grew worse during the day, and despite the interventions of "a number of physicians," she passed away in the early evening. Riker's uncle, although "an uncommonly rugged man," fell ill and perished even more suddenly, within just a few hours of showing symptoms. "Well do I remember that gloomy night, time will scarcely efface the impression," Riker recorded in his life's history. His family had hoped to stay put, but the "sudden and mournful providences" led his father to pack them up and head to Westchester County, where friends offered them a place to stay. The Riker family remained away from the city until early October.[48]

The Riker family included just two of the increasing number of victims who fell during the overnight period of July 15–16. The board of health's daily report on the sixteenth listed a total of ninety-four fatalities. "The Cholera spreads & proves more fatal," John Pintard admitted, signaling the beginning of his shift from skeptic to believer in the disease's power. The patrician noted the outbreak approaching the "comfortable abode" where he, his wife, their daughter, her husband, and their children lived. The Pintards held a meeting in which they considered leaving the city. They decided not to. The patriarch would not shut his bank down and leave depositors without access to their funds, and the rest of the family would not go without him. He worried about his wife, however. She had grown "more agitated" by the scene of gravely ill people being transported aboard biers into a nearby hospital and hearses continually rumbling down the streets.[49]

Vibrio grew even more vicious and exacted a severe toll on residents who remained in the city. Mortality fell to sixty on July 17, but heavy rains that day fueled a dramatic increase and spawned infections in multiple areas of the city. On July 21, the report of daily deaths peaked at 104.[50] Editors of the *Evening Post* seemed flummoxed. They had been publishing the board of health's daily reports alongside their skeptical commentary, but as the outbreak approached its apex, they did so without dismissive language. The word "humbug" disappeared from their editorial observations.[51]

The Five Points neighborhood experienced the worst of the surge as the deadly bacteria found its way into the Collect Pond, which lay underneath the impoverished residents and supplied their drinking water.[52] Since the early 1800s, impoverished people had found some of the most affordable housing options available to them in an area near the five corners formed by the intersection of Cross, Orange, and Anthony streets. The neighborhood's inhabitants, largely African American and Irish American, hoped to avoid cholera just as much as the more affluent did, and many did set out in multiple directions. A surge of people fleeing from New York during the latter half of July was reported in Boston, Massachusetts; Philadelphia, Pennsylvania; Poughkeepsie, New York; and Paterson, New Jersey, whose residents described the new arrivals as "vagrants," "abandoned women," and "the poorer classes."[53] If fear of the malady alone was not enough to drive people out of the Five Points, city officials ordered many to be removed from dwellings where cholera cases occurred and burned bedding, clothing, and other personnel possessions.[54]

Unsympathetic elites saw this new wave of fatalities as conforming to preconceived notions. The board of health pointed to the Five Points' growing

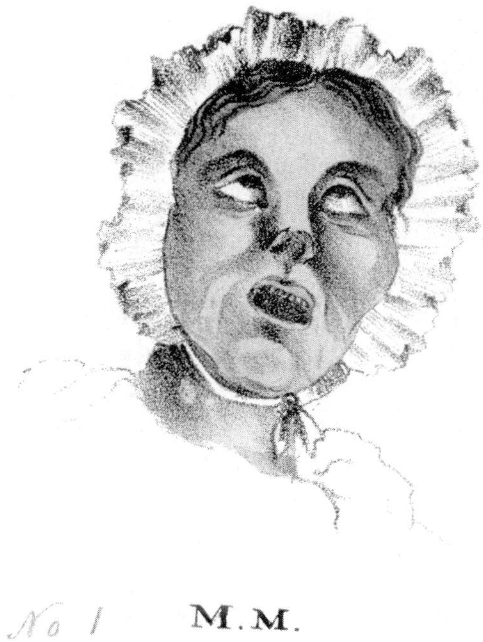

Victim No. 1, from *Illustrations of Cholera Asphyxia: In Its Different Stages. Selected from Cases Treated at the Cholera Hospital, Rivington Street* (1832) by Horatio Bartley. (Printed by S. H. Jackson, New-York.) Hand-colored lithograph. The New York Historical, 80486d.

mortality as showing "the immense importance of cleanliness and temperance," taking for granted that many New Yorkers understood the neighborhood to be rife with filth and drunkenness.[55] The *Morning Courier and Enquirer*, vacillating from its earlier claims of cholera's nondiscriminatory direction, called the Five Points "a sink of iniquity, which our authorities should cause to be immediately vacated."[56] A letter in the *Evening Post* stated that the notorious neighborhood was filled with "a race of beings of all colours, ages, sexes and nations...beneath the nature, almost, of the vilest brute."[57] John Pintard callously described the pestilence as sweeping away "the very scum of the city" and expressed his hope that the quicker it did so, the sooner the outbreak would end.[58] Thomas Masters, a wealthy merchant and future director of the Bank of the Manhattan Company, informed his daughter in Amherst, Massachusetts, that he and her mother felt secure in the city because God protected "all who live orderly and regularly and in well ventilated situations." That was not the case with Five Points residents, where deaths occurred among "the lowest class whom nobody knows."[59]

The struggle against cholera remained dire in Bellevue. As many as nine hundred impoverished inmates remained in the almshouse for weeks after *Vibrio* found its way into the complex. These were presumably the elderly, physically disabled, orphans, and others who could not be released on their own recognizance or simply had nowhere else to go.[60] City officials could not find places to evacuate them, and the scourge continued to afflict them severely.

Dr. Isaac Wood, the resident physician, himself became severely ill and left his post by July 15.[61] He recovered, lived to be an elderly man, and related the traumatic experience to an interviewer in 1866. "Forty bodies laid in the dead house at one time, the undertakers not being able to make coffins fast enough to bury them," Wood recalled. He added that he was "obliged to step over the dead and dying, who were lying in rows on the floor, the nurses not having time to prepare beds, as the patients were taken so suddenly."[62] The remaining doctors utilized a variety of heroic therapies, including bleeding, administering copious doses of calomel, and injecting a concoction of warm water and tobacco juice into the veins of their patients. The results were not good.[63] By July 20, a total of 221 inmates had perished, a little over a quarter of New York City's entire mortality of 847 up to that time.[64]

The press never painted a full picture of what happened behind Bellevue's walls. The cases and deaths that occurred there appeared as a separate column in every board of health daily report, but outsiders only saw raw numbers and no details of the terror there. The editors of the *American* did not even want the board of health to include the total case and fatality counts in its daily reports, claiming that the outbreak within the facility stood "entirely distinct" because it had "no connection with the city."[65] They imagined that its location three miles from city hall and its walled off facilities made it separate from the general population, but they ignored Bellevue's role as a place where the city deposited its impoverished and unwanted.

Judith Roosevelt witnessed municipal authorities at work rounding up the poor as the death toll mounted. "The wretched beings lying about the streets are taken up and carried to the different hospitals," she wrote to her son Samuel on July 18. Two "nearly starved" and sick vagrants were removed from Desbrosses Street, where she lived. "We are all well [and] our neighbors are well and our friends generally have been so far favored that they have not been afflicted with this terrible complaint," she remarked. "We feel encouraged that the disorder will soon cease [and] that God will in mercy spare us that the people may soon return to their homes," she stated, yet reassuring her anxious son that "if contrary to our expectation the sickness should grow worse you may expect to see us with all the family."[66]

The letter must have crossed paths with her son. He had already left for Manhattan to implore his mother and father to go back to Hyde Park with him. When he arrived at his parents' home, he found them recalcitrant. They insisted on staying, and he returned home on the morning of July 20.

In his comfortable house, Samuel Johnson opened the pages of the *Evening Post* published on the day he left Manhattan and read the first entry of the obituaries: "DIED. This morning, of a short illness, Judith, wife of Peter Roosevelt, Esq. The relatives and friends of the family are invited to attend the funeral to-morrow morning, the 21st July, at 9 o'clock, from the corner of Desbrosses & Greenwich streets."[67] When he had last seen his mother, she had appeared in good health and spirits. She died a few short hours later and would be buried before he could return to say goodbye. Her cause of death was not given in the notice, but Samuel must have known instantly that cholera had taken his mother.

If Samuel had any doubts, they were quickly dispelled after he arrived back in Manhattan to be with his grieving father. "Elizabeth and myself hastened down immediately to the city & house of pestilence," he later told a friend. He lauded his wife for her bravery as "she would not be absent from me but would share the danger." From his father he must have learned the details. "In a few hours this most violent of sicknesses which the world has ever seen, had completed its work of death," Samuel said of cholera's assault on his mother. The scourge had been a topic in his correspondence since its appearance in Canada, not just to his mother, whom he had practically begged to leave Manhattan, but to his friend as well. "Little did I think when last I wrote to you, and spoke of that dreadful disease, which has since made desolate so many a home, little did I think I should so soon be called to mourn over its ravages in my own family circle," he cried.[68]

Cholera had shown itself to be the "extensive danger" that Johnson and so many other affluent and middle-class Americans thought it would not be. The cases were far from the "few" he imagined, and the alarm continued long after he thought it would pass. Mourning within family circles—rich and poor, free and enslaved, propertied and dispossessed—had just begun in the United States.

4

Terror on Arch Street

INCARCERATION'S FATAL CONSEQUENCES IN THE NORTHEAST

PATRICK CANE ARRIVED in the United States from Ireland in 1817, traveled from city to city looking for work, and served time in various jails and almshouses between jobs. Arrested in Philadelphia on July 10, 1832, Cane did not survive the duration of his one-month sentence in Arch Street Prison. Susan Hunter had regularly been in and out of trouble for vagrancy, and on August 3, 1832, she found herself incarcerated in Arch Street. She perished two days later. On the same day, police sent a destitute couple, Jane and John Welsh, to the same prison. Jane immediately died, while her husband became gravely ill. The impoverished Welshes, Patrick Cane, and Susan Hunter had lived with constant threats of incarceration. Their crime of being poor, however, amounted to their death sentences in the summer of 1832.[1]

Cholera quickly ripped through Arch Street Prison. On July 29, a recently jailed woman came down with symptoms of the disease, and within four days numerous female inmates became sick. Cholera spread to the men's wing of the institution, and the dead began to pile up. On August 4, the coroner sent two cartloads of coffins, while the inmates clamored for release. "In the same room were mingled the dead, the dying, the sick, and the well," described Dr. Samuel Jackson, secretary of the Philadelphia Board of Health Special Medical Consulting Board. "The prisoners became frantic with despair, and threatened the lives of the officers and attendants."[2] An investigation found that amid the chaos, "no accurate enumeration of the deaths during this terrible catastrophe" could be made but suggested that during those dark days of late July and early August the scourge had taken more than a quarter of the 310 inmates to their graves.[3]

Arch Street prisoners experienced an especially intense period of terror amid cholera's ravages of the Northeast. The disease continued to strike New Yorkers through August, hitched a ride with many of those fleeing its wrath, and found its way into the water supply, food, and dwellings of an increasing number of susceptible people. It traveled up the Hudson and along the Erie Canal, caused sporadic fatalities in New England, spread more thoroughly in New Jersey, and erupted in Philadelphia. Scores of travelers, urban residents, and small-town inhabitants fell to the disease. Wherever it went, people with the means to flee did so, thus keeping the pathogen in constant motion into the fall. The poor had a more difficult time outrunning the pestilence, and those shuttled into makeshift hospitals, almshouses, and prisons were made into sitting ducks.

The Philadelphia Sanatory Committee had a plan to deal with the poor even before cholera arrived in the city. On July 4, the commission explained to the public that it was "morally certain" that Philadelphia would see "many cases . . . among persons destitute of the means of support." A series of temporary hospitals to meet the coming emergency was therefore necessary, not simply to treat the poor but to protect the public from observing "heart-rending scenes" and "to obviate the panic which a few such spectacles would inevitably produce."[4] For the next three weeks, however, only a few cases and fatalities suspected of being cholera occurred in Philadelphia.[5]

Then the outbreak escalated. The board of health reported several new cases of "malignant cholera" on July 29. Significant rainfall occurred the night after the announcement, breaking a period of drought, and infections took off.[6] A total of twenty-one cases and eight deaths occurred over a two-day period that ended on the thirtieth.[7] "Our time of alarm has at length come," John Lamb wrote to his sister on the last day of the month. "Every family that can find the means to go and the places for their reception is clearing out from the fair city of Philadelphia."[8] On August 3, the board of health reported 125 cases and forty-one deaths occurring over the previous twenty-four-hour period.[9] Even heavier rain fell on the fourth. Daily mortality peaked at seventy-four and seventy-three on the sixth and seventh, respectively, marking the deadliest forty-eight hours of Philadelphia's pandemic experience.[10] Flight from the city during those dark days was substantial.[11] "No words of mine can give an adequate idea of the panic which prevailed at that time in the city and country," Dr. Hiram Corson later recalled. "People fled from the city as best they could."[12]

The delayed escalation of Philadelphia's outbreak can be explained by the effectiveness of the city's Fairmount Water Works in separating drinking water from sewage. The city had dammed the Schuylkill River in 1822, built steam engines to pump the river water to a reservoir on top of Fairmount Hill, and then let gravity send the water to a pump house in the center of the city. From there, iron pipes relayed the water into homes, businesses, and public fountains across the city. Schuylkill water, taken from above Philadelphia and thus free from seepage from the city's privies and cesspools, was used to fight fires, clean streets, quench thirst, and prepare food.

Municipal works, however, did not reach the suburbs, which had yet to be incorporated into the city proper. Southwark and Moyamensing, both below South Street, particularly lacked access.[13] With the heavy rains of July 29 and August 4, ideal conditions emerged for *Vibrio* to wind its way from the intestines of a few infected people into the privies and cesspools of the poorest and most densely populated neighborhoods and through the soil and into the well water that supplied impoverished people in underserved neighborhoods.

The disadvantaged population that remained faced intense medical policing. City officials combed the most disreputable parts of the metropolitan area, dragging impoverished people who appeared ill to one of the eighteen cholera hospitals and sending the still healthy into temporary huts constructed near a graveyard along the Schuylkill River.[14] "I shall never forget that grand moving-day," one Philadelphian recalled after observing the process. "Oh what a sight!—men, women, and children, black and white, barefooted, lame, and blind, half-naked and dirty, carrying old stools, broken chairs, thin-legged tables, and bundles of beds and bedclothing to their summer retreat on the common!"[15] One neighborhood described as having a population of "low blacks with a slight inter-mixture of whites" remained vacated and fenced up during the outbreak.[16]

The poor offered some resistance, especially to forced hospitalization. Protestors blockaded entrances to the hospitals and threatened medical personnel with bodily harm. On August 5, physicians called on the city for protection, specifically for themselves and more broadly for the reputation of the city and nation. "Though we were fully aware of the most unreasonable and disgraceful popular prejudices which existed in Europe at the out breakings of cholera," the doctors decried in an appeal to the sanatory committee, "little did we suppose that in our enlightened Republic, and especially in the City of Philadelphia... that we should be subjected to the most opprobrious abuse and insult." Municipal authorities complied, stepped up law enforcement around the hospitals, and vowed to punish anyone who disturbed public health measures.[17] The efforts appear to have worked; no further disturbances were recorded after the fifth.

The press, both local and national, relayed and amplified the physicians' message. The Philadelphia *Inquirer* condemned the crowd's actions as the work of "ignorant persons... under a strange prejudice against the doctors and the mode of the treatment in these institutions."[18] The New York *American* published the Philadelphia physicians' appeal with a preamble expressing the editors' dismay that "scenes of incomprehensible ignorance and prejudice, on the part of the lowest mobs" could appear in an American city as they had in Paris.[19]

New York City, of course, had not been immune to such protests. Impoverished people hid their sick friends and loved ones from officers sent to retrieve bodies, while stories circulated that the gravely ill lay unattended or, worse, subjected to medical experimentation and dissection, even before they died. The city's hospitals had, in fact, become the butt of a joke that circulated widely in the American press. One "young lady, a teacher of a flourishing school," so feared ending up in what was widely regarded as a place where the poor were sent to die that she supposedly did not go anywhere without a label affixed to her clothing that read, "If Miss L—should be taken with the Cholera in the street, don't take her to the hospital, but to her boarding house, No. 214—street."[20] More direct action occurred as well. In early August, mobs stopped litter bearers from carrying patients into cholera hospitals, and in one case, a gang assaulted an alderman and a physician as they attempted to tend to the sick.[21]

One of the most publicized protests against forced hospitalization occurred in the thriving Erie Canal city of Utica, New York. By late July, boats traveling along the busy waterway had been carrying cholera-stricken people. On August 7, Utica's officials grew concerned enough about a local outbreak that they constructed a temporary hospital to receive patients. On August 13, the city's board of health confirmed cases not only among the poor and supposedly debauched but also among "the temperate" and "those in comfortable circumstances [and] comparatively free from pressing anxieties."[22] "A sudden terror prevailed and frightened our inhabitants," one resident revealed. "All that could take themselves off deserted their homes."[23] Some three thousand out of a population of around eight thousand had reportedly fled within days of the initial announcement.[24]

Utica's less affluent residents, especially Irish immigrants, then became an even larger proportion of the population that *Vibrio* could prey upon. City officials rounded up the ill who had no one to care for them. As hospitals filled, enough medical attendants could not be found.[25] Cholera "swept the inhabitants off by scores," one resident told his friends, adding that the board of health "would pay most any price for nurses."[26]

The Irish viewed the hospitals as murderous centers of incarceration rather than as places of healing. On September 1, 1832, Barney Keating and several other Irish-born Americans marched to the cholera hospital, forced their way into it, and caused physicians and nurses to flee. The police rushed to the scene, arrested the ringleaders, and dispersed the remainder. The Utica *Observer* did not mention Keating by name but claimed the group he supposedly led was "possessed of an idea that their countrymen were not fairly dealt by when carried to the hospital." Newspapers across the country ran the *Observer*'s vague summary of the event and described it as a "riot" by "foolish and silly" Irishmen.[27]

This story was incomplete at best. In an article that circulated mainly within Utica, the weekly *Sentinel and Gazette* quoted Keating as saying that he and his cohorts attacked the facility and its personnel "because they killed all the Irishmen who were taken there to be cured of the cholera."[28] Keating would later deny his leadership role in the fracas but admitted trying to get into the facility after learning that his "friends and countrymen were confined" and suffered "a great remissness and want of attention on the part of the Nurses."[29] Utica's Irish population saw hospitals much the same as impoverished people in other US cities did: as places where people were taken against their will, subjected to torturous remedies, hastened to deaths that would not have otherwise happened, and then hurried into graves without customary funeral rites.

In Utica, Irish resistance had an impact. On September 3, the board of health enacted new ordinances. First, nobody could be taken to the hospital without a physician's certificate, and second, individuals seemingly near death, or in a "collapsed state," were not to be admitted. The latter ordinance certainly reflected an unstated capitulation to the Irish's lack of faith in heroic medicine and their desire to see that their deceased received proper burials.[30]

More permanent institutions of US towns, cities, and counties—almshouses or poorhouses—essentially became hospitals during cholera's sweep through the mid-Atlantic. New York City's Bellevue was far from the only such place where medical policing led to an influx of *Vibrio*-carrying inmates and consequent mortality of tragic proportions.

On the east bank of the Hudson River, roughly halfway between New York City and Albany, the Dutchess County Poorhouse in Poughkeepsie became the scene of an explosive outbreak. Authorities in the city of some six thousand people organized a board of health in early July, began to police boat traffic for ill passengers, and stepped up enforcement of vagrancy laws.[31] On July 10, officers rounded up a poor man who lay ill on Union Street and sent him to the poorhouse, located a mile east of the town center. He died within a few hours of his arrival.[32] On the fifteenth, an African American man collapsed after a violent attack of vomiting and diarrhea. The board of health ordered officers to transport the man from his domicile—a cellar beneath a burned-out home—to the poorhouse. The man died within a day of his arrival, while a woman who lived in the same place went with him to serve as his nurse. She soon sickened and passed.[33]

Civic leaders struggled to maintain a perception that Poughkeepsie was healthy. On July 15, the board of health issued a statement declaring that none of the five recent deaths were due to the novel disease. Editors of the two local papers, the *Independence* and the *Journal*, reassured readers in their July 18 issues that their city remained safe, even with an influx of refugees from Albany and New York City. Residents, the *Journal* urged, should "disregard utterly the thousand idle, extravagant and unfounded stories which are put afloat respecting the health of this village."[34]

One day later, however, the board of health had to admit that the scourge was at work in their supposedly healthy community. They announced that Nell Dubois had come down with "Spasmodic Cholera" and been taken to a makeshift hospital. Dubois died within hours of her arrival. Two days later, Peter Herrick and Benjamin Mackey perished after a rapid progression of symptoms. Editors of the *Journal* declared the victims "to be of extremely intemperate and dissolute habits" and their deaths to have "produced no alarm."[35]

Residents' anxieties increased despite such depictions. "The alarm is very great, so much so that people from the country dare not come in," one Poughkeepsian informed a New York City correspondent.[36] Dr. Hunting Sherrill, a local physician, recalled widespread anxiety and found himself "very much engaged in attending the increased number of patients" who thought they had the premonitory symptoms.[37] Residents pointed to the cellar where the first cases had occurred as the culprit in producing disease-causing miasma. Sherrill described it as filled with "blacks, and indigent degraded whites," living "promiscuously mingled" and "indulging in vice and dissipation, and surrounded by filth."[38] The board of health demolished the property and forced its inhabitants to find new places to reside.[39]

Cases in the city became frequent after July 28. That day, the board of health announced that Jacob Mace, "a man of intemperate habits," perished from "Malignant Cholera." The unfortunately named secretary of the board, Mr. A. J. Coffin, informed the public that they would receive daily reports thereafter. That evening, Seldon Blakely died of the same disease that took his neighbor Mace, prompting officers to visit the location to "remove the inhabitants from that section of the town."[40] Many ended up in the poorhouse.[41] Editors of the *Journal* applauded such vigilance and expressed hope that municipal authorities "will not relax in their exertions."[42]

Those exertions set the stage for a sudden and horrific outbreak in the county poorhouse. At 6:00 p.m. on August 2, an individual came down with symptoms; by 8:00 p.m. the following day, ten people had died and another dozen lay gravely ill.[43] "The disease seemed to make a general attack upon a great number at almost the same time," recalled Sherrill, who put the total number in the facility at 190.[44] The scourge continued its deadly work, taking a total of forty-nine lives in its first five days in the establishment.[45] It was not done yet.

Readers of American newspapers received a highly problematic description of the tragedy in Poughkeepsie. Editors of the Dutchess County *Republican*, in a widely circulated article, assigned the blame squarely to the poor. The overseer, they claimed, had been absent the day before the malady appeared, and during that time, "many of the paupers entered the garden and stripped the cucumbers from the vines, eating them as they were picked, and also ate large quantities of green apples, beans, &c." The poor and obviously hungry inmates, the editors charged, "paid dearly" for consuming proscribed cholera-causing foods.[46]

There was, as was so often the case, much that the article left hidden. The editors surely knew that Poughkeepsie officials had been clearing impoverished neighborhoods and sending residents to the poorhouse. The editors also had to know that the inmates had been abandoned. The superintendents of the institution had fled at the beginning of the alarm and gone with their families to safe places some twenty miles away from the city. The overseer left in charge was not merely absent for a day but refused to even go into the main house of the facility.[47]

The board of health stepped in to deal with the emergency. Poughkeepsie's officials had difficulty finding doctors and nurses, as locals proved "unwilling to risk their lives" and as "panic . . . possessed the public mind." They managed to employ a corps of nurses from New York, allowed some inmates to leave on their own recognizance, and constructed huts on elevated ground where the incarcerated could stay in "comfort as well as safety."[48]

Even with these measures, *Vibrio* persisted into early September, sweeping away a total of ninety-six inmates before burning out. Over 50 percent of the facility's incarcerated population died from the disease.[49] An estimated 175 cholera deaths occurred throughout Poughkeepsie—private residences of the city plus the poorhouse and makeshift hospital—meaning that 54 percent of the fatalities occurred in a place of incarceration. As the outbreak began to wind down in mid-August, one local newspaper admitted that cholera seemed to have taken a higher proportion of the population in Poughkeepsie than it had in other places, but the editors emphasized that the bulk of mortality occurred in the poorhouse and that "scarcely a temperate person has been removed by the disease, unless through neglect of the premonitory symptoms."[50] The press once again repeated the narrative of cholera's selective predation and erased the real horror experienced by incarcerated, hungry, and abandoned people.

Compared to Poughkeepsie, Newark seemed to endure the pandemic rather well. From July 6 until early September, only sixty-five of the eleven thousand inhabitants of New Jersey's largest city perished. Still, small numbers should not hide what was a nightmare for the city's poor. On July 9, an African American man who had left New York City four or five days earlier came down with symptoms of the disease and was immediately transported to the Essex County Poorhouse, which stood within Newark's city limits. The man managed to recover.[51] On the eleventh, an Irishman named John Sharkey, who lived alongside twenty to thirty people crowded into a four-hundred-square-foot dwelling, fell to the disease.[52] When others showed symptoms, municipal authorities sent them off to the poorhouse, while forcing the apparently healthy to relocate to a crowded shanty.[53]

By the next day, the Essex County Medical Society counted a total of nine cholera deaths in Newark. All but two lived together in the decrepit dwelling in which Sharkey had died.[54] On the night of July 15, vigilantes torched the vacated dwelling, and firefighters made no effort to stop the blaze.[55] One observer "found the panic very great," with people remaining shut up in their houses and with officers incinerating the bedding of the sick and deceased "in the middle of the street."[56] The county tried to meet the growing challenge of the outbreak by constructing a makeshift hospital on the poorhouse's grounds, about a quarter of a mile away from the main building.

It was too late and ineffective. *Vibrio* had already infiltrated the place. On July 19, Henry Cinderbox, a twelve-year-old boy and inmate of the institution, came down with violent symptoms, which were reported to follow his consumption of "unripe apples" after spending the day standing barefoot in water. He died on the twentieth.[57] His younger and older brothers as well as a seven-year-old female inmate also became ill but recovered.[58] On July 31, the eight-year-old James Clark escaped his incarceration but did not make it far. He was returned to the facility's hospital after being found in a collapsed state, having endured a severe episode of vomiting and purging. His mother and father had just died of the scourge a few days earlier, and the grieving and certainly traumatized child may have been trying to find his two-and-half-year-old sister, who had been separated from him and sent to live with another family. He would never find her. She died on August 1. James never recovered from the ordeal and perished in October.[59] Cholera, meanwhile, continued to infect those in the poorhouse through the remainder of the summer.[60]

The horrid circumstances that occurred in the Essex County institution received little detail in Dr. Samuel H. Pennington's official report of the outbreak. He provided the New Jersey Medical Society with the final count of sixty-five total fatalities in Newark, but he did not disaggregate deaths that occurred in the poorhouse from those that occurred in the city's neighborhoods. He furthermore explained away the deaths with the usual victim blaming, as occurring among people living "dissolute lives" who paid no attention to a proper diet, had intemperate habits, and gave in to an "anxiety of mind, fear and all depressing emotions."[61]

Pennington highlighted only one exceptional episode of the outbreak. Three cholera deaths within the "respectable" Becroft family occurring over a two-day period was, to the doctor, "the most melancholy and distressing scene of desolation which its whole history in Newark presented."[62] The Becrofts' unexpected suffering deserved his sympathy, while inmates of the poorhouse were understood to fall into the class of people predisposed to the disease. The terror of being incarcerated in a place where a deadly disease lurked received no acknowledgment.

Cholera also took a frightening toll among inmates of Philadelphia's almshouse, an institution not connected to Arch Street Prison. On July 29, the malady appeared in the establishment, which typically held more than one thousand orphans, widows, elderly, disabled, and mentally ill. The Guardians of the Poor, who oversaw the facility, moved healthy inmates to the partially constructed Blockley facility on the west side of the Schuylkill River and left the infected to be treated in the old almshouse.[63] Mortality grew in both places, with a peak of eighteen fatalities reported on August 8.[64] Another twenty-five inmates passed away over the next five days, leading the *Daily Chronicle* to resort to the well-rehearsed narrative of how cholera chose its prey. The editors exonerated the institution's doctors, who could not save paupers suffering from pre-existing diseases and "gross intemperance."[65]

Victim blaming hid a grim reality. The Guardians of the Poor later explained that while "the disease raged in all its horrors," nurses and their assistants in the old almshouse drank themselves into a stupor and left the sick abandoned. "Such was the appalling nature and extent of the disease," they added, "that fear overcame every other consideration, and it was found impracticable to keep the nurses to their duty or to obtain, at a reasonable price, proper persons to attend the sick."[66] Guardians appealed to the Sisters of Charity for help. Five nuns came from Philadelphia's convent, and another eight came from Baltimore's.[67] *Vibrio* continued to infect those kept at the old facility and at Blockley into early September. By then, the scourge had taken the lives of ninety-two inmates.[68]

While public health measures propelled *Vibrio* into poorhouses, cholera had a more mixed record when it came to prisons within the Northeast. Officials avoided a major outbreak in New York City's Bridewell jail by releasing petty offenders and dispersing inmates convicted of more serious crimes to other facilities after an initial case had occurred.[69] The scourge did not even get into Auburn Penitentiary in upstate New York, New Jersey's state prison in Lamberton, or Pennsylvania's Eastern State Penitentiary in Philadelphia.

Cholera also avoided a Massachusetts state prison just outside of Boston in Charlestown, although a stomach bug of some sort certainly alarmed the public. One hundred and eighteen inmates, almost all at once, began vomiting and having diarrhea on August 5. City officials immediately suspected that their turn with cholera had begun, and physicians rushed in and administered "active remedies." By the evening of the sixth, every patient was convalescent. With no fatalities, physicians ruled out "Spasmodic cholera."[70]

The Boston area, in fact, went rather unscathed during the pandemic. Two sudden deaths occurred in Boston on August 15 and were quickly diagnosed as a malignant form of the novel disease. Alarms reverberated throughout the city and surrounding towns, but nothing came of it.[71] Nine fatal cases diagnosed as cholera occurred on Eliot Street during the second week of September, but there was no significant spread beyond the confined location.[72] Some more cases occurred during the last week of October on Broad Street, resulting in a reported fourteen deaths.[73] An investigation published eighteen years later counted seventy total cholera deaths during the summer and fall of 1832.[74]

Vibrio took more lives in New York's Sing Sing Prison than it did in the entire Boston area. Completed on the banks of the Hudson thirty-five miles north of Manhattan just four years before the pandemic, the facility housed 939 inmates as of June 25. On that day, officials stopped accepting new prisoners. They essentially hedged their bets that cholera was a contagious disease that might tear through their facility once introduced. Despite such efforts, an inmate became sick on July 17 with what the attending doctor described as "all the appalling symptoms" of cholera.[75] The next day, five more prisoners showed signs of the disease and two perished.[76] How the disease got into the prison is unclear, but once it did, it haunted the place for weeks to come.

Prison officials countered rumors and reassured the public. One of the first accounts described inmates growing "much alarmed at the appearance of the distemper" and demonstrating "symptoms of insubordination."[77] The superintendent reported to the governor that he and his staff remained in control. They administered prompt treatment of inmates with premonitory symptoms, suspended hard labor in the marble quarry, eliminated foods thought to be conducive to cholera, and kept healthy prisoners out in the fresh air during most of the day. "Considerable alarm exists among them," the superintendent admitted about the inmates, but "they acquiesce with entire cheerfulness in the new arrangements and there are no appearances of insubordination."[78]

It stretches the imagination to believe that Sing Sing's inmates endured the outbreak with cheerfulness. No riot occurred, to be sure, and daily mortality never exploded as had happened in other places. Nevertheless, cholera's slow grind added up. Poor hygienic conditions and perhaps contaminated food, rather than infestation of the common water supply, kept *Vibrio* in circulation in the large facility for over a month. During this time, prisoners were under constant inspection for signs of illness. The slightest diarrhea could lead them directly to the prison hospital, where a team of doctors administered laxatives and cathartics to help the body eliminate the morbid matter, bled their patients to restore humoral balance, and followed up with camphor suppositories and blistering.[79] Prisoners understandably proved unwilling to consent to such treatment, hid their symptoms the best they could, and were then blamed for their own demise when they succumbed to the malady.[80]

Between July 17 and August 14, at least one person died of the disease daily, with a peak of seven fatalities reported on August 4. No deaths occurred on August 15, but cases lingered, and mortality continued for a few more weeks. By September 4, a total of 103 prisoners, or 11 percent of the inmate population, had perished.[81] Sing Sing's staff and administration escaped unscathed, except for one of the guards, Mr. Van Wart, who succumbed to the disease on August 27.[82]

Vibrio terrorized the inmates of Philadelphia's Arch Street Prison more instantly and intensely than those in Sing Sing. Before the outbreak began, an average of twelve to fifteen individuals per day were sent to Arch Street, which held untried vagrants and disorderly individuals, prisoners convicted of petty crimes, and some debtors. On July 30, the police directed a total of twenty-four into the prison, an increase almost certainly due to the zeal of public authorities trying to keep cholera's preferred victims away from the general public. Seventeen cases and five deaths occurred between July 30 and August 3. The first victims were described as newcomers, who came down with cholera within twenty-four hours of arriving. These initial victims likely carried *Vibrio* with them into the prison.[83] With 310 inmates crowded together under poor hygienic conditions, the deadly bacteria easily traveled from person to person.[84]

The prison's staff and physicians quickly became sick and overwhelmed. By the end of the day on August 4, eighty inmates lay "dead, dying or suffering," and staff members found it difficult to walk through the facility without stepping on a victim.[85] On the same day, an attending physician came down with symptoms and had to leave; a watchman died after a short struggle with the disease; and the chief prison keeper became "bewildered with fatigue" and fell into "a state of derangement."[86] After sunset, the keepers forced the inmates back into their locked sleeping quarters. The two cartloads of coffins arrived from the coroner, and prison staff conveyed the corpses out a back entrance.[87] Living prisoners clamored for release as their jailmates continued to suffer and die around them during the night. "They twice, in a furious and mutinous manner, rushed towards the keeper to inquire," a later investigation revealed, "'if they were to be kept to die there?'"[88] The keepers refused to open the doors until the early morning hours of the fifth for fear the prisoners would do anything to escape.[89]

Additional medical personnel and law enforcement arrived at the same time. Among them was Dr. Jesse Reading Burden, a member of the Philadelphia Board of Health Special Medical Consulting Board. At 6:00 a.m., Burden found dozens of prisoners "lying on the floor in the different stages of the disease." Throughout the day, he and other officials sorted inmates. They dispersed fifty of the ill to several of the makeshift hospitals, released petty offenders and untried vagrants on their own recognizance, and sent serious offenders to the holding cells of the city courthouse. Some heathy prisoners chose to stay and serve as nurses and orderlies in return for wages. One African American man, convicted of assault and serving a term of six to nine months, earned a pardon for helping dispose of corpses. Amid the work, nobody could keep up with counting the number who had died during the previous twenty-four hours, and the board of health's official report released at noon that day contained no statistics from the prison. The work continued into the next day, when Dr. Richard Harlan arrived and found "the suffering and agony of dying wretches . . . an awful sight to witness."[90]

With Arch Street Prison cleared of most of its inmates, the outbreak within its walls subsided. Between the seventh and the eleventh, twelve more prisoners perished in the facility, bringing the official total to forty-four fatalities. That number, though, did not include several people, including those who died in the prison during the overnight period from the fourth to the fifth, ill inmates who perished on their way to or shortly after arriving at the hospitals, and others who carried *Vibrio* with them and died during their brief stint of freedom. The Philadelphia Society for Alleviating the Miseries of Public Prisoners investigated and offered estimates that ranged from sixty-two to eighty prisoners succumbing to the scourge.[91]

The horror in Arch Street Prison could not be completely hidden from the public, although the press certainly stuck to a narrative that cholera purposefully chose its degraded victims. With the dead piling up and the public aware that something was happening, the *Inquirer* had to admit on August 6 that "the condition of the prison yesterday morning was frightful in the extreme."[92]

Any sympathy was short-lived, however. The editors of the city's *Journal of Health* callously said of all who had died, "humanity could hardly regret their end."[93] The *Courier* described the inmates as "the very scum and refuse of the population."[94] The *United States Gazette* claimed the prisoners' stomachs were "always inflamed with raw whiskey, and their limbs embrowned and embossed with filth and sores."[95] They then said the quiet part out loud: "Death is generally terrible to every one; but when the *removed* are moved, when the feelings of the living are spared, his sting is blunted."[96] The poor, in other words, had been sent away, just as city leaders had originally planned, to protect the public from the pandemic's unpleasantness.

Those who experienced cholera's terrors and felt death's sting had names. They were Patrick Cane, Susan Hunter, Jane Welsh, John Welsh, and many others whose identities and lives have not made the annals of history. Cholera tragically cut short the sentences of countless Americans incarcerated in temporary hospitals, almshouses, and prisons during that deadly summer of 1832.

Far from being the "scum" who cholera would inevitably take, they were people who died under horrific conditions, not because of their supposed moral failings. Municipal authorities in America's towns and cities had criminalized their poverty, shuttled them away from public view, put them in the worst possible circumstances to experience *Vibrio*, and explained away their demise as the unsurprising outcome of a pathogen that supposedly acted as predicted.

5

A Preacher, a Banker, a Judge, and a Quaker

CONVINCING THE NORTHEASTERN ELITE

ON AUGUST 11, 1832, twenty-year-old Ann Van Wart left her New York City family home with her mother and father and spent a delightful seventeen-day visit with their friends in West Orange, New Jersey. She recorded days filled with nature walks in the Watchung Mountains; religious and social events at St. Mark's Episcopal Church; picnics and teas with other evacuees and locals; and a captivating tour of a nearby canal where she marveled at the locks and other engineering feats that symbolized the progress of her nation.[1]

The scourge was not out of her thoughts, however. While standing atop a ridge on August 13, Van Wart recorded seeing the outline of Manhattan in the horizon and wondering about friends "whom I may never again see this side of eternity." She prayed to God to prepare her family "for the change which awaits us." During church service on August 26, the minister preached so strongly about the pestilence that Van Wart transcribed his harrowing words into her journal. Cholera "is now spreading its devastating influence and fast depopulating our largest cities," the minister charged, because "God is not acknowledged." He further warned, "God visits all orders and degrees of men, the rich and the poor, the base and the honorable, the public benefactor and the bane of society." It must have been with some trepidation that she returned to the city on August 28, not knowing who among her social set had lived or died and whether the disease awaited her own family.[2]

As Ann Van Wart understood, cholera, supposedly a predator of the poor and dissolute, could defy expectations. The pathogen had forced affluent Northeastern families to ask themselves difficult questions. Should they flee? Could they rely upon medical professionals and their treatments? When would life return to normal? Why did people like them become subject to such a loathsome illness? The ordeal that these questions posed played out in numerous households, and the variety of answers can be seen through the of four select individuals: the Reverend Charles Grandison Finney, arguably the most famous evangelist of nineteenth-century America; John Pintard, a trustee of the Bank for Savings in New York City; Charles Ewing, a Trenton resident and chief justice of New Jersey's Supreme Court; and Deborah Norris Logan, a Quaker historian who lived in suburban Philadelphia. Their experiences showed that cholera could convince some well-to-do and respectable people that it would not conform to what they expected.

The Reverend Finney picked a terrible time to move to New York City. During the first part of 1832, he had been working in Providence and then in Boston, moving from church to church and preaching to various audiences. The prospect of having his own pastorate and giving his family some stability appealed to him.

Back in 1821, Finney, a young lawyer working in Upstate New York, had a conversion experience and decided to dedicate his life to Christ. He received his license as a Presbyterian minister two years later, achieved regional fame with his captivating sermons, and received a regular barrage of invitations to evangelize cities and towns throughout the Northeast. Lewis and Arthur Tappan, wealthy silk merchants in New York City, followed Finney's theology, one that rejected Calvinism's emphasis on original sin and predestination by telling individuals that they had the power to give up wickedness and gain salvation. They shared his vision of a perfected society, one in which individuals abandoned alcohol, observed the Sabbath, repudiated slavery, and shunned the myriad other evils that kept them from prayer and conversion. The reformist Tappans wanted nothing more than to have Finney exert his efforts against sin in their city, and they got their wish.

In May 1832, the thirty-nine-year-old Finney started preaching to massive audiences in Manhattan. Together with other like-minded elites, the Tappans bought Chatham Street Theater, turned it into a church, and paid the reverend handsomely to serve as its pastor. The theater, located near the vice-ridden Five Points area, had a bawdy reputation that attracted inebriated patrons. But rechristened as the Chatham Street Chapel, with no pew fees needed to attend services, the church would become a focal point of evangelical reform efforts. To sweeten the deal, the Tappans provided funds to Finney to relocate his entire family—his twenty-eight-year-old wife Lydia, four-year-old daughter Helen, two-year-old son Charles, Jr., and three-month-old son Frederic—into a home at 177 Grand Street, a few blocks away from the church.

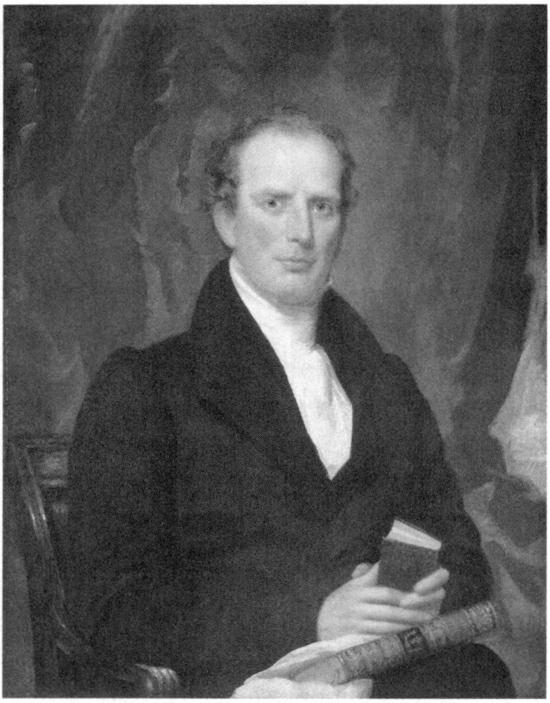

Charles Grandison Finney, by Samuel Lovett Waldo, 1834. Oil on hardwood panel. Allen Memorial Art Museum, Oberlin College, 1916.6.

Just as the Finneys got settled, cholera arrived in their neighborhood. "This awful desolating judgment will no doubt sweep through the length & breadth of the Land," Lydia wrote to her parents on July 15. The Finneys had by then sent Helen to stay with friends in New Haven and had twice packed up their belongings for a retreat to Lydia's parents in Whitesboro, a small village outside of Utica. A "sense of duty" to their new church, Lydia explained, kept them in the city. "We may do good to a greater extent now than at any other time."[3]

On the morning that Lydia started her letter to her parents, the Finneys witnessed harrowing scenes on their way to the church. They "saw a corpse just put into a coffin only a few doors" from their house. They passed a hearse as they walked, as well as a carriage loaded with caskets. Charles added a postscript to his wife's letter: "Our healths remain tolerable—People dying all around us. O that we may be also ready, & may the peace of God be with you forever."[4]

While Finney remained in the city, his patron Arthur Tappan, among many other elites, left and was publicly ridiculed for doing so. On July 23, the merchant added a note to his usual newspaper advertisement, declaring "that notwithstanding the alarm on account of the Cholera, the principal stores continue open, and the city may be visited without any apprehension of danger."[5] The *Morning Courier and Enquirer* skewered him for his hypocrisy of encouraging people to come into a disease-ridden city while he had fled.[6] The Catholic newspaper the *Truth Teller* lambasted the Protestant in harsher terms. "He is now rusticating with his family, well clothed and fed, and no doubt beyond the influence of the dreadful pestilence, which is at this moment threatening all in the city of New York," the editors decried. "Shame! Shame!"[7]

Finney continued his work in the city as the pestilence took increasing numbers of people who were thought to be safe from it. The deaths in Reverend George L. Hinton's family proved particularly shocking. On Tuesday, July 24, the Hinton family was sitting at the dinner table when two-year-old George, Jr., suddenly became sick. He died within five hours. George, Sr., and his twenty-three-year-old wife, Sara, became ill as they watched their young son die, and they followed him into the grave by sunset the following evening. The youngest Hinton, an infant named Howard, held on until August 3 but died due to swelling of the brain, a condition that may or may not have been related to a cholera infection.[8]

News of the Hinton family's extinction could not have escaped Finney's attention. The *Evangelist*, financed by the Tappans, reported the passing of Reverend Hinton and lauded the man as one who "devoted himself with unwearied assiduity, to the sick."[9] Just a few days after the widely reported tragedy, Reverend Thomas H. Skinner penned a letter to his close friend and colleague Finney. "If Satan by any means could get you to expose yourself to the dreadful pestilence which rages around you," Skinner wrote from New Haven on July 29, "he and his would rejoice, but ... others throughout this land would be left in tears." Finney's confidant further argued that the charge of "cowardice" against those who fled "sounds in every ear not like religion but a devilish sophism." People who stayed did so, in other words, because they feared public shame more than they feared God. "Do dear Brother leave the city at once," Skinner implored.[10]

Finney took Skinner's advice. He had planned on traveling upstate later in August to visit his parents and retrieve some of his wife's belongings from her family's farm. He moved those plans up and took Lydia, Charles, Jr., and Frederic with him. By August 11, they had settled in with Lydia's brother George Andrews in the village of New York Mills, just west of Utica. "The panic became great, and a great many Christian people fled into the country,"

Finney recorded in his *Memoirs*. The reverend recollected cholera being "especially fatal" near his Manhattan home and seeing "five hearses drawn up at the same time, at different doors within sight."[11] The Finneys remained in the small upstate village into early September. Charles, who suffered from chronic tuberculosis, had been ill since leaving New York City and unable to preach, even if he had dared venture into the nearby cholera-ridden towns and villages along the Erie Canal.

Like other evacuees, the Finneys received steady reminders of the ongoing scourge.[12] They learned of Susan Hallock's shocking death, for example, from Lewis Tappan, who, unlike his brother, stayed in the metropolis through the outbreak. Hallock, a thirty-year-old mother of three, had joined the Chatham Street congregation in June after hearing Finney preach. On Friday, August 17, she had "premonitory symptoms" and took the medicine that her husband, a doctor, had prescribed. The next morning, however, she experienced "violent diarrhea & vomiting" and perished by 2:00 p.m.[13] William Green, Jr., another of the reverend's patrons, wrote to him later in the month that his city friends were all well and urged him to return in early September. Green, though, had no illusions that the pandemic would retreat across the nation. "God is going to scourge our whole country," he predicted.[14]

While Finney had retreated, John Pintard stayed put. On July 18, the day after the Pintard family held a council and decided to stay, they had a scare. A six-year-old grandson suffered a stomach ailment, requiring the attendance of their family physician, John Wakefield Francis. The doctor administered castor oil and brought his patient to recovery.[15] Pintard, nonetheless, took note of Francis's change of demeanor from being skeptical about the outbreak to being "alarmed."[16] A few days later, John Pintard's wife, Elizabeth, decided to go stay with relatives in Princeton. He knew, though, that relocation would be a gamble, as the scourge seemed to be spreading throughout the region. "Where is safety," he asked rhetorically in one of his several letters to his daughter. "A hard question to answer."[17] Elizabeth, in fact, changed her mind, declaring she would have "no peace of mind" being apart from her family.[18] Instead of fleeing, the Pintards relied upon a prudent diet free of vegetables and fruits, frequent walks, and medical advice that included, among other things, taking "a teaspoonful a day in water of purified charcoal powder... as a detergent."[19]

Pintard, meanwhile, continued to attend to his duties at the savings bank. The banker complained to a friend that he did not like to be around crowds of "human bodies... teeming with exhalations," but the institution needed to stay open so that laid-off workers could access their money.[20] He remained one of the few trustees who stayed in the city and felt it his duty to protect against "artful" individuals fraudulently laying claims to the funds of the bank's deceased depositors.[21] "Perhaps according to my advanced years," he bragged to his daughter, "I am doing as much good as any man in town."[22]

The growing death toll began to humble him. On July 24, the banker took his morning walk and became "a little appalled" to see a crowd gathered around the body of a "good looking" mechanic. The man had collapsed on his way to work and became one of the many scooped up by health officials and carted off to a cholera hospital. "These are times when we may emphatically exclaim in the midst of life we are in death," Pintard penned to his daughter.[23] On his evening walk on the twenty-seventh, he passed a Catholic church. "It was melancholy to notice the number of new graves, dug... to hold 3 & 4 coffins," he described.[24] He almost certainly read about the demise of the Hintons and revealed to his daughter that he had some doubts about the doctrine of noncontagion after three physicians he knew had perished.[25] On August 1, the scourge took his neighbor across the street, Mrs. Magdelana Bristed, the eldest daughter of John Jacob Astor, arguably the nation's wealthiest man. Most newspapers did not list Bristed's cause of death, but Pintard knew it to be cholera.[26]

As the outbreak continued, its meaning to the banker changed. Back in July, Pintard had cheered the scourge for sweeping away the "scum" of the city, but by mid-August, he came to see it as a broader collective punishment.[27] Since the founding of the American colonies, "we have experienced nothing like this modern strange pestilence," he declared. The pandemic had become, in his mind, an instrument "in the hand of the Almighty to chastise guilty nations & call them to reflection."[28] At the end of the month, with the number of cases subsiding, he even gave grudging praise to Catholics and criticized his fellow Protestants for their religious failures. Pintard had observed on numerous occasions Irish mourners arranging private hearses to retrieve bodies from the hospitals so they could conduct funerals more dignifying than the swift burials city officials tried to enforce. "Whatever be the errors of the Roman Catholics, we must give them credit for their zeal & faith," he remarked to his daughter. "God help us Protestants, I wish that we manifested more of both."[29]

Charles Ewing never got the chance to see the pandemic abate and reflect on its meaning. On August 4, 1832, the fifty-two-year-old man began to feel discomfort that would have brought instant dread to anyone at the time.

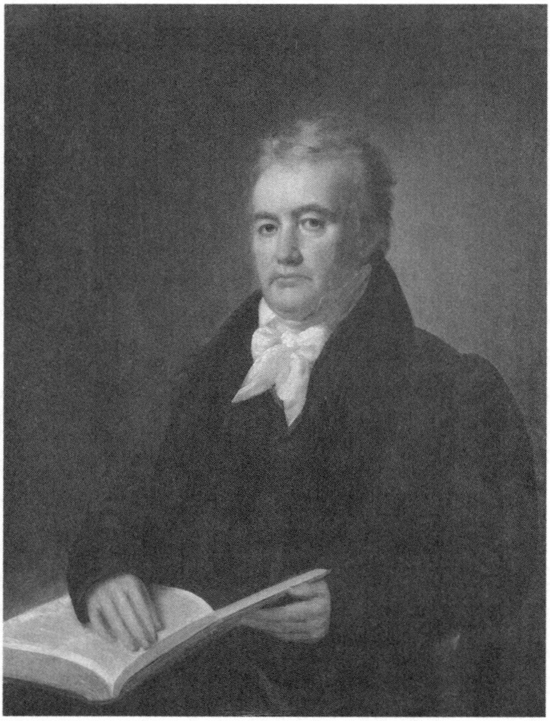

John Pintard, by William Jewett, 1832. Oil on wood panel, 36 × 27 1/2 in. The Louis Durr Fund. The New York Historical, 1928.1.

His stomach turned with nausea, and an uneasiness gurgled through his intestines. Perhaps he thought something he ate did not agree with him and that the discord in his bowels would soon pass. Or maybe he allowed himself to consider that his suffering might be the beginning of a deathly ordeal with the prevailing malady. Even with the pandemic at its height in the Northeast, Ewing may not have immediately leapt to this conclusion. He was the chief justice of the New Jersey Supreme Court after all, a well-respected, temperate, and otherwise healthy man.[30] He had been told repeatedly that people like him had nothing to fear.

If Ewing had such confidence, *Vibrio* soon disabused him of it. His symptoms grew worse, with vomiting and diarrhea rapidly dehydrating him, painful cramps seizing his body, and his consciousness fading on Saturday night. He died at 3:00 a.m., Sunday, August 5. By the end of the day, his corpse had been interred during a rushed funeral in Trenton.

News of Ewing's death spread quickly. On the sixth, the press in New Jersey as well as New York City and Philadelphia received bulletins announcing that cholera had taken the judge's life. Editors of New York's *Commercial Advertiser* publicly expressed their shock. "So far as a . . . robust constitution, equanimity of mind, and scrupulous regularity of life, may be considered guaranties against the mysterious pestilence . . . ," they opined, "the life of Judge Ewing might have been deemed to be insured."[31] New Jersey resident Silas Canfield read the newspaper and logically concluded, as many others must have, that cholera did not discriminate as much as he presumed. He privately confided to his brother, "this will strike terror through out the state—it is not confined to the intemperate alone."[32]

Questions about Ewing's dietary prudence immediately emerged after his death. The Salem, New Jersey, *Messenger* reported that on the night before the judge died, he feasted on "a hearty dinner of the good things of the season, including GREEN CORN."[33] The New York *Commercial Advertiser* found no reason to doubt the *Messenger*'s claim and found it useful in promoting proper behavior in New York City: "Those who choose to eat it," the editors said of green corn, "should remember that they assume by so doing the risk of committing suicide."[34]

Charges against Ewing for his supposed indulgence were quickly countered. His son took offense at the New York *Commercial Advertiser*'s uncritical acceptance of his father's alleged indiscretion. The editors published an apology for "the pain" the story had inflicted on the Ewing family and printed the son's letter describing his father as "temperate and prudent at all times." The judge also "without exception, excluded from his table" green corn and all other fresh produce of the season.[35] Trenton's *New Jersey State Gazette* also came to Ewing's defense and made a rare public expression of the anxiety elites privately felt. "If one so uniformly correct, prudent and temperate is subject to an attack of cholera," they warned, "who among us can be considered safe."[36]

The deceased judge would have to wait some time, however, to receive a eulogy that would fully exonerate him. Samuel Southard, New Jersey's attorney general and Ewing's good friend, accepted the invitation to deliver remarks at his funeral, but the ongoing outbreak in Trenton put those plans on hold.[37] Southard joined the general exodus from pestilential places and fled to Schooley's in the hills of western New Jersey. A "black cloud . . . is hovering over our Country," one of Southard's friends wrote to him on August 23, making it unadvisable to hold Ewing's memorial service any time soon. People would be afraid to come, and few would attend. "Those fears are too serious to be disregarded and prudence dictates the propriety of avoiding large collections of people until they can meet without apprehension," his friend advised.[38] Southard remained at his rural retreat into early September.

Deborah Norris Logan never considered fleeing. The seventy-year-old Quaker was the editor of William Penn's correspondence, the first female member of the Historical Society of Pennsylvania, and the widow of the former US Senator Dr. George Logan. Earlier in her life, she had had hosted George Washington, John Adams, and Joseph Bonaparte (Napoleon's older brother) at her Stenton estate, five miles north of Philadelphia's center.[39] Her detailed diary was a rich and witty chronicle of the events of her time, with the pandemic of 1832 figuring prominently. She had thought seriously about the disease before it arrived, and what she read about it convinced her that it preyed indiscriminately on all ranks and that it would be best for her to stay put in her mansion. There she would be near medical help should she need it.[40]

Logan believed cholera was contagious. She condemned her relative and local mill operator Thomas R. Fisher for "poking about among the cholera patients in New York" during an early July trip into that city and returning to Philadelphia "absolutely sick." "Had he inoculated the city," Logan recorded of Fisher, "he would have deserved to have passed the remainder of his days either in the Hospital or Penitentiary."[41] When cases escalated in Philadelphia in late July, she claimed "contagion is too apparent to be doubted."[42] Its explosion among the imprisoned population in early August confirmed her beliefs. "I had almost more excitement than I could bear from hearing accounts from the city of the awful progress of the cholera," she recorded on August 6. "Its ravages in the Arch street Prison are dreadful. People, in crowds are leaving the town."[43]

Her Stenton estate kept her distant from the seat of infection, but she worried the pathogen would reach her family regardless.[44] Her adult son Algernon made a trip into the city on August 8 to meet with some associates and on the way back visited his ill cousin Hannah Norris. Norris had fainted, supposedly from cholera, and after a doctor promptly bled her, she managed to recover.[45] Logan disapproved of her son's travels. His activities filled her mind with "vague apprehensions and fears" for she believed he would contract the disease. "He would be displeased if he saw this page," she recorded in her diary, "but it is dictated by a mother's anxiety."[46] To her great relief, her son returned safely and did not subsequently come down with the disease.

Logan continued to think no one was safe, as evidenced by an odd inclusion in her diary on August 9. "A most excellent citizen . . .," she recorded, "has died of the reigning disease in New Jersey; Charles Ewing Chief Justice of that state."[47] It is unclear whether she knew him personally, but regardless the notice of his death in her preferred newspaper, *Poulson's American Daily Advertiser*, caught her eye. *Poulson's* published the news along with a warning about the scourge to people just like her: "no station however lofty, and no habits however regular, can turn away the messenger of death in its dreaded progress through our land."[48]

For the remainder of August, cholera gave Logan mixed signals. The disease was a "most awful scourge . . . ," she wrote to her friend on the nineteenth, "that hurries its victims with frightful violence into their graves." Yet fatalities did not escalate to the extent they did in New York, leading her to think Philadelphia's preparedness had mitigated its virulence.[49] On August 21, *Poulson's* reported that cases had declined to such an extent that city officials could close four of the makeshift hospitals.[50] This was "the best news" to Logan. Yet the next day, a man died of the disease in Nice Town, a suburb just a mile south of her home. Logan described him as "a person of wretchedly intemperate habits" but clung to her contagionist views. The dead man's mourners stayed up all night with the corpse, and she refused their request to borrow her carriage for the funeral procession.[51]

One week later, Logan learned of five fatalities among six cases in Germantown. "'Tis a most frightful disease," she recorded in her diary. "After death, the relaxation of the muscles creates a motion in the limbs for some time, like Galvanism."[52] On August 30, she referenced the continued abatement of the outbreak in Philadelphia and the return of evacuees but lamented the death of a physician who attended the sick in Germantown. She further noted that "Maria Powell, a young married woman that we know, has it in Nice Town."[53] On the last day of the month, Logan referenced the death of a boarding house keeper in Germantown whose death within twelve hours of her first symptoms prompted the rapid evacuation of her tenants. Positive news, though, continued to emerge from Philadelphia, where people had "no fear of its increase."[54]

New Yorkers received increasingly positive news in late August as well. On the twenty-second, the New York City Board of Health reported twenty-two daily fatalities and announced "that the city may be safely visited by strangers, and that those who have left it from fear of the disease, may return without danger."[55] On August 27, merchants of the city, including Arthur Tappan, signed a circular letter declaring that the outbreak had to "a great degree abated, and promises to pass away altogether." The pestilence had retreated and only remained among those who it was supposed to inflict in the first place, the "intemperate, acting in defiance of repeated admonitions" as well as the "dissipated and profligate."[56] The board of health helped the merchants' cause by discontinuing its daily reports on August 29, when the reported number of daily deaths dropped to just six. "This is very right," the editors of the *American* claimed, because daily mortality reports "keep the timid from town, and continue the illusion of our living in a 'city of the plague.'"[57]

Ann Van Wart arrived back the day after the board ceased its daily reports. She, like thousands of other evacuees, experienced a feeling of safety and pleasure. "So short, so quickly did time pass when beguiled with improving and interesting conversation," she recalled while on her way home. Any anxiety she had about her return soon dissipated. "How delightful to meet our dear friends after a long separation," she recorded with a sense of relief. She did not mention losing anyone particularly close to her, and her subsequent journal entries did not suggest that she or anyone in her family had a bout of the nasty disease, even though it continued to lurk in the city through the month of September.

Other evacuees were not so fortunate. When the board of health ceased daily reporting, it had tabulated a total of 2,951 fatalities. Over the next few weeks, several hundred more people would die, many of them returnees confident in the reassurances they had received about their safety.[58] By the time the outbreak ceased, cholera had taken an official total of 3,515 New Yorkers to their graves.

Charles Grandison Finney was nearly one of them. On September 28, a couple of weeks after his family's return, he sat in the Chatham Street Chapel, where he was being formally installed as pastor of the Second Free Presbyterian Church. As the services proceeded, Finney's stomach started to churn and he felt pressure in his bowels. Soon after his arrival home, the unmistakable violent vomiting, purging, and cramping began. A next-door neighbor became sick the same day but did not make it. America's most well-known evangelist clung to life through the night.

Finney somehow survived. His body managed to withstand both *Vibrio* and the counterproductive therapies that his doctors employed. He remained incapacitated for months nevertheless. He did not receive visitors until the end of October and would not preach again until the spring of 1833.[59] In the following years, he published his sermons and lectures, became the president of Oberlin College, and solidified his stature as one of the most important religious figures in US history. He lived until 1875, just short of his eighty-third birthday.

He reflected that he was fortunate to have done so. "I was then in New York City," Finney later said about the 1832 outbreak, "an eye-witness and more than an eye-witness of its terrific power. My own system experienced its withering shock. A man of the strongest constitution occupied a room adjacent to mine; was attacked the same hour that I was, and within a few hours was a corpse. Its powerful sweep was appalling."[60]

John Pintard remained unscathed by the disease but agreed with Finney's assessment of cholera's power. His daily observations of the traumatic experience led him to recant his earlier dismissive attitude. The seventy-three-year-old Pintard told his daughter that, even if he lived two more decades, "I shall never forget the solemn impressions of the late dreadful month of July, when the face of heaven appeared to be obscured with a somber shroud of pestilence & death."[61] On August 31, he strolled along Bowery and Chatham streets, observed crowded stores, and lamented the shoppers' carefree behavior. "So soon we forget the terrors & solitude of the last 2 months," he remarked.[62]

The banker had continued reminders of the awful summer. On October 1, Pintard, who had long since retired from the presidency of his insurance company, noted the death of John Slidell, president of the Traders' Insurance Company. He commented that Slidell was the city's third executive in that industry to lose his life to the global killer.[63] The following summer, seeing cholera resurging in the United States and anxious that it would return to New York City, the banker secured a rural retreat for his family. Back in early July of 1832, he had called evacuees "Cowards." Within a year, he knew better that cholera struck the "high & low" and the "prudent as well as imprudent." "We shall be . . . better prepared than last year," he assured his daughter. It would be one of the last letters he would write to her. She died on October 1 in New Orleans after suffering from a short, unidentified illness. Her father lived until 1844 and reached his eighty-fifth year before succumbing to old age.[64]

Judge Ewing did not get to enjoy his retirement as did Pintard, but he did finally receive a postmortem defense of his character. On November 14, Southard, who had recently been elected governor, stood at the pulpit of the Trenton First Presbyterian Church and addressed an audience of dignitaries. He gave his deceased friend effusive praise and made sure that posterity would remember him as anything but the expected cholera victim. Southard remarked that Ewing had "a constitution, firm and healthful: habits, the most temperate and cautious: prudence, the most watchful; a whole character most pure." Everyone believed, according to Southard, "that the destroyer would pass by and leave him, at least, unscathed." But it was not to be—the mysterious scourge, without any exciting causes or premonitions, took Ewing to his grave within twenty hours. Southard even gave the judge credit for taking the emergency seriously. "He did not disregard its approach, nor make light of its terrors," Southard said of Ewing's attitude about cholera, "for he had reflected; and he knew that it was guilty madness, not manly courage, to brave the power of Him who wielded it."[65] The deceased judge thus rendered judgment. Elites foolhardily dismissed the scourge, believed in their own invincibility, and did not prepare to meet their maker.

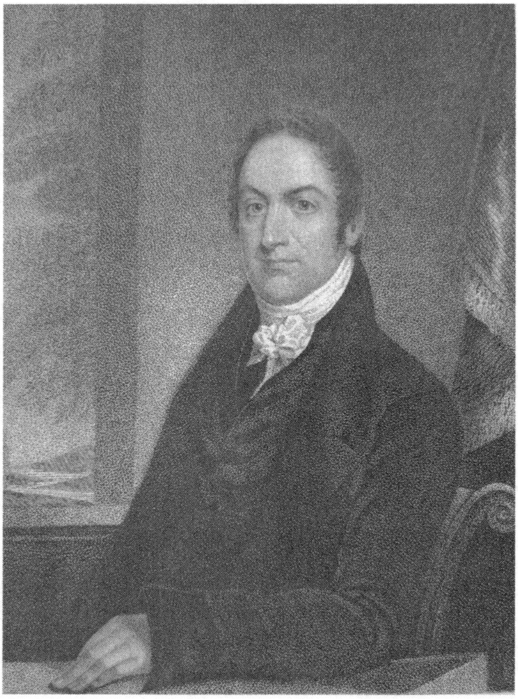

Charles Ewing. Engraving in James B. Longacre and James Herring, *The National Portrait Gallery of Distinguished Americans*, Vol. 2 (Henry Perkins, 1835).

Unlike most cholera victims, Ewing had a praise-filled inscription on his tombstone, which one can still visit in Trenton's First Presbyterian Church cemetery. "In integrity, pure and incorruptible; in manners, affable, dignified, and polished; in morals, spotless,..." his weather-worn monument declares, "he won, in an eminent degree, the respect, love, and confidence of his fellow-citizens." The engraved words state he had happy "domestic relations" and "endearing virtues" and that he "practiced the precepts of the Christian religion." While the text celebrating his life can barely be read today, whoever wrote it wanted to spare him from eternal embarrassment by specifying his cause of death. "In the vigor of his mental and bodily powers, surrounded by blessings, cheered by the approbation of his fellow-men,..." the inscription concludes, "he was attacked with a violent disease, which suddenly terminated his life on the 5th day of August, A.D. 1832, in the 53d year of his age."[66]

Deborah Norris Logan knew that Ewing was no mere exception and that cholera demonstrated its power more universally than portrayed. A tenant farmer on her property, Mr. John Peiffer, had been in Philadelphia selling his milk on the morning of September 20, began experiencing cholera symptoms during his return home, and then died shortly after midnight.[67] The Quaker historian recorded in her diary on the morning of the twenty-second, "The earth is closed over the poor fellow who industriously cultivated its surface. He has left a modest, humble & industrious wife and a train of little children to stem the misfortunate of life! I know not how to express the shock of seeing such a wrench from existence!"[68] The day after the funeral, she retreated into her library to work. " 'Thy Mercies are new every morning,' " she prayed. "And it is a great one that this desolating Plague has not yet entered our dwelling. May it still be averted from us!"[69]

It would be, but not before taking the lives of more people she knew. Deaths in the nearby Bowman family made her mind "a prey to harassing anxieties" and confirmed her "dread [of] this formidable disease."[70] Henry Bowman had avoided Philadelphia since August 1 but resumed his periodic ventures into the city on September 5, the day after the city's board of health announced it would discontinue daily reporting of cases. Deborah Bowman, his nineteen-year-old daughter, wrote in her diary on the thirteenth, "A serene and beautiful

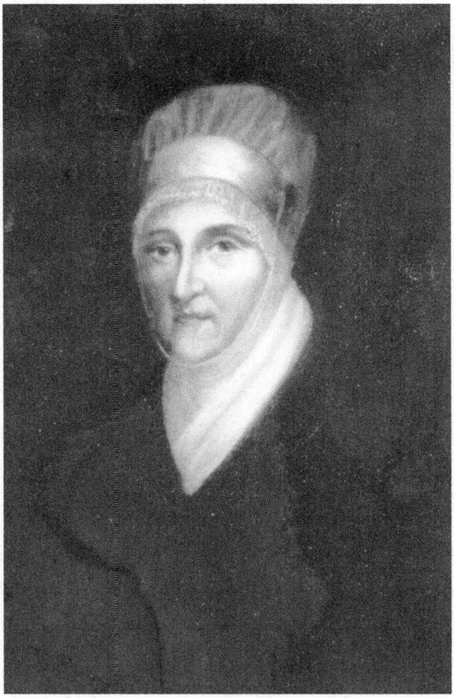

Deborah Norris Logan, copy after Charles Willson Peale, 1816. Courtesy of the National Society of The Colonial Dames of America in the Commonwealth of Pennsylvania at Stenton, Philadelphia.

day Our Dear Father quietly departed this life between 1 and 2 O'clock last night in a resigned and sweet manner." He died of cholera.

Her father's death was the last entry Deborah Bowman penned in her diary. Her mother, Tabitha, fell to the pandemic on September 21; her twenty-three-year-old sister, Margaret, succumbed on the twenty-fourth; and Abram, an African American man who worked for the family died a few days later. It is unknown whether Deborah came down with the disease, but she would not live to see her twenty-first birthday. She passed away in March 1834. A surviving sister came into possession of Bowman's diary and added a conclusion to it: "My dear lovely sister Deborah never recovered the shock of the loss of her parents whom she most tenderly loved."[71]

More tragedies occurred within families that Logan knew well and had none of the predisposing characteristics of the malady's expected victims. On September 24, the Quaker historian learned that George Kiel "was seized with Cholera upon his return from market and was not expected to live thro' the night."[72] The man, who resided just north of Germantown, was buried on the twenty-sixth, and Logan lent her carriage to his family for the funeral.[73] He, like Peiffer, had left a widow and young children, which affected Logan greatly. "I am sorry so very much has been said of its attacking only the intemperate and dirty," Logan said of cholera to her friend. She continued to believe in contagion and described the deceased she knew as "honest, industrious, useful citizens."[74]

Unlike so many other elite people, Deborah Norris Logan never bought into the delusive notion that cholera respected her privileged status and would stay away from her. The Quaker historian instead stayed away from cholera, remained safe in Stenton Mansion for the duration of the pandemic, expressed sympathy for peoples who succumbed to the disease, and reached the age of seventy-seven at the time of her passing in 1839.

As the late fall chill set in, cholera ultimately subsided in the Northeast. Newspapers, boards of health, and other authorities reported more than seven thousand fatalities in the region (table 5.1).[75] The deceased, to be sure, included a disproportionate number of impoverished people as the wealthy fled to safe locations, but the pathogen demonstrated its ability to strike indiscriminately. Finney's near-fatal experience that he recalled in his later years, Ewing's controversial death, Pintard's private thoughts on the disease, and Logan's entries into her personal diary revealed cholera's persuasive powers.

The public narrative went unchanged, however. The New York City Board of Health, for example, published a post-outbreak analysis in November in which the city's doctors reported that "drunkards and prostitutes" accounted for most of the fatal cases they attended. "As a class of people, the low Irish suffered most," the physicians concluded, "being exceedingly dirty in their habits, much addicted to intemperance, and crowded together in the worst portions of the city."[76]

Samuel Jackson, consulting physician to the Philadelphia Board of Health, agreed. In his final report, he described the hundreds of fatalities occurring in the city and its nearest suburbs as overwhelmingly consisting of incarcerated

Table 5.1 Reported Cholera Mortality in the Northeast, 1832

Location	Deaths
Vermont	6
Boston, MA	70
Massachusetts, excluding Boston	15
Connecticut	38
Rhode Island	17
New York City, NY	3,515
Albany, NY	416
Poughkeepsie, NY	175
Sing Sing Prison	103
Utica, NY	177
Rochester, NY	135
Buffalo, NY	144
New York State, excluding above	743
Newark, NJ	65
Bulls Island, NJ	50[a]
New Jersey, excluding above	330[b]
Philadelphia, PA	935
Malverne, PA (Duffy's Cut)	57[c]
Pennsylvania, excluding above	90
Total	7,081

[a] These represent Delaware and Raritan Canal workers who were not counted in New Jersey's total and will be discussed in chapter 7.

[b] Some Delaware and Raritan Canal workers who perished in Princeton, Trenton, and other cities and towns are in these totals, but many who died in work zones are not.

[c] These pertain to workers on the Philadelphia and Columbia Railroad to be discussed in chapter 7.

and hospitalized people as well as Irish and African American populations crowded in the Moyamensing and Southwark neighborhoods. *Vibrio* thrived in those neighborhoods, which were not served by the Fairmount Water Works and where local wells filled with the deadly bacteria after the drenching rains of late July and early August. Jackson, though, reflexively resorted to the standard explanation. The pandemic's victims, he described, were "the worst portion of our population" and of "the lowest order and most abandoned habits."[77]

Finney, Ewing, Pintard, and Logan knew there was more to cholera than its supposedly selective predation. They would have agreed with James Riker, Jr., whose family had escaped New York in mid-July after the painful losses of his grandmother and uncle. "In the beginning of October the cholera having nearly left the city, we returned home," Riker recalled. "Business gradually regained its former briskness, but a gloom hung over the community which time alone could dissipate. Few were the family circles left unbroken by the fatal epidemic, few the hearts that were not bereaved."[78]

6

Ms. Maury's Prophecy

VIRGINIA IN THE PANDEMIC'S GRIP

ANN MAURY CLAIMED to be "a true Prophetess." The English-born woman arrived in the Old Dominion in 1831, along with her Virginia-born father, James Maury, who had been recently dismissed as US consul at Liverpool. It was a tumultuous time in the state. Nat Turner had led a revolt of his fellow bondsmen in Southampton County in August that killed fifty-eight white men, women, and children. Local and state authorities quickly put down the rebellion and executed about 120 participants, including Turner. The revolt frightened white residents to the core. Some citizen groups petitioned the state government to come up with a plan to emancipate all 469,755 people held in bondage and deport all people of color, even the 47,349 who were then free. They wanted Virginia to be a free state for white people only.[1] Others saw no end to slavery and called for the policing of enslaved people and free people of color to be significantly increased.

The debate that ensued during the winter of 1831–1832 enthralled Ann Maury. She sat in the gallery of the state legislature and listened to speeches, she read opinions published in the state's newspapers, and she exchanged her views on the subject with her correspondents. She was no abolitionist. Her family's trans-Atlantic business—Maury Latham & Company—made its fortune from importing American goods produced by enslaved laborers into British markets. The twenty-nine-year-old, however, sided with a group of largely young and newly elected legislators who favored a scheme of gradual emancipation and colonization of people of color to Africa, Haiti, or the American West.

They would not prevail. Virginia's enslavers effectively countered even a gradual abolition plan as an attack on their "private property." The state's economy would continue to depend heavily, as it long had, on captive labor.

During the debate, Maury claimed to have made a ghoulish connection. She read with interest the news of cholera's global spread, particularly as it arrived in England. As she informed Dr. James Morris—a family friend, physician, and planter of Louisa County, Virginia—she understood the novel disease "to confine its attacks on the poor, dirty & aged." In part for that reason, she did not want her elderly father to go back and live in Liverpool anytime soon.[2] Instead, she, her brother Matthew, and their father decided to make their new home in New York City. The scourge halted their move. In early July, they veered off course to wait out the pestilence at Schooley's Mountain, New Jersey.[3] There, in early August, Ann read troubling news. "I see by the late papers that [cholera] is raging in Norfolk & Portsmouth among the colored population," she confirmed to Morris. "I have always thought it would be severe among them," she declared, recalling, "indeed I told some of the members of the Virginia Legislature last winter that the Cholera would cross the Atlantic before long, & would save them the trouble of legislating about the poor Negroes for it would sweep them off."[4]

Maury's grim prophecy may have been just a sick joke, but to those who wanted to continue profiting from captive labor, the pandemic was nothing to laugh at. Enslavers agreed that the scourge would threaten their financial interests because of its predilection for African American victims. They held to racist views of African Americans as a helpless people who would only survive the disease with the paternal care of a superior and less vulnerable white race. As it did in so many other places, though, the pandemic unfolded in Virginia in unscripted ways.

The assumed vulnerability of people of color became a topic of public discussion before *Vibrio* crossed the Mason–Dixon Line. "The black population of the southern states are supposed to be particularly obnoxious to the disease," the editors of New York's *Morning Courier and Enquirer* declared before admitting that cholera was present in their own city. "Their food and habits of life, their want of cleanliness, &c., resemble, in a great many particulars, the Hindoos, among whom the Cholera first made its appearance."[5] The Baltimore *Gazette and Daily Advertiser* and Richmond *Constitutional Whig* republished the *Morning Courier and Enquirer*'s piece as a warning to enslavers.[6]

One Northern paper that had the audacity to suggest that people of color in Canada had more resistance to the disease received a quick and thorough rebuke.[7] The New York *American* pointed out that "there were hardly two dozen persons of color in Quebec—but at New York, Albany, &c. these are attacked and die—like other people."[8] "We have taken some notice of the matter here in New-York, where there are 14,000 colored persons," editors of the city's *Journal of Commerce* informed its readers, "and the result is that blacks are as liable to cholera as whites and that as many die in proportion to their number."[9] The Charleston, South Carolina, *Courier* relayed the observations of their Northern peers and warned enslavers, "A mistake on this subject might lead to disastrous results."[10]

Medical advice flowed from north to south as well.[11] New York physician Christopher C. Yates published a treatise marketed to Southern customers. His *Advice to the Planters of the South*, with its noncontagionist stance and recommendation of heroic treatment, stated the obvious to its intended readers: "Humanity as well as interest pleads for suitable care and protection to your slave population."[12]

A public letter dated August 18, 1832, from Dr. Nathaniel Chapman of Philadelphia circulated more widely. Chapman, whose advice Dr. William Bradley Tyler of Frederick, Maryland, solicited, went against the grain somewhat by downplaying the idea that premonitory symptoms would give enough notice of the onset; individuals should expect a rapid onset of symptoms that would require immediate attention. The Philadelphia doctor, however, advocated the standard heroic interventions of bleeding, cupping, calomel, and opium. If properly treated, most cases, he claimed, "will almost invariably yield to these remedies." He bragged that "a triumph over the disease is pretty certain."[13]

If Southern enslavers did not get the message from the press, their Northern correspondents privately told them they had much to fear.[14] Benjamin Wright, writing from New York City, for example, gave a stark warning to John Hartwell Cocke of Virgina. "I dread...for the Southern States," the Northerner declared to his Southern friend, "if this disease once gets among the Slaves, I should fear it would sweep of[f] one quarter of them."[15]

As warnings from the North circulated, *Vibrio* proliferated in Norfolk. "Joe died on Wednesday morning the 25th of July supposed with the Cholera after being attacked about seven hours," a Norfolk master succinctly and privately recorded about his deceased captive.[16] The press did not note the death, nor did it mention that two other enslaved people had died the day before.[17] Other acute cases followed, and city authorities said nothing for about a week. Perhaps they were unsure if the novel cholera had arrived, or perhaps they remained hopeful that, if it had arrived, it would soon pass.

It did not. On August 2, the Norfolk Board of Health began the morbid process of informing the public of cholera's toll, with eight cases and four deaths occurring over the previous twenty-four hours.[18] During a rainy start to August, the deadly bacteria found its way into more of the residents' drinking water. The city did not have a central works, and easily polluted wells and springs continued to serve the bulk of the population. Cisterns, brick tanks that collected rain runoff from roofs, may have offered the propertied class some protection, but even these could be at risk of contamination since sometimes they were built below ground.[19] The number of fatalities steadily climbed, reaching twenty during a twenty-four-hour period that ended on the ninth.[20]

Residents lost confidence that the Norfolk Board of Health was accurately reporting the extent of the outbreak. The number of daily burials significantly surpassed officially declared cholera fatalities, leading the press to publish daily interments as a more accurate measure of the number who died. On August 16, mortality peaked at twenty-six.[21] Thereafter, the number of cases gradually declined and reached such a low level that the city ceased issuing daily reports on September 11. By that time, the board of health estimated from the record of interments that four hundred people had died of cholera.[22] The Southern city of some ten thousand people lost 4 percent of its population, more than doubling the per capita death rate of New York City.[23] The numbers in Norfolk would have been higher, as they would have been in other cities, had many residents not fled.[24]

Those who stayed faced a dire situation. Eliza Vickery, for example, described on August 10 a "gloomy" scene of hearses making repetitive trips down the rain-soaked road and nervous residents asking each other, "how are you & how is your family," no longer as a matter of formality but instead as a serious question in which the answer was in doubt. "You can read in the *voice* & *countenance* of the Speaker the intense anxiety, with which they listen to hear, *all is well*," she explained.[25] "Our physicians seem worn down, & much jaded," she noted ten days later. "I have but little confidence in what man can do, in this disease." Some whites she knew had perished, but the pathogen more easily found its way to the free and enslaved people of color. "They look so desponding & so cast down & so many of them in mourning both of countenance & dress," she observed. So far, she and her family as well as their enslaved servants had escaped.[26] "Every one seems spiritless & it is uncommon to see a cheerful face," she bemoaned at the end of the horrible month.[27] Four white people she knew recently died, and the city's doctors remained in high demand and greatly fatigued.[28]

One of those tired physicians was Dr. John Galt Williamson. He and his peers had received Dr. Chapman's suggested treatment at the height of

Norfolk's outbreak and immediately employed it. "I am sorry to say," he privately informed his uncle, a doctor in Williamsburg, "it has not been very successful, owing probably to the greater malignancy of the disease here than in Philadelphia." He furthermore refuted any notion that cholera would take a lesser toll on US cities. "In proportion to our population," he stated, "it has been at least as bad here as in any country whatever."[29]

William Kennon seemed to agree. He evacuated the city on July 25 and returned by the middle of September to what he called an "ill fated place." His brother, a physician, who remained the entire time, filled William in on harrowing stories of "death & annihilation," which he then relayed to his fiancée, Nancy Randolph of Richmond. Cholera commenced on the day he left, William wrote, and "like an invading army it went on, killing all who came within its death scope. We who were removed, from the scene were strangers to the havoc it made." Perhaps trying to impress his fiancée with his poetic yet morbid prose, William declared that "it spared none in its march [and] like a winged wolf it devoured the young, the gay, the witty, & the wise & my acquaintances one by one have, dropped off." The disease paid no attention to sex, age, or condition.[30]

Powerful public voices, however, made sure to summarize the pandemic according to the script that they had written in advance. The Norfolk Board of Health segregated black and white fatalities, which always showed the former dying in larger numbers than the latter despite the city being roughly divided in half between the two races. The press, while ignoring the fact that large numbers of white people had left, emphasized the disparity and blamed black people for their own victimization.[31] "The mortality, it will be seen, continues to be confined, in Norfolk, with very few (and those not alarming) exceptions, to the blacks," the *Herald* asserted. The editors attributed this "to their inattention to cleanliness and diet" and "to their perversity in concealing the premonitory symptoms." Enslaved people had supposedly been hiding their symptoms from their captors until it was too late, while free people of color had great "repugnance to being put 'under the doctor's hands.'" The *Herald* further instructed its readers as well as those of all "our southern towns" that "timid" African Americans could not care for themselves because they "instinctively" shunned "their unfortunate fellows as they would the embrace of death, on the slightest alarm of the cholera."[32]

The board of health reinforced this interpretation. As it ended daily reporting, the board declared, "the mortality among the white population... has been but little, if any greater than what is common at the same season of the year." Then it added, "the great mortality among the colored people may in a great degree be accounted for from their habits and imprudence."[33]

City officials, in their final assessment, gave numbers to support their view. Of the four hundred fatalities, the board estimated that three hundred were African American and one hundred were white, without explaining their reasoning and ignoring the fact that large numbers of the latter had fled. They furthermore made sure that it was recorded that white people who had perished were those expected to do so. Only about twenty white people who died were "persons of any distinction," and they perished due "to neglect of the symptoms, or previous debility of the system produced by other diseases." The remaining eighty were "either strangers, or persons dwelling in obscurity."[34] Mortality among African Americans did not need any further explanation for the white public, who had been bombarded by a clear message: cholera strongly preferred people of color, especially those who did not live under or would not submit to the paternal protection of enslavers.

Eliza Vickery did not share the board of health's gloss of what Norfolk experienced. Sporadic deaths, especially among white returnees, continued for about a month after city officials stopped counting fatalities.[35] A spike in early October prompted Eliza to write to her sister-in-law to tell her she was safe, and in doing so, she did not hide the terror that she had faced. "Really it was a time of such intense excitement & deep feeling with such horrible scenes," she reflected, "that I feel I can *never forget* it, no *never*!"[36] The day after penning those lines, *Vibrio* took the life of Mr. John Holt, who had been Norfolk's mayor for the last twenty years.[37]

After erupting in Norfolk, cholera circulated in towns and villages near the mouth of the James River. Local spread occurred in Portsmouth, Hampton, and Suffolk as well as among personnel stationed and working at Fortress Monroe.[38] Smithfield, a small village some thirty miles up the James from Norfolk, sustained a heavy blow. Twenty-five out of the village's four hundred people died between August 26 and September 10, and more fatalities certainly would have occurred there if a "great many families" had not fled as the crisis unfolded.[39]

Vibrio nonetheless took its time before escalating in Richmond. On September 7, Robin Hill, a young worker enslaved by the tobacco factory proprietor David Barclay, came down with a suspicious disease and died quickly. The physicians declared Hill's illness to be cholera, and concerns rose through the city. Barclay tried to get ahead of the story and wrote directly to the Richmond Board of Health that Hill did not have the disease. He "had been long subject to fits," and on the morning of his death, he had eaten "a quantity of pears."[40] The board investigated, agreed with the doctors that a case of "Malignant cholera" had occurred, and announced the news to the public later the same day.[41]

Barclay's efforts had failed, and the tobacco industry ground to a halt. Richmond, a city of about seventeen thousand people at the time, led the world in processing the product for the global market and depended on enslaved laborers, many of whom had been hired to them by rural planters.[42] Hiring agreements obligated employers to provide adequate food, lodging, and medical care and thus subjected them to liability if an enslaved worker suffered a debilitating injury or preventable death. Employers did not want to bear that risk during a cholera outbreak, while anxious owners conversely did not want to lose human captives whose surrendered wages provided valuable income. The tobacco barons generally complied with the requests of planters to send the workers back to them.[43]

For white residents, though, the outbreak seemed trifling and discriminatory for over two weeks. The Richmond Board of Health began daily reporting on September 11, but up to September 21, it had counted only twenty-five fatalities. Fewer than three deaths per day hardly validated cholera's reputation as a lethal pathogen. "The cholera is slowly on the increase in our city," the *Enquirer* informed its readers on September 21, but with the qualification that "cases are scarcely more malignant than they have been" and "are found manageable, if taken in time."[44] On the same day, Richmond's *Southern Religious Telegraph* told its readers that the pandemic had only come to the city in a "comparatively mild form" and residents had reason to hope "that its victims will not be numerous."[45]

More was going on than most people realized. The city opened two hospitals at the onset of the outbreak, but in Richmond, as elsewhere, people avoided them. Enslavers had a disincentive to use public hospitals because they would be obligated to pay five dollars for the first day and three dollars for each day after that for each of their hospitalized bondsmen or bondswomen. The board of health also had a difficult time getting daily reports from city physicians.[46] The editors of the *Whig* scolded the city's doctors for their "neglect" and for making the board's reports an inaccurate reflection of the outbreak's extent. Physicians, though, remained uncompliant.

The press went to the sexton's reports to get a better gauge of what was unfolding. The *Compiler* tabulated interments at the public graveyard, a burial ground near the poorhouse where the corpses of inmates, free people who could not afford a funeral, and deceased slaves often ended up. They deduced that from September 11 to 21 sixty-two cholera deaths had occurred, based on excess mortality. Ten or more cholera victims, the *Compiler* speculated, had been buried in other places.[47] Seventy-two fatalities certainly dwarfed the twenty-five that the board of health had reported, and the calculations led the body to base its daily reports thereafter on interments at the public graveyard.

Still, *Vibrio* appeared to infiltrate the city only slowly. The bacteria likely found its way into some local wells or springs that served the poor and enslaved or perhaps spread among them through contaminated food and poor hygienic conditions. *Vibrio* probably had yet to get into the city's central water supply—a city-owned and -operated works that pulled water from the James upstream, pumped it into a reservoir, ran it through a series of sand and gravel filters (the first in the United States to do so), and then sent it through iron pipes into the heart of the city. The waterworks served thirty-one fire plugs and a number of hydrants of business owners and private residents who had paid the hook-up fees.[48] People who had this water described it as "pure" and "sweet" and considered it an improvement to their property values.[49] Filtering, of course, would not have removed bacteria, but drawing water upstream away from the city's sewage runoff would have offered protection and explained why the disease escalated rather slowly and why it disproportionately struck the poor and enslaved.

As the week of September 23 began, Richmonders came to understand that they were in for a more severe blow than previously thought. In its first issue of the week, the *Whig* noted the death of "Mr. Hardie, a respectable Shoemaker, and his wife." "Confined heretofore to negroes almost entirely, the cholera begins to embrace whites," the editors declared. The editors reported on "a brief walk" that they took, where they observed "corpses of unknown blacks proceeding to burial," a funeral procession for the Hardies with their orphaned children marching behind the casket, and soldiers from the state guard armory carrying a dying comrade to the hospital. Despite scolding physicians earlier, the editors praised them. They could be seen throughout the city, "galloping in the haste of Aids de Camp, on a field of battle" and giving their services "equally at the call of white and black, of rich and poor." The *Whig* professed that cases were beginning to occur over a wider array of neighborhoods.[50]

It got much worse over the course of the week. It rained on the twenty-fourth, and *Vibrio* proliferated, possibly getting into the central water supply. One hundred-sixty-seven burials took place at the public graveyard during the week of September 23 through 29. The *Whig* bemoaned that proportionately

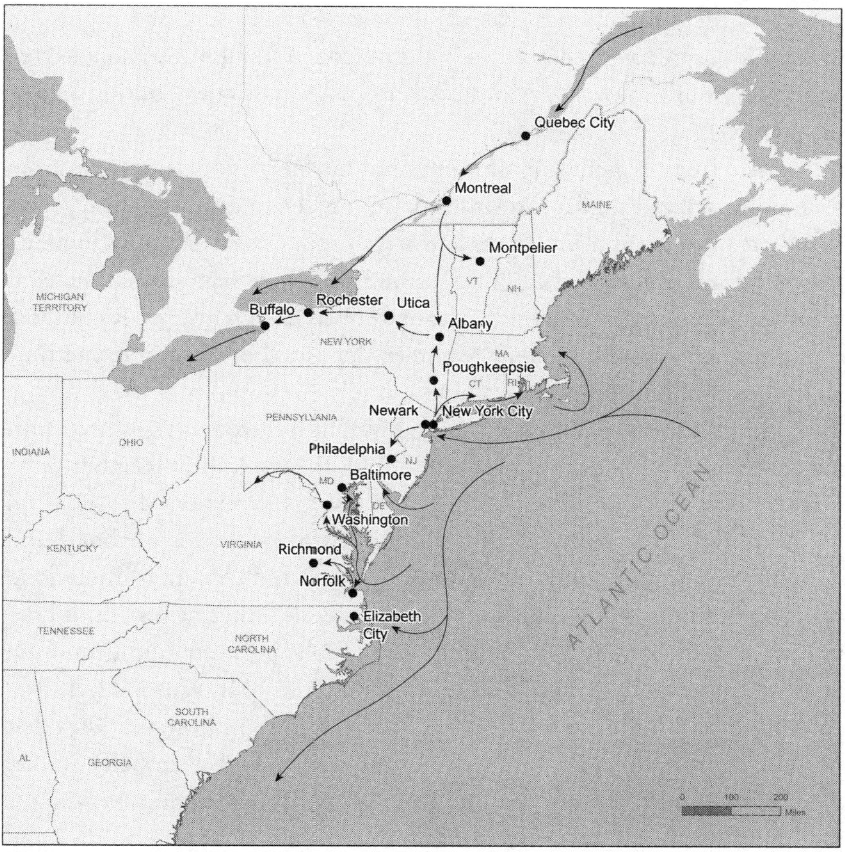

The Pandemic in the East, 1832. Map by Franchesca Rodriguez, Geospatial Center, Stony Brook University.

their city's one-day high of thirty-five burials on September 28 among an estimated in-residence population of 15,000 exceeded New York's single-day record of 104 among, what the editors guessed, was an in-residence population of 150,000.[51] The *Whig* was correct in making the claim. If readers did their math, which the paper invited them to do, they would have figured that Richmond experienced 2.3 deaths per thousand, while New York's peak equaled a loss of 0.7 deaths per thousand.

The numbers, of course, did not capture the true extent of the horror. Richmond resident James V. Willcox, Jr., who had been in Philadelphia several weeks earlier when that city experienced the worst of the disease, wrote to his Pennsylvania cousin and claimed that "no place... has suffered more" than his home city. "It is painful to witness the distress here," he added in his letter of September 26. "Nothing else seems to be talked of by the living." He had passed by the public burial grounds three days earlier and "saw a grave in which 18 corpses were deposited." The sexton told him he had interred between fifteen and twenty African Americans in mass graves during each of the previous days.[52]

Frank Harris, a merchant who operated his business twenty miles from Richmond, relayed similar information. "You will have seen from the papers that there has been as many deaths as thirty or thirty five a day in Richmond," Harris informed his brother, "but I assure you there has been as many as ninety of a day buried frequently as I learn from my friends living in Richmond, a friend of mine told me he saw eighteen deposited in one pit at one time without coffins & covered up."[53]

Vibrio continued to afflict Richmond well into October. The sexton buried another 139 victims of the disease during the week of September 30 to October 6. A series of deaths of elite people received notice. Mr. Anderson M. Waddill, "an extensive merchant and tobacco dealer in Lynchburg" and "a highly respectable and respected man," contracted cholera in Richmond while on business and never made it home.[54] Mrs. Catherine Austin, "a kind mother and affectionate wife," succumbed to "the prevailing Epidemic" on September 27, and then seven days later her husband, "Mr. Wilson H. Austin, an honest and industrious man," followed her to the grave. They left "two little orphans to the humanity of the wide world."[55] Isabella Stalker died "after a short illness" on October 4, just days after her wedding.[56] "Mr. A.T. Shepherd, a young gentleman of great moral worth esteemed and beloved by all who knew him," died on the same day.[57]

The following week saw mortality fluctuate between five and twelve.[58] Then, on October 15, only one interment occurred, and the board of health declared the outbreak had ended. "But one death reported today," the *Whig* exclaimed. "The cholera is extinct here. We shall cease reports from this time. Richmond is not only safe to visit, but now the safest place."[59]

Richmond's total losses are shrouded in mystery. The *Compiler* reported that an excess of 408 burials had taken place at the public graveyard, with 79 percent of the deceased being people of color and 21 percent being white people. The editors believed that fifteen more cholera victims had been buried at the Old Church graveyard, six at the Rocketts' burial ground, eight at the Old Academy, and twelve corpses sent for burials outside the city. (The race of these extra burial victims was not noted.) The total then amounted to 449. The editors referred to twenty-nine deaths that occurred in the penitentiary, but they did not believe these properly belonged to the city's total, since the institution was beyond municipal limits.[60] Also excluded from the count were several people who died after the *Compiler* came up with the numbers. *Vibrio* lingered on in the city through the remainder of October and took an untold number of lives before it ultimately fizzled out.[61]

That people of color suffered disproportionately more than white people led some observers to question a key belief about cholera's preferred victims. How could the poor, especially enslaved African Americans, die in such large numbers when they had very little means and opportunity to consume alcohol? That is the question that a subscriber to the *Whig* dared to ask. The poor and enslaved, the subscriber asserted, "have not generally the means of establishing and keeping up a regular and habitual system of intemperance." Enslaved people, he further posited, "are the most temperate lower class of people in the world, *from absolute necessity!*" They only received alcohol occasionally at harvest time and at Christmas, and never in quantities that produced intoxication. The connection between cholera and alcohol, he argued, "falls entirely to the ground."[62]

A Richmond resident let his similar view be known to New York's *Journal of Commerce*. "The assertion that intemperate drinkers are most liable to Cholera, does not hold good here," the resident wrote in a letter dated October 6. "Of that description of whites, none or very few have been attacked here, but it has fallen on the temperate and decent portion of whites, and seven eights of the blacks who have died were not intemperate. Many of them had no means whatever with which to procure liquors."[63] Editors in a variety of cities and towns found the information noteworthy and republished it.[64]

The *Southern Religious Telegraph* countered the widely circulated letter and made sure to let readers know that cholera behaved as it was supposed to. Its editors pointed to the supposed fact that an elderly and debilitated man was the only member to have succumbed to cholera out of more than a thousand who belonged to the Richmond Temperance Society. They added that no member of the two Presbyterian churches perished either. The scourge's preferred victims, they insisted, were the impoverished and enslaved. "It appears to us impossible to persuade a people, whether white or black, who are ignorant, uncultivated, and shut out as it were, from the privileges of civilized life, *to be temperate* and *prudent* in their habits," the *Telegraph* claimed. "Their recklessness is inseparable from their condition."[65]

Two weeks later, the editors published an obituary without acknowledging its obvious and tragic irony. The Presbyterian minister, Reverend Joseph Barr, died on October 28 after "he was taken violently ill of cholera." They lauded the man as an exemplary Christian and did not even bother attributing his death to a momentary act of imprudence.[66] They let their previous interpretation of the outbreak stand without any reflection.

The *Whig* also defended the idea that cholera discriminated. "We are afraid that the black population of the United States . . . are destined to more than decimation," the editors warned their fellow Southerners. "Poor wretches! nothing can exceed their alarm, but their fanatical rejection of the means of safety." They then printed a story based on racial stereotypes to illustrate their supposed inferiority: " 'Mus'nt *drink*, exclaimed Pompey! how the doctors know *that*! none but God can know whether drink hurt!' Caesar was greatly scandalized at the notion of the Cholera being circulated through the air. 'In the air! said he—how the Doctors know *that*—none but God Almighty could know that!' " The story was meant as a lesson to white masters to "exercise the most unremitting vigilance, and the most determined police over their habits" as the disease seemed destined to engulf the entire nation.[67]

Such racist assumptions underlay Ann Maury's prophecy. She remained sheltered at Schooley's Mountain into the fall, informing Dr. Morris that she spent her time by taking "many pleasant walks & rides in every direction." Her brother Matthew occupied his time playing billiards, flirting with women, and reading. He, nevertheless, found it "rather dull" and wanted to be in New York City, "making money all the time."[68] He left on September 1—three weeks before his sister and father were ready to take the risk.[69]

Matthew did not die from cholera, but he suffered from what were likely side effects from the treatment. Not too long after he arrived in New York City, he had what Ann described as "a slight attack bordering upon cholera." We cannot know, of course, whether *Vibrio* infected him, but he did as he was supposed to and immediately called for a physician. The doctor "subdued" the symptoms, but several weeks after treatment, he continued to look quite ill. "The blood does not seem to circulate properly," Ann informed Dr. Morris, adding "his hands & feet are always cold & numb & he is pale."[70] Matthew remained debilitated well into 1833, most likely from bacterial infection following bleedings, mercury poisoning, and the adverse effects of opium. Not until August 1833 could Ann tell Dr. Morris that Matthew "has entirely recovered from the chilliness of his hands & feet & other unpleasant symptoms that followed the cholera."[71]

Cholera could not change Ann's mind about its nature, however. The scourge, to be sure, exacted a heavy toll on Virginia's African American population, but the disease's behavior might have led one to rethink preconceptions. Except in the Norfolk area, the state's numerous rural plantations, where the vast majority of people of color lived, largely came out unscathed. The state's newspapers continued to herald cholera's discriminating nature, but there were skeptics whose voices emerged from the noise, and there were numerous obituaries of people who were not supposed to die. Maury did not budge. In November, she again ghoulishly claimed to Morris that cholera did the work that the legislature should have done—ridding the state of people of color.[72]

African American voices obviously did not figure into either Maury's private, macabre musings or to the public discourse that dehumanized them. How they understood their experience during the calamitous times was not a concern to those whose voices the archival record privileges. Upon closer inspection, though, there is evidence that people of color resisted white supremacy and demonstrated that they were not the degraded and deserving victims of a disease that purposefully targeted them.

African American actions speak volumes when their words are missing. Their supposed failures to submit to white medicine were similar to the Irish immigrants' resistance in Northern cities. Neither group wanted to subject themselves to medical treatments that at best made them feel even more ill and at worst accelerated their demise. The "fanatical rejection" of these measures was understandable for a people who rightfully had little reason to trust those who deprived them of freedom and equality, and in hindsight their resistance benefited their health far more than the coercive care that white enslavers provided.

Words do exist, moreover, in retrospective accounts of African American survivors. Born enslaved in 1812, John Jasper worked in a Richmond tobacco factory in 1832, became a Baptist preacher in 1840, and after the Civil War and his emancipation, led one of the largest congregations in the state capital. The "cholera year," he told his biographer, deepened his faith. "This disease was so disastrous among the colored people," he recalled, "that it caused a very large number of them, as they used to say, 'to sit out to pray,' believing that the last day was not far off." White people considered their response "not at all intelligent, but rather superstitious," Jasper recounted. For him, however, "a great good was the result and many were added unto the church."[73]

Another enslaved worker, Henry "Box" Brown, also had a religious experience during the epidemic. Of 1832, he recalled, "I began to grow alarmed respecting my future welfare, as a great eclipse of the sun had recently taken place; and the cholera reaching the country not long after, I thought that perhaps the day of judgment was not far distant, and I must prepare for that dreaded event."[74] White masters had been telling themselves that, if left alone, men like Jasper and Brown would serve themselves up to cholera because of

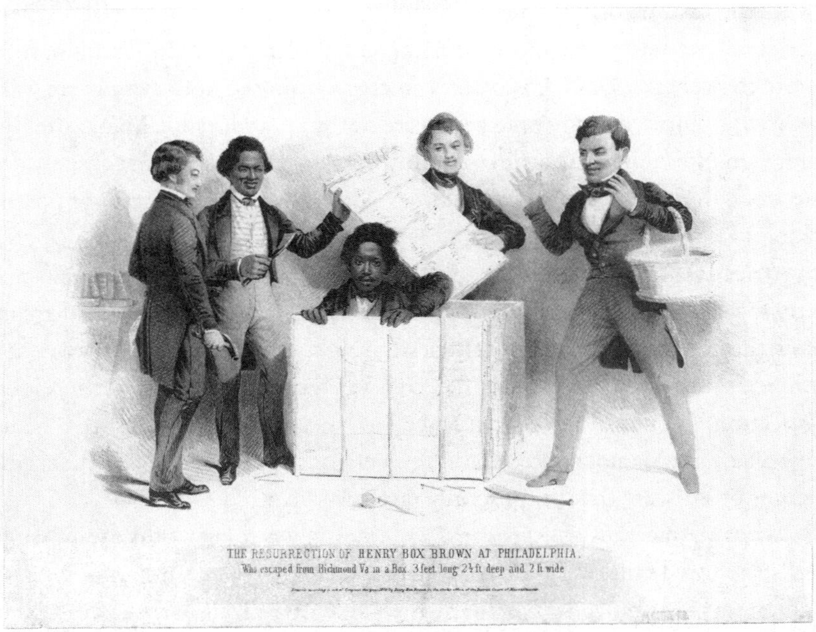
THE RESURRECTION OF HENRY BOX BROWN AT PHILADELPHIA.
Who escaped from Richmond Va in a Box 3 feet long 2½ ft deep and 2 ft wide

The Resurrection of Henry Box Brown at Philadelphia, 1850. Lithograph by A. Donnelly. Library of Congress Prints & Photographs Division, LC-DIG-pga-04518.

their foolish behaviors and should have their bodies closely policed and under the strict control of the superior race. Cholera taught Brown the opposite lesson. Dying enslaved was not the way he wanted to go. He looked for ways to escape and ultimately mailed himself in a crate to a Philadelphia abolitionist in 1849, thus earning his nickname, "Box." He thereafter had his life story published, became a well-known anti-slavery lecturer, and lived as a freeman until his death in 1897.

James Williams remembered the pandemic through a similar lens. Born enslaved in Virginia in 1805, Williams was separated from his wife and child in 1833 when his master moved him to an Alabama plantation. In 1837, he escaped on foot, made it to the North, and the following year moved to Liverpool to avoid capture. Before he fled the United States, abolitionists published his story, one in which his brother's resistance to white supremacy stood out. The brother, whose name was not given in the written account, joined the Baptists and was taught to read and write by his wife, a free woman of color from Philadelphia. He began to preach and emphasized in his sermons "that all are of one blood." In 1832, he delivered an even more revolutionary message. "During the cholera at Richmond," Williams recalled, "my brother preached a sermon, in which he compared the pestilence to the plagues which afflict[ed] the Egyptian slave-holders, because they would not let the people go."[75]

Williams, Brown, Jasper, and countless other African Americans survived the pandemic with strengthened belief in equality and deepened faith in ultimate justice. It was a justice far from what Ann Maury had prophesized, wherein cholera sacrificed people of color to rid white people of the guilt of enslavement. Tragically, the justice that Williams envisioned would be delayed for several decades. Instead of causing a nationwide reflection on the country's original sin, powerful public voices cast people of color in the role they had scripted for them from the beginning. They were made to be dehumanized prop players whose mortality held up an imagined story about a loathsome disease's selectivity.

7

"Poor Exiles of Erin"

IRISH LABORERS IN MID-ATLANTIC WORK ZONES

ON SEPTEMBER 3, 1832, Charles F. Mercer, president of the Chesapeake and Ohio Canal (C&O), penned an ominous letter. He had just returned to his Leesburg, Virginia, home after traveling up and down the Potomac. In C&O labor camps, he saw men "turning black and dying in twenty four hours." Surviving workers fled in horror. He wrote to his board of directors that hospitals, doctors, and medicine were immediately needed to treat ill workers. The company should also assume the expense because contractors who directly employed the men could not afford to do so. The C&O needed to demonstrate to its largely Irish-immigrant workforce that, if they stayed on the job and got sick, they would be well cared for. If the board did not enact his plan, Mercer warned, financial ruin would be in store.[1]

Mercer's internal company correspondence contrasted sharply with a public message he addressed to the editors of Washington, DC's *National Intelligencer*. The scourge's presence along the Potomac had received notice in the press, and Mercer went into damage control.[2] "The reports ... of the cholera and of its mortality along the line of the canal are greatly exaggerated," his anonymously published letter declared. He stated that only two cases of sickness had occurred along a twelve-mile stretch of the canal above the Point of Rocks, Maryland, and those were not cholera. At Harpers Ferry, cholera could not be denied. Fourteen deaths had occurred near there, but these had been "confined to shanties." On his journey back home, he claimed to see no cases and to discover that "the general health of the valley of the Potomac had ... never been so good as during the present autumn." He further assured the public that the company was taking effective measures. By providing hospitals and nursing, he indicated, "the laborers will be sure of being properly taken care of, if the disease returns; and by ceasing to be fatal, it will lose nearly all its terrors for the living."[3]

Mercer's efforts to control the story faced an uphill battle. Boosters of the C&O, a joint venture of private and public investors including the states of Virginia and Maryland as well as the cities of Alexandria, Georgetown, and Washington, dreamed of an artificial waterway that ran from the Atlantic and through the Appalachians to the Ohio's headwaters. Conflict with private landowners, cost overruns, and labor shortages had caused disappointing progress over the previous four years, and after getting off to a promising start in 1832, a pandemic posed another impediment to the C&O. Mercer, a man of high repute who served as a military officer in the War of 1812, as a US Congressman (1817–1839) from his home state of Virginia, and as leader of the C&O since 1828, tried to make the case that minor occurrences of cholera in work camps could be contained there and that nearby towns would stay safe. Stockholders could rest assured that construction would continue.

As he did, Henry Boteler, a C&O investor and physician, wrote to the company's board of directors from Shepherdstown, Virginia. The disease had spread up the line another ten or so miles to Williamsport, Maryland. Between August 31 and September 4, the scourge had taken thirty lives, and Irish workers were not willing to stay at the worksite. The "poor Exiles of Erin are flying in every direction," he decried, adding "by the last of this week you will not have a working man on the whole line."[4]

The flight of workers from the canal zone threatened the C&O's development, but the company's pain paled in comparison to that of their labor force. Not just the C&O but also New Jersey's Delaware and Raritan Canal (D&R) and Pennsylvania's Philadelphia and Columbia Railroad (P&C), both of which were under construction in 1832, depended almost exclusively on Irish immigrants. In all three cases, cholera exacted a terrible price on workers, which company leaders, often in league with nativist newspaper editors, struggled to keep hidden.

Even before cholera arrived, constructing canals and railroads were some of the most hazardous jobs in the United States. Irish immigrants, some before boarding ships to cross the Atlantic, chose this work because contractors offered to pay for their transportation and promised higher wages than what they could earn in the cities and on farms. Uprooting trees, digging artificial channels, blasting through hills, and diverting water, though, led to frequent crushed appendages, drownings, and infections. Malaria-carrying mosquitos multiplied in the altered environments, while typhoid- and dysentery-causing bacteria easily made their way from latrines into the waters that men worked in and drank from. Germs also spread quickly in the hastily built shanties, in which fifteen to twenty men slept on wooden planks bunked on top of each other.[5] When *Vibrio* entered these conditions, the pandemic exposed inequalities that Americans had been told did not exist in their country and exacted mortality that they thought impossible.

Two years into the building of New Jersey's D&R, the pandemic hit. A venture of a private joint stock company, the artificial waterway was to run from the Delaware River, just below Trenton, eastward to New Brunswick, where it would connect to the Raritan Bay and the Atlantic Ocean. A twenty-mile feeder branch was to extend northward from Trenton along the Delaware to Bulls Island, making the D&R a giant "Y" that would create a shorter and cheaper waterway for Pennsylvania coal to get to New York City. The D&R's president, naval officer Robert F. Stockton, who fought against the Barbary pirates in 1815, had sunk much of his family's fortune into the project and taken out loans from English banks. In 1831, with construction lagging, the state ultimately stepped in and forced Stockton's company to merge with the Camden and Amboy Railroad. Once on more secure financial footing, the D&R appeared to be ready to make substantial progress in 1832.[6]

Cholera brought work on the D&R to a halt. On July 18, ten workers came down with the disease at a site just east of Princeton. Seven died quickly. Cases subsequently broke out at other work camps. Two weeks into the emergency, Stockton hired Dr. S. Howell to investigate and take the necessary steps to treat the sick and allay panic. The doctor, however, found that some contractors perished, others suspended work, and laborers fled. "The dispersion of the remnants of these unfortunate people rendered it unnecessary for me to execute your humane instructions," he informed Stockton.[7] The company, though, did establish a hospital in Princeton for stragglers who wandered into the small college town.[8]

Residents and relocated evacuees from cholera-scourged communities were not pleased. "Great uproar has been occasioned by some cit[izens] who are rusticated here," the Reverend James W. Alexander wrote from Princeton. They had "condemned" the town's board of health for agreeing with the company to locate a hospital in their midst.[9] Benjamin Rice, a Presbyterian minister, was among the chagrined. He had fled New York in mid-July, only to find himself surrounded by the cholera victims he had hoped to escape. "It is God's Judgement upon a wicked world and marks the profligate with a certain & fatal aim," Rice said of cholera's supposed selection of "drunkards & prostitutes."[10] Some theological students, while not immune to such prejudice, nonetheless volunteered to nurse the ill, even after the college had sent most students home.[11]

Trenton also saw an influx of fleeing Irish laborers. Ten or twelve workers arrived in the state capital on August 1 looking for work, and others followed over the next couple of weeks as canal construction remained suspended.[12] Some found jobs building the city's new waterworks, but the scourge erupted there too. Laborers who had no one to care for them ended up in the city's makeshift hospital, where death was almost a certainty.[13] The city allocated a portion of its cemetery for Catholic graves, but many of the dead were hastily buried and even abandoned at various points along the canal.[14]

A grotesque, yet disputed, example of an unceremonious treatment of the dead occurred just outside of Trenton. Four decaying corpses had allegedly been found along the Delaware River. The first account identified the deceased as Irish canal laborers who made it back to their shanty just in time to die. This initial report also claimed that "some colored persons," after receiving "a large reward," buried the victims in a single pit and then burned the shanty down.[15] A second account indicated that the man who found the bodies was a passerby who "happened to look" into the shanty and see three bodies. A fourth corpse—that of a female—lay outside of the dwelling. The passerby called neighbors to help. They dragged the deceased woman into the shanty and called a doctor, who rendered his opinion that cholera had taken them. This later report diverged from the initial account by claiming that, instead of being buried, the deceased had been consumed in the flames of the torched shanty.[16] Both versions circulated in newspapers from Maine to South Carolina.

The *New Jersey State Gazette* tried to make sure that no one would believe the stories. The *Gazette*'s editors claimed to have asked several people who lived near the site, and none of them knew anything about the alleged fatalities. They declared the whole episode "to be destitute of truth" and one concocted from "newspapers at a distance."[17]

Civic leaders did not try to hide their disdain for cholera's supposedly preferred victims. Newspapers rarely named deceased Irish workers. A Philadelphia paper noted that James Lowrey, Alexander Kelly, and Josiah McDonald drew their last breaths in the Princeton hospital, while the *State Gazette* recorded that contractor James Williams, a "native of Ireland," succumbed to the disease. Initial accounts, however, explained that cholera found canal workers "food for the disease" because of "their filthy habits" and crowded living arrangements.[18] The Trenton Board of Health described initial cases and fatalities in the city as being among laborers who were "mostly though not wholly of the intemperate class."[19] As fatalities continued through mid-August, the Trenton Board of Health tried to dismiss "exaggerated reports . . . respecting the unhealthfulness of our city" by pointing out that the majority of deaths were among those most expected to die. Of the laborers who found their way into the city, the board declared, "every attention have been paid them that humanity required" but most perished because of their intemperance and arrival to the hospital too late to receive effective treatment.[20]

Public silence would reign in the immediate aftermath of cholera's scourge of the D&R. Neither company officials nor news editors offered even a rough estimate of how many workers had perished.[21] Governor Peter Vroom vaguely referred to the project's cholera struggles in an October address, but he couched his reference in language that covered up the disease's terrors more than illuminating them. Vroom admitted the "sickly season" curtailed the D&R's "operations," but approvingly claimed "they are now progressing onward with renewed activity." The outgoing governor, to be sure, did not entirely gloss over the pandemic. "Gloom sat upon every brow, and fear found an entrance into every heart," he said of the scourge's impact on his state. "The pestilence swept away a number of our citizens." He inevitably lauded Charles Ewing and accorded the pandemic meaning that the judge's death had threatened to contradict. "If the pestilence that has just passed by, shall prove the missionary of temperance . . . ," Vroom concluded, "it will not have come in vain."[22]

There is no record of Robert F. Stockton saying anything publicly about the numerous Irish immigrants whose lives cholera cut tragically short. The D&R became fully operational in 1834, cutting the time it took for Pennsylvania coal to reach New York City from two weeks to a few days. Stockton's wealth and prestige grew. During the US war with Mexico, he served as commander of the United States' Pacific squadron and afterward received the honor of having Stockton, California, named for him. He served New Jersey in the US Senate from 1851 to 1853, returned as president of the D&R, and oversaw its operations during its especially prosperous years of the American Civil War. He died in 1866, and his remains were entombed in a clearly marked grave in Princeton.[23] Several generations would pass before the sacrifice of Irish laborers on the D&R would become publicly acknowledged.

Workers on the Philadelphia and Columbia Railroad experienced the pandemic's deadly circumstances in an even more mysterious way. Chartered in

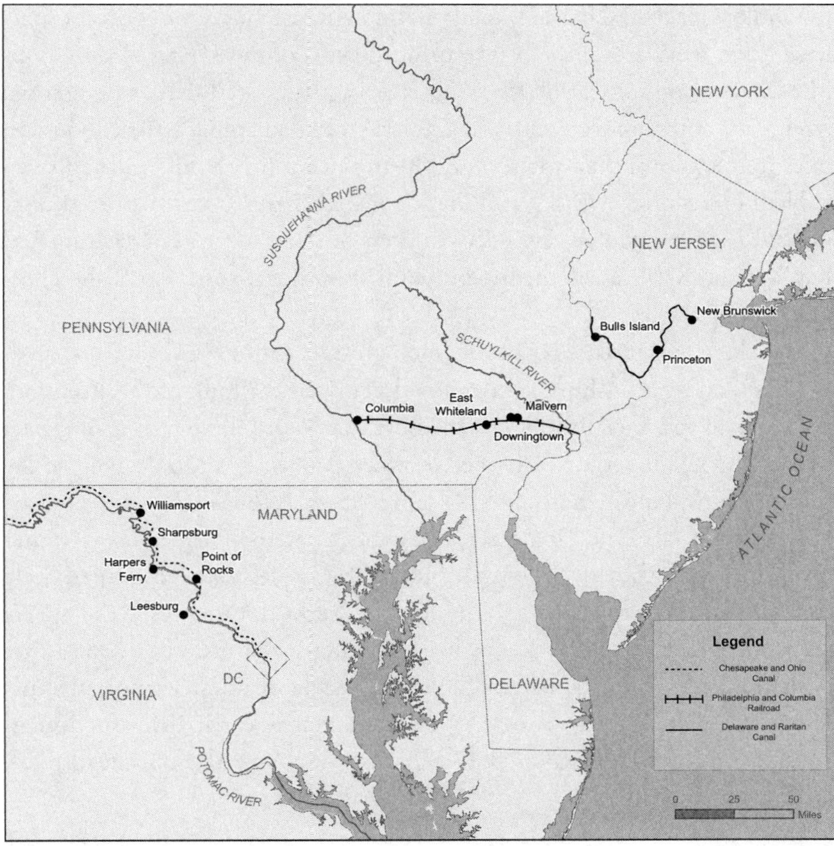

Cholera in Work Camps, 1832. Map by Franchesca Rodriguez, Geospatial Center, Stony Brook University.

1823 as a state-owned enterprise, the P&C was to run over eighty-two miles from the Schuylkill to the Susquehanna. While horses were used at the time to pull trains of relatively few cars along wooden rails, steam-powered engines traveling on iron rails were seen as the future of transportation, especially across the rugged terrain of Chester County, Pennsylvania.[24] There, in the summer of 1832, a largely immigrant workforce uprooted trees, carved off sides of hills and mountains, built embankments, and laid tracks. The P&C's camps were perhaps somewhat healthier than those in canal zones, as railroad construction involved varied topography rather than the low-lying and poorly drained riverine environments. Nonetheless, wherever dozens of men shared small and unhygienic living spaces with latrines near water sources, an environment ripe for an explosive growth of *Vibrio* existed.

Cholera reached Chester County in mid-August, but few details about its presence in worksites made it into print. Editors of the *Village Record*, published in the county seat of West Chester, vaguely stated that "a pestilential dysentery... more mortal than the Cholera in Philadelphia" struck about ten miles to the west of their town, along "a strip of country a mile wide and two and half miles long."[25] The West Chester *Temperance Advocate* reported "that several cases" erupted among P&C workers in the same general vicinity and that William B. Mitchell, the superintendent of the railroad, established hospitals "along the line."[26]

A sudden and intense outbreak among residents of East Whiteland, with no identified relationship to the railroad, received the bulk of the attention. In this small town, eight miles to the north of West Chester, nine of eleven people who fell ill with cholera died between August 17 and 25.[27] Four of the deaths occurred in the household of James Speer. "*All were intemperate, and* ALL ARE DEAD," the *Temperance Advocate* exclaimed. "The house or rather hovel, in which they lived, with all its contents, was burned immediately after the bodies were buried."[28] The *Village Record* did not name the Speers but reported that cholera victims lived in a house "of little value" and that locals torched it and its material contents "as the readiest way of effectual cleansing."[29] "It felt like a bomb; whizzed, burst, carried destruction in around, and all was still again," the *Village Record* observed about the disease's quick work.[30]

But did something more sinister than cholera infections occur? The *Chester County Democrat*, also published in West Chester, said so and attributed some of deaths in the area to murder. "An affair of a very interesting nature, lately occurred near our Borough, which has occasioned a great excitement," the editors declared in their September 11 issue. A respectable yet unnamed man who had "long since" settled in an unidentified Chester County neighborhood became suspected of welcoming into his home someone who had been in an "infected district" of upstate New York. Neighbors panicked and drove the man and his family from their home. The family wandered from house to house looking for shelter until a shoemaker took them in. A mob gathered around the shoemaker's home, bribed someone inside to unlock the door, rushed in, killed the owner, and then burned the dwelling "that they might effectually destroy, (in their own language) every trace of the *infection*." The next day, bones of incinerated victims could be seen in the rubble, while suspects were reportedly arrested and bound over for trial. The editors concluded, "It is not the first instance wherein selfishness, in these trying times, has obliterated justice and destroyed the best sensibilities of the heart."[31]

Devoid of specifics and without any known corroborating evidence, the account might have been made up. No record of the suspects being tried has been found.[32] Editors across the United States, however, expressed little skepticism about the story's veracity. Baltimore's *Gazette and Daily Advertiser* took up the article in its October 23 issue, giving it the title "Humanity Disgraced." The editors prefaced the piece, "what detestable savages, do we read of in the following narrative; surely they seem to have forgotten that there is justice on earth and vengeance in heaven."[33] An abbreviated version titled "Unparalleled Barbarity" also circulated widely. This version repeated the same basic facts but declared the event to be "a horrid account of murder and incendiarism, equaling in enormity, if the details are void of exaggeration, the most barbarous cruelties practiced among hostile savages."[34] Nashville's *National Banner* published the full account, while suggesting that the occurrence of the crime threatened "the honor of the American name."[35]

As the scandalous tale circulated, the *Village Record* wanted readers to move on from the pandemic. The October 3 issue included a poem expressing joy that the "pestilence cloud has passed over" the mid-Atlantic.[36] Its verses alluded to the return of patrons to theaters in New York and Philadelphia, and then declared, "Tears & smiles—cholera or no cholera, the world will roll on, we believe, much after the old fashion."[37]

But cholera had not gone away. A resurgence of the disease in Chester County occurred in late October among P&C workers. Superintendent William B. Mitchell expended $1,030, according to a state commission's records, in October and November to procure "physicians, medicine, and a temporary hospital" for sick laborers.[38] The state authorized the extra expenses but proved less generous to Philip Duffy, a contractor who was building a section of the line near East Whiteland, through what is today the town of Malvern. "This man has been rather unfortunate during the last fall, nearly one half of his men died of Cholera," Mitchell explained to the commission. The superintendent, while disparaging the Irish-born Duffy as a "perfect master of the art of complaining with or without cause," nonetheless called for him to get paid an extra $500 to cover additional expenses. The state denied the request.[39]

The October outbreak only faintly made it into the news. The *Democrat* made no reference to cholera appearing again in Chester County after it published its scandalous article, while the *Village Record*, in its November 7 issue, informed its readers that only eight fatal cases had occurred about two weeks prior "on the Railway, in East-Whiteland township." The paper indicated that many workmen fled, leaving a "humane" blacksmith behind to nurse a man, who succumbed to the disease. The blacksmith subsequently "blew his horn, and called in some neighbors who aided to bury him." An unnamed contractor, almost certainly Philip Duffy, came back "after a day or two, set fire to the shanties and burnt them down." The *Village Record* felt compelled to publish news of the outbreak "to prevent exaggeration" and let readers know cholera's spread was of limited scope and passed quickly. "All along the line we learn, it now is, and has been, through the summer, with the few exceptions noted, remarkably healthy," the editors disingenuously claimed. "Confident hopes are entertained that, next season, the whole line of Railway from Philadelphia to Columbia, will be in full operation."[40] Such a spin smacked of a cover-up dictated by P&C officials. The half of Duffy's crew who died certainly numbered more than eight, and the truth about their demise would remain buried until the twenty-first century.

One week after their reluctant admission that cholera had returned, the *Village Record* followed up with an attempt to exonerate Chester County's reputation. Noting the wide and continuing circulation of the *Democrat*'s story of incendiary killings, the editors claimed that the original was "an Allegory, or species of wit" that they did not understand when it was first published. The murdered individuals supposedly represented members of the Masonic order, who at the time had come under suspicion as conspirators against the American Republic. The *Democrat*, if the anti-Masonic *Village Record* was correct, intended to show the dangers of such prejudice.

Only one known newspaper found the *Village Record*'s explanation worth noticing.[41] "We took it for an honest story of blood and fire and murder," editors of New York's anti-Jacksonian *Spectator* admitted. But they claimed it as a poor example of political humor with an obscure meaning.[42] The Jacksonian Pottsville *Miner's Journal*, which was the source of the abbreviated "Unparalleled Barbarity" version, issued its own retraction and condemned the original authors. Whoever wrote it, the editors charged, should be ashamed for perpetrating "a stupid burlesque" that deceived "hundreds."[43] Many Americans at the time and later historians have seen it as evidence of a violent response of scared people confronted with a deadly scourge.[44]

Compared to the experience of people in southeastern Pennsylvania, that of Irish laborers constructing the C&O Canal occurred with more visibility. Cholera cases began to pop up in the Lower Potomac Valley in mid-August. Washington, DC, usually a ghost town during the hottest and muggiest part of the year, became even more so. Congress had already begun its usual recess; federal officers fled; President Jackson and his family headed to Tennessee; and few of the city's affluent class remained. Heavy rains later in the month spread the pathogen widely, and working-class people bore the brunt of mortality.[45] A total of 459 people had lost their lives to the malady by the time *Vibrio* burned out in the fall.[46]

The catastrophe extended up the Potomac, a fact that the C&O's internal correspondence revealed in stark contrast to Charles Mercer's deceptive letter of September 3 to the *National Intelligencer*. Panicked contractors and engineers sent urgent messages to the board of directors describing a mass exodus of workers amid the rapidly multiplying number of deaths.[47] "Humanity is outraged by some of the scenes presented," an engineer described on September 11. "Men deserted by their friends or comrades, have been left to die in the fields, the highways, or in the neighboring barns & stables: in some instances, as I have been told; when the disease has attacked them; the invalid has been enticed from the shanty & left to die under the shade of some tree." The engineer reported that residents of Sharpsburg, Maryland, tended to the sick and dying, but "nearly every person who has been with the dead bodies or has assisted in burying them have paid the forfeit with their lives: and now it is scarcely possible to get the dead buried."[48]

Cholera made sure that the company could not keep it out of the press. "Report says that as many as three, four, five and six dead bodies have been seen in a single shanty at one time," the Hagerstown *Torch Light* claimed in its September 6 issue. Four bodies had been brought into Hagerstown for interment in the Catholic burial ground, but civic leaders feared traffic into their community and demanded that the company bury the bodies "on some suitable point of the canal."[49] "The disease yet prevails severely on the line or in the neighborhood of the Chesapeake and Ohio canal," Baltimore's *Niles Weekly Register* reported. "The panic was awful, and the sufferings of the people, chiefly newly arrived foreigners, exceedingly distressing. The bodies of many laid on the roads unburied for days—being abandoned by their late relatives or associates."[50] An "old correspondent" wrote the editors of the New York *Commercial Advertiser* describing that as he traveled through the canal zone, he found "the graves of the dead laborers... in rows by the road side, melancholy mementos of the passing fiend."[51]

By September 24, with outbreaks abating but not yet gone, President Mercer went to work presenting the C&O as a safe place for workers. To accommodate sick laborers, he rented some cabins and paid a contractor fifty dollars to build "a large and commodious shanty" near Harpers Ferry. He employed attendants, purchased medicine, and implemented a plan in which workers paid part of the expenses by having twenty-five cents withheld from their monthly pay. He expressed confidence, which his board undoubtedly wanted to hear. "As to the obstructions occasioned by the cholera," he claimed, "they spring partly from the mortality of the disease, but yet more from exaggerated reports of it, at a distance, deterring laborers from coming on the line." It was his "arrangements . . . for the sick," Mercer asserted, that would bring contractors and workers back to the Potomac.[52]

The *National Intelligencer* again served as a vehicle for the company to promote its efforts. The newspaper published Dr. James P. Quinn's favorable letter, dated October 10. Quinn, a Harpers Ferry resident, claimed, "Cholera has almost entirely disappeared from this section of the country." He added, "efficient and responsible contractors" had resumed "full operation" in their construction efforts.

Quinn's argument was misleading. The doctor downplayed the nightmare that had occurred over the past several weeks. "Rumor, with her thousand tongues," he asserted, "has been busy in exaggerating the mortality that attended this dreadful disease, on the line of the canal." Then he deceptively reported that at Harpers Ferry only three cases of cholera occurred, and those were more than a month ago. Quinn could not have been counting the dozens of deaths among workers in the camps near the canal. The doctor also claimed that workers did not go "without relief," contrary to what internal company communications and newspapers had earlier reported about the sick being abandoned. Quinn heaped praise on Mercer but offered no condolences to the Irish immigrants.[53]

Cholera, moreover, was not at the end of its career, as Quinn suggested. Between October 10 and 20, nine cases were reported around Williamsport, with four of these ending in death. A "few cases and deaths" also occurred "several miles below the town."[54] The pathogen also spilled over to Halltown, Virginia, a village less than four miles away from Harpers Ferry. Sixteen people in a town of just one hundred residents were taken to their graves in a matter of a few days.[55] Local spread also picked up in Hagerstown, Maryland, during the middle of October and caused at least thirty-two fatalities there.[56] The pandemic eventually passed the Potomac Valley, in part due to a lack of nonimmune victims and cold weather, which inhibited the survival of *Vibrio* in local water supplies.

The scourge left the C&O in a financial pinch. Some contractors could not find enough labor, failed to complete the work within the time allotted to them, and breached their contracts.[57] An exasperated Mercer asked for a government bailout. "The fatal disease which has spread alarm throughout the world," he pled to Maryland's legislature, had forced a general suspension of construction. The dream of connecting the Chesapeake Bay to the Ohio River and bringing "population and wealth" to the towns along the Potomac was in jeopardy. He did not mention the fact that workers died, never mind how many perished, but he did promise that contractors would resume their work and do so with an abundance of labor as cholera had disappeared.[58] The state came through and infused cash into the company, allowing it to continue its operations.

Well into the summer of 1833, though, construction lagged behind schedule. In its annual report, company officials admitted to their stockholders that disease had impacted progress. "But for the prevalence of the cholera," officials claimed, a navigable channel would have been completed all the way to the head of the falls at Harpers Ferry by May 1833. Still, the report downplayed the number of deaths, as the pathogen's "mortality in the valley of the Potomac bore, indeed, no proportion to the terror which its approach inspired."[59] The pandemic's visit to the Potomac thus became officially recorded as a trifling affair, just as many Americans had believed it would be before it ever began.

Despite what Mercer and other powerful people dismissively said, the disease that Irish workers saw during that terrible summer and fall of 1832 was fact, not rumor; the terror they felt was genuine, not imagined; and the dangers they believed themselves to be in were real, not exaggerated. Immigrant bodies, in large and unknown numbers, lay in and alongside much of the infrastructure being built in Jackson's America. Not until more recent times have their losses been acknowledged.

In the 1970s, the state of New Jersey had to do something with the D&R, which by then had become defunct and polluted. The canal had thrived for much of the nineteenth century and aided the growth and industrialization of Trenton and New Brunswick. In 1871, however, the Pennsylvania Railroad (PRR) gobbled up the D&R along with the Camden & Amboy Railroad, neglected needed repairs, and then gave the canal to the state in 1933. New Jersey planned to repurpose the artificial waterway as a state park. In 1973, state historians prepared a report that concluded fifty victims taken by cholera in 1832 were buried at Bulls Island. At one time these graves had crude headstones, but they had disappeared over the years. The remains of countless other laborers, the historians claimed, "were buried in unmarked graves along the banks of the canal." Today, the Delaware and Raritan Park hosts more than a million yearly visitors who enjoy hunting, fishing, canoeing, jogging, picnicking, and other recreational activities.[60]

Irish heritage groups made sure that the park would be thought of as more than a recreational site. On St. Patrick's Day 2003, the state dedicated a granite memorial "honoring the hardships and triumphs" of the Irish workers who

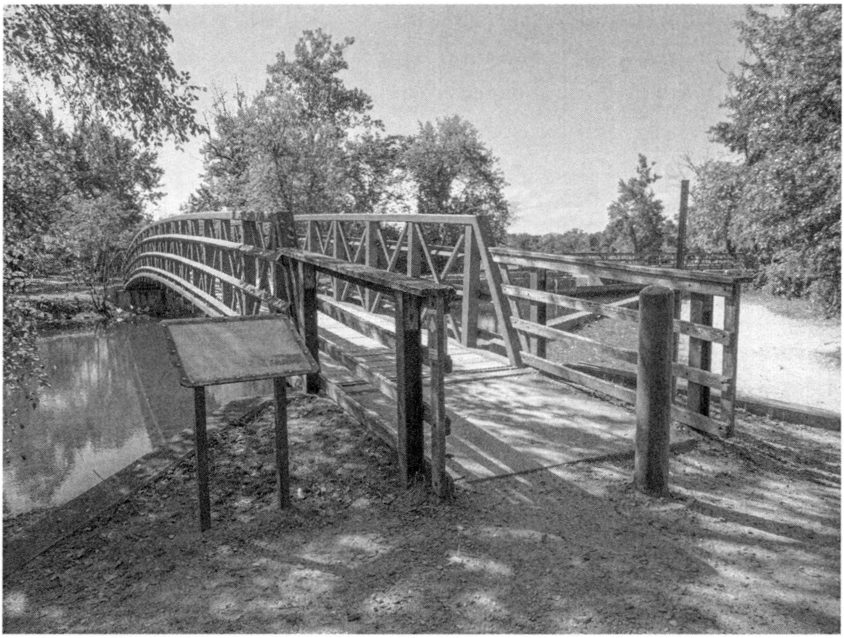

Dug by Irishmen Plaque. Before crossing the bridge over the canal near Princeton, New Jersey, today's visitors to the Delaware and Raritan State Park can learn about cholera's dire toll on immigrant workers in the 1830s. Photograph by Kristia Adams.

built the D&R. Placed at Bulls Island near the unmarked graves, the monument stands in opposition to the story that powerful people told about cholera's victims in 1832.[61] In Princeton, the Somerset County Ancient Order of Hibernians placed a plaque in the park that called the working conditions of Irish workers "appalling." Hundreds died, according to the plaque, with many being "buried in the fields where they died." The workers, it recorded, deserved praise for building "our nation's first great transportation systems."[62]

Commemorating the deceased P&C workers has entailed more complexity. The route that they constructed became a major thoroughfare of the PRR, and after that company's demise in 1968, it served as a well-traveled route for Amtrak and Southeastern Pennsylvania Transit Authority (SEPTA) trains. A mass grave of railroad workers claimed by cholera in 1832 is believed to exist in the vicinity of the Northwood Cemetery in the town of Downington.[63] Today, a team led by brothers and historians William Watson and J. Francis Watson is engaged in locating the grave, reburying the deceased with proper ceremony, and marking the site with a Celtic cross.[64]

The Watsons' interests stem from their prior success at Duffy's Cut, the location where the contractor lost half of his crew. They had inherited from their grandfather, a former PRR executive, a file that contained a variety of sources pertaining to the mass grave, which the company compiled between 1909 and 1932. The sources—dating back to the nineteenth century and including letters, newspaper articles, and reminiscences of railroad workers—led PRR officials to conclude that fifty-seven workers had been buried at Duffy's Cut.

The Watsons made some startling discoveries. They found that Duffy had hired fifty-five men and two women straight off the ship the *John Stamp*, which arrived in Philadelphia in June 1832. Shipping records contained the names of these individuals, but no genealogical records turned up documenting their existence after their arrival. The Watsons believed they had died of cholera and set out to locate their remains. Between 2009 and 2014, the Watsons' team exhumed and analyzed seven skeletal remains buried at Duffy's Cut. Surprisingly, each had been buried in a coffin and bore marks of a violent death. One skull, for example, had a clear blow of an ax, while another had a hole indicative of a bullet fired from a small-caliber, low-velocity firearm.[65] Vigilantism rather than cholera appears to have been the cause of death for at least some of the Irish workers.

The physical evidence proves that violence had taken place, but it does not match the "Unparalleled Barbarity" story that circulated in the press in 1832. The evidence clearly indicates that the outbreak at Duffy's Cut occurred in late October, over a month after the shocking account of murder and incineration was first published. These findings do not suggest that those who were killed worked on the P&C.

Nevertheless, a crime that had been successfully covered up occurred at Duffy's Cut. The Watsons suggest that a local law enforcement group enacted a quarantine on the workers and that they caught at least seven individuals trying to escape. After they executed the escapees, they put them in coffins to hide their violent demise, took them back to the worksite, and had them buried in the fill in a different location than the mass burial of cholera victims. The *Village Record*'s dismissive reporting of the outbreak was thus part of the cover-up. It is a perfectly plausible explanation, but one for which corroborating evidence has yet to be discovered.

What of the remaining bodies? Geophysical testing provides evidence of multiple remains in the fill that supports the current rail line. The proximity to the active railroad tracks has prevented further excavations.[66]

The Watsons' team succeeded in giving the seven murdered workers the proper burial that so many of their contemporaries were denied. Through forensic and archival work, they were able to identify two of the victims.

One was John Ruddy, originally from Donegal, and the other was Catherine Burns of Tyrone. Their remains were flown back to their respective ancestral homes, and each received a funeral and grave marker.[67] The five remaining victims were reburied at West Laurel Hill Cemetery in Bala Cynwyd, Pennsylvania. A Celtic cross stands as a memorial to the fifty-seven

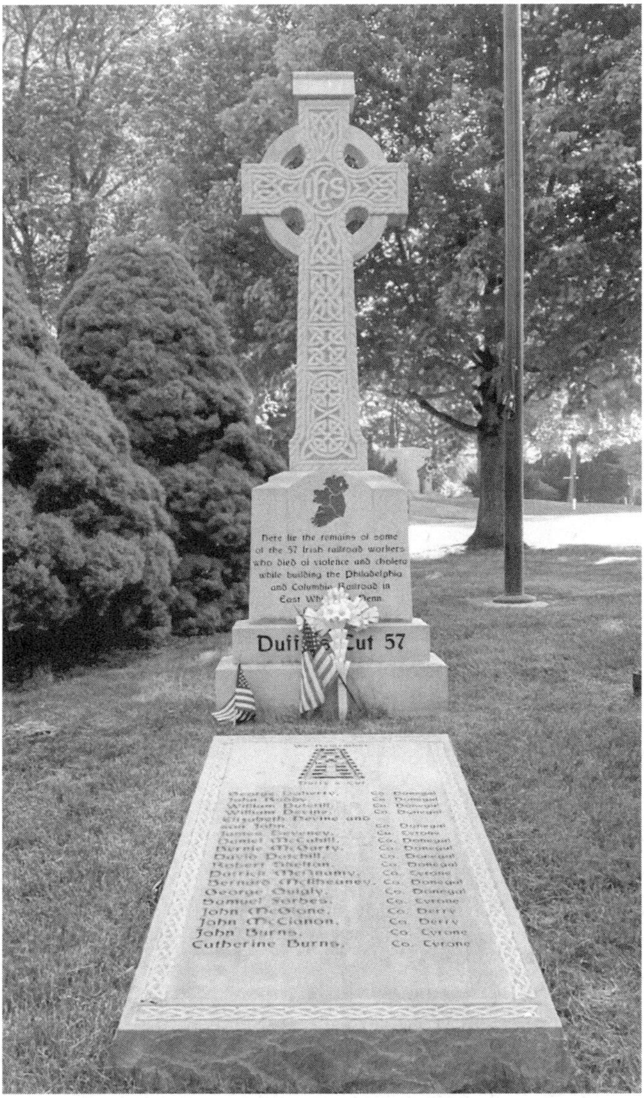
Here lie the remains of some
of the 57 Irish railroad workers
who died of violence and cholera
while building the Philadelphia
George Quigly, Co. Donegal
Samuel Forbes, Co. Tyrone
John McGlone, Co. Derry
John McClanon, Co. Derry
John Burns, Co. Tyrone
Catherine Burns, Co. Tyrone

Duffy's Cut 57 Monument. Before the list of the names of the deceased, the etching reads, "Here lie the remains of some of the 57 Irish railroad workers who died of violence and cholera while building the Philadelphia and Columbia Railroad in East Whiteland, Penn." Photograph by William Watson.

immigrants whom Duffy employed directly from the docks, with a limestone ledger listing the names of twenty individuals whom the Watsons are "reasonably certain died at Duffy's Cut."[68]

None of the Irish workers whose lives came to an end building the C&O were ever named. The canal failed to live up to the dreams that Charles Mercer had for it. It never went through the Appalachians as planned, and the Baltimore and Ohio Railroad dominated transportation profits. The C&O became defunct by the end of the nineteenth century. Today, the canal area is a US national park that offers recreational activities for visitors. This park would not exist without the labor of Irish immigrant workers, many of whose bodies remain entombed in the canal's earthen embankments and nearby fields. No known historical markers commemorating their sacrifice exist.

So little is known about the immigrants who perished building the D&R, P&C, and C&O because company officials and news editors allied to diminish, dismiss, and even cover up the ravages of cholera. Voices of the Irish remain silent in the sources available to reconstruct the history of their labor during that deadly summer and fall of 1832. Erin's exiles deserve to be remembered as more than the intemperate and dissolute props that nativists seemed to need to assuage fears of a global killer.

8

"So Much for Freedom"

DISMISSIVENESS AND DEATH IN BALTIMORE

"I WAS ALL ears, all eyes," a man recounted about his life as an enslaved teenager in Baltimore. People around him, in those early years of the 1830s, discussed the topics of the day, especially abolitionism. The literate fourteen-year-old was not sure what abolition meant until he read about it in discarded issues of the Baltimore *American*. Its proponents, the *American* disapprovingly reported, had inundated Congress with petitions to end slavery in the nation's capital and to prohibit interstate commerce in human bodies. "There was HOPE in those words," the man later recalled.[1]

At the same time, ominous news of global pestilence circulated throughout Baltimore. On June 6, 1832, the arrival of the *Brenda* drew the attention of health officers. The ship had departed Liverpool on April 24 with a clean bill of health, but between the first of May and the twenty-third, nine passengers died of "dysentery or cholera" and five others perished from other illnesses. Although no one became ill during the last two weeks of the voyage, authorities kept the ship at the lazaretto for disinfection. Rumors could not be contained, and news that cholera was in Baltimore spread beyond the city itself.[2] Although no local outbreak immediately occurred in June, residents were still anxious. Following news that Quebec and Montreal had fallen into the pandemic's grasp, terrible reports of the disease's impact in New York, Philadelphia, and Norfolk filled Baltimore's papers throughout the summer. Some residents did not wait for the disease to appear in their midst and fled to rural retreats.[3]

It was a frightening yet auspicious time for the enslaved teenager. "I remember thinking that God was angry with the white people because of their slaveholding wickedness, and therefore his judgements were abroad in the land," he recounted, echoing what had become a widespread belief among African Americans. "Of course it was impossible for me not to hope much for the abolition movement when I saw it supported by the Almighty, and armed with DEATH."[4]

Fear never seemed to grip Peter Hoffman Cruse, an editor who worked at the *American* until his move to the *Patriot and Mercantile Advertiser* in 1832. Suspicious cases began to pop up in early August throughout the city, with a concentration of fatalities among free people of color living in the Ruxton Lane neighborhood.[5] These victims, a racist Cruse explained to his friend John Pendleton Kennedy, were "birds you might expect in such a nest." They were mired in "filth" and addicted to eating watermelons, a cheap fruit that was widely associated with poverty and condemned for its supposed association with cholera. Kennedy, a Baltimorean who left the city, invited Cruse to join him beyond the Blue Ridge Mountains, but the editor asserted, "I see no cause for alarm to the temperate and prudent."[6]

With the outbreak escalating during the last week of August, Cruse remained confident. "As yet, the *discrimination* of the disease is marvelous," he informed his friend, "for, as you will have seen by the reports, the black people are almost its exclusive victims."[7] The editor referred to the Baltimore Board of Health's report of interments for the week ending August 27 and declared, "the deaths among negroes [are] out of all proportions." What was more, of the seventy-eight people of color who had perished, seventy-five were free and only three were enslaved. "So much for freedom," the proslavery Cruse gloated to Kennedy.[8] The following day, words similar to his private ones appeared in print. The *Patriot* castigated free people of color as "exposed, indigent, ignorant, and incurably imprudent" and claimed that they could not resist the "temptation" of eating cheap and "unwholesome fruit." "If death is an evil to them," the newspaper declared, "freedom so much abused can be no blessing." [9]

The enslaved teenager, of course, did not see it that way. Six years later, he escaped bondage and went to live a long and healthy life in freedom. His name was Frederick Douglass. Meanwhile, cholera would put the white supremacy of Cruse and other white Baltimoreans to the test and challenge their preconceived notions about its supposed selectivity.

Baltimore's turn with the global pandemic began on August 4. Then, a seven-year-old white girl suddenly died, leading the city's leading physician, Horatio Gates Jameson, to investigate. Jameson, a University of Maryland–trained doctor, had made his expectations already known with a treatise he wrote back in the spring. He echoed the widely held belief that cholera stemmed

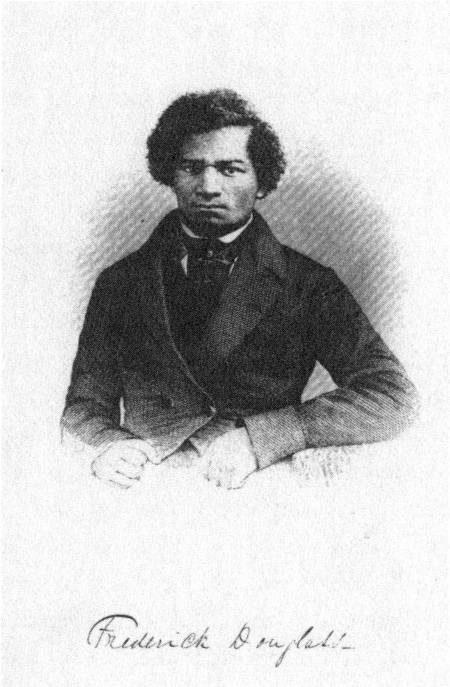

Frederick Douglass. Frontispiece of *My Bondage and My Freedom* (Miller, Orton, and Mulligan, 1855). Schomburg Center for Research in Black Culture, Photographs and Prints Division, The New York Public Library, 5161080.

from atmospheric causes and became malignant among the most degraded of peoples. "Providence shields the better part of the human race from this scourge," he declared. Health, for him, as for so many in the medical profession, had political and moral dimensions. "Enlighten the heathen, reclaim the drunkard, breakdown lordly power, infuse the spirit of freedom and self-respect throughout mankind, . . . and much will be done," he advocated as the proper prevention for cholera.[10] The seven-year-old's death after having the well-publicized symptoms of the novel malady then caught the doctor off guard. "She was of respectable parentage, and in a neighborhood where cholera was not likely," he later explained.[11]

Jameson quickly became convinced that an outbreak was beginning in his city. An "old colored man" came down with the telltale signs of the disease the same day as the girl, and then "a white boy" perished a few days later after having the same symptoms.[12] By the ninth, Jameson and like-minded physicians became so concerned about growing numbers of illnesses that they implored Mayor William Steuart to have the board of health begin reporting cases and deaths. Some doctors remained skeptical, however, and insisted that the mayor issue a public pronouncement declaring the city free of the disease. Municipal authorities decided to do and say nothing, at least for the time being.[13]

Cholera's growing presence in the city was a poorly kept secret. Resident James Hawkins privately wrote to his associate that twenty-two fatalities had occurred before August 13 and that the city's silence only fueled rumors of an even deadlier situation. "With respect to our city I am really at a loss what to say, a majority of our board of health have refused to make any publication (a most unfortunate decision)," Hawkins complained while lamenting the negative impact such rumors had on commerce.[14] Another Baltimorean privately suggested the board's silence had to do with where the cases were concentrated. "As yet there are not cases of cholera reported by the board of health," Henry Wells wrote to a physician friend in the southern part of the state, "altho[ugh] there are several cases in Ruxton Lane—you know the place well as being one of the most filthy in Balt[imor]e."[15]

Wells's private thoughts echoed those of Peter Hoffman Cruse. In his August 15 letter to Kennedy, he revealed, "There has been a great effort here, on the part of the merchants, to keep matters as quiet as may be." He and his fellow editors fell in line, and he was just waiting to see if "the danger passed over" or became so obvious that the board would have to start making daily reports. He personally believed "that the visitation may be light" and might spread no farther than predominately black neighborhoods. He would stay put. "I am perfectly well, very studious, and shall be glad to see my friend when calm & security can return with them," he reassured Kennedy.[16]

Others were not so confident. "The Cholera is raging here with considerable virulence," a letter from Baltimore dated August 11 declared. "The public are considerably excited, and there appears to be a disposition . . . , on the part of some, to leave the city." Philadelphia's *United States Gazette* published the letter, although its editors acknowledged, perhaps sarcastically, that the "authorities" in its sister city had yet to announce the disease's presence. "Considering the method pursued in New York and in Philadelphia, of telling the truth, and the whole truth, relative to the pestilence, we are bound to believe that the writer of the letter is in an error."[17]

There was no error. The outbreak grew and became painfully obvious to Baltimoreans who remained in their city. On August 16, Methodist minister Reverend Thomas H. W. Monroe returned to the city after being away at a revival. He found "a considerable state of alarm" and saw a hearse retrieving a man who had become ill at 2:00 a.m. and had died by noon. "Wherever we go, nothing is talked of but the *Cholera, the fearful and the dreaded Cholera*," he recorded in his diary. Over the next four days, Monroe observed a stricken woman of color being taken from her dwelling; visited a dying "temperate" woman; learned that a "respectable," sober, and churchgoing neighbor had come down with the nasty illness; baptized two dying children; buried an "intemperate" woman who left her widower with four small children; and observed a physician being called upon numerous times to come deliver aid. "The pestilence is doubtless spreading, and gathering fresh force," he concluded, as he prepared for his sermon on Sunday, August 19.[18]

Finally, on Monday, August 20, the board of health issued a statement tepidly acknowledging that an outbreak had started. This was hardly news to anyone. "At length the Board of Health in Baltimore, after disingenuously (we had almost used a harsher word) concealing the fact of the existence of Cholera in that city, have made a report," editors of the Lynchburg *Virginian* quipped.[19] Baltimore's officials revealed that fifty-four deaths "under the denomination of cholera" had occurred over the previous week and announced their commitment to making daily reports.

They also assured the public that the disease was behaving in their city just as it was supposed to. Twenty-five of the deaths, the board explained, "were colored persons, and with few exceptions, all were either of intemperate habits or had been imprudent in their diet." The following day, the board reported fatalities of seven people of color and six white people over the previous twenty-four hours and noted, "scarcely an exception occurs to the fact that cholera has only become malignant in persons of very intemperate habits, or who had been greatly imprudent in the use of fruits and vegetables."[20]

In addition to diminishing the emerging tragedy by victim blaming, the board of health used a sleight of hand to obscure the outbreak's true extent. For instance, they omitted from their reports the deaths of impoverished people whom city officials had sent to the Calverton Almshouse. In 1822, Baltimore bought the Smith family country estate of Calverton and converted it into an asylum for orphans, vagrants, alcoholics, paupers, and the insane. By mid-July 1832, when city officials stepped up municipal cleaning efforts, the number of inmates there swelled to five hundred. Indigent and infected people were deposited there in early August, and *Vibrio* mushroomed in the facility during the month. The board ignored the situation, perhaps believing that the institution's location three miles outside of city limits did not require them to reveal the grisly statistics. Only a scant reference to cholera's presence at Calverton made it into public print. "Several fatal cases have occurred at the Almshouse in Baltimore County about three miles distant," the *Gazette and Daily Advertiser* reported on August 21.[21]

Knowledge about the situation in Calverton circulated through unofficial channels, nevertheless. Monroe recorded in his diary on August 24, "It is said that the inmates of the Alms House are dying by scores."[22] That same day, Cruse wrote to Kennedy, telling him that Calverton's gravedigger and his assistant had succumbed to the disease, as had numerous inmates. The editor privately described the deceased as having "the worst description of battered constitutions" and referred to the situation as "melancholy and disgusting enough."[23] "The mortality at Calverton Alms-House is horrible and astonishing," Cruse told his friend four days later. "I am authoritatively informed that...108 have already died."[24] In a letter three days later, Cruse referred to "hideous mortality" occurring that "beggar description."[25]

Baltimore's papers did not bring up the almshouse until cholera abated there.[26] Cruse's *Patriot* revealed on September 6 what its editor had only privately written about and did so as evidence of the scourge's supposed discriminating nature. "The Alms House, situated some miles from Baltimore, has been the scene of an impressive and awful warning to drunkards," the *Patriot* opined. "Of about 500 inmates (the number on the 15th July), 475 were intemperate persons; this accounts for the extreme mortality of the cholera there, which numbered 125 victims, one fourth of the whole."[27] Fatalities ultimately reached 133 before the pathogen ran out of victims, but the board of health never included those deaths in the city's official reports.[28]

Meanwhile, cholera did not explode within Baltimore's city limits as some might have expected, at least not until the end of August. Between the twenty-first and thirtieth, the board of health reported a death toll that fluctuated between a high of twenty-nine and a low of ten.

During this time, Reverend Monroe saw signs that cholera was conforming to expectations. "Several deaths in my own neighborhood," Monroe recorded on August 22, but "in almost if not every case Cholera is the result of intemperance, imprudence in eating vegetables, fruits & neglect of diarrhea."[29] On Sunday the twenty-sixth, the minister learned that a man who lived opposite of one of his parishioners had recently died, as had a woman in the neighborhood of another parishioner. The latter had allegedly said the night before that "she was not afraid of the Cholera—went to market and purchased & [ate] watermelons & cantaloupes—and before morning was a corpse!"[30] When the board of health noted that daily fatalities jumped from thirteen the day before to twenty-three fatalities in its report for Monday, the twenty-seventh, Monroe attributed this to the "dissipation, idleness & riot" of Sabbath breakers.[31]

Civic leaders focused on Ruxton Lane as the source of persistent pestilence. A city committee described a sewer that ran through the neighborhood as "merely covered with slight boards, removeable and removed at the pleasure of every individual," with "privies . . . erected over it." The raw sewage then flowed onto the surface of Light Street and drained down into the Patapsco Basin.

Miasma theory remained the unquestioned explanation for the outbreak. "The whole enlightened medical profession concurs in the opinion that the miasma generated by such places as this," the committee claimed about Ruxton Lane, "is one of the most nourishing aliments of disease." The sewage's "putrescent exhalations" supposedly wafted through the air and sickened Baltimoreans. The *Gazette and Daily Advertiser* published the committee's report and described the impoverished neighborhood as a place of "much mortality, misery and crime." The editors added, "the advent of the disease was hastened, its continuance encouraged, and its virulence increased by the condition of Ruxton Lane and other similar places."[32]

By following their noses, Baltimoreans were directed away from the source of what made so many of them sick. The Baltimore Water Company, a private corporation, supplied a portion of the city by way of a canal that delivered water from the Jones Falls River before it entered the heart of the city and then drained into the Patapsco River. The company's waterworks on the corner of Calvert and Centre streets received the water and pumped it to elevated reservoirs, which then piped the water to fire plugs and some homes and businesses. During most summers, the reservoirs ran dry and machinery broke down, leaving residents to rely on other sources. The company did not even bother connecting poorer districts.[33]

The poorest of these districts was Ruxton Lane. Residents there utilized Western Fountain, more popularly known as Clopper's Springs. At this site, water originally flowed directly out of a stream bank that drained into the Patapsco, but by 1832, the area around the springs had been reclaimed, the location had been domed over, and pipes had been inserted to funnel water down to the wharf. Western Fountain unfortunately stood in the direct line of drainage from the neighboring Ruxton Lane. It was in the perfect location to receive the neighborhood's sewage.[34] Baltimore's most impoverished, with nowhere to go, drank the free yet deadly water available to them.

Cruse saw cholera as confirming his views of black inferiority. He had to inform Kennedy that Miss Harriot West, a mutual acquaintance who belonged to their social circle, "had a very severe attack, and was for more than twenty-four hours in a very doubtful state." Cruse was pleased to tell his friend, however, that cholera did not make an "exception" out of her and that she was on her way to recovery. The editor admitted that cases had become more widely distributed throughout the city, but he maintained, "the preponderance of death is in the dirtier or lower streets, or in such as are inhabited by vile livers." He did not have to tell Kennedy, but he did anyway, that "Most of the deaths are among blacks."[35] Four days later he emphasized that among people of color, cholera preferred those who had freedom, leaving unsaid the widely held racist view that black people could not care for themselves and needed slavery to enjoy health and happiness. "The cholera never enters my head, except when I see the bill of interments," he claimed. "Among *polite* people, it is hardly spoken of."[36]

The scourge had a way of making its presence known even to those who wanted to ignore it and a way of changing the minds of those who, at first, thought it discriminated. Heavy rains on August 28 caused a spike in cases.[37] By the thirty-first, the daily deaths had reached thirty, the highest to date. "This is an alarming and unexpected increase of mortality," Reverend Monroe recorded in his diary, "calculated to produce a complete reaction in the minds of those who fancied the disease was passing away."[38]

Ninety people perished over the next three days, keeping the minister busy visiting the sick, administering funerals, and consoling the bereaved. On September 1, he received a letter from a friend and fellow preacher, exhorting him "to be courageous, and have faith in God" and, if he perished, "let it be at the post of duty." Monroe remained determined to stay, although "it may truly be the post of danger—death is now—& has been for days—all around me—and I have had perhaps more than an ordinary share of nervous fear & excitement." He resolved, "nothing but the imperious order of Divine Providence would remove me from this scene of alarm, of danger, and of death." The next day, he went from home to home, arriving at some houses after it was too late. "How awful is the stillness of the night," he declared that evening. "Nothing to be heard but the distant tread of the watchmen, going their nightly rounds—and the ever and anon the rumbling of the *dead cart*!"[39] Thereafter, the reverend did not associate intemperance or imprudence with cholera's lethality.

Another Methodist minister—Dr. Lewis G. Wells—also remained quite busy during the outbreak. Wells, a free man of color, began preaching in the Methodist Episcopal Church in the 1820s, while at the same time working as a porter at Baltimore's Washington Medical College. There, he devoted several years to the study of medicine and subsequently served as a physician for members of his community, although he was not allowed to graduate with a medical degree.[40]

As cholera ripped through Baltimore, the thirty-one-year-old Wells worked tirelessly. "The doctor told us what to eat and what not to eat; how to cook it and how not to cook it; what to drink and what not to drink," Frederick Douglass recalled about Wells's efforts. It was just the sort of advice that Cruse thought people of color would not follow unless in bondage to white masters. The Methodist physician warned his temperate congregants against becoming too confident. "But, my hearers, it is the Lord's will," Douglass quoted Wells as saying, "this scourge will come to them that drink and them that do not drink."[41] As the number of cases escalated, African Americans observed the doctor "riding up one street and down another, administering to the sick and dying."[42] Dr. Horatio Jameson also witnessed Wells attend to his patients and described his treatment of vigorously rubbing the stricken to relieve them of cholera's excruciating cramps and employing the standard heroic technique of bleeding at the onset of symptoms.[43]

Wells, like so many other doctors during the pandemic, put his life at risk and paid the ultimate price. In the early morning hours of September 1, the Methodist physician arrived back home exhausted, and cholera quickly set in. His family members tried to rub away his cramps, and Wells tried to bleed himself but could not manage to do so. Jameson and one or more of his colleagues were called to the Wells house in the early morning and found the doctor in a collapsed state. "Being in an agony of suffering," Jameson recorded, "we gave him a large dose of laudanum, telling him, however, at first sight, that his case was too far advanced to admit of the slightest hope of recovery." He died an hour later. The African American doctor became another of cholera's victims, perhaps due as much if not more to heroic medicine rather than the disease itself.[44]

People of color and even some white people mourned his death. The *Republican and Commercial Advertiser* published Wells's lengthy obituary two days after his passing. His eulogizer, identified by the initials "A.B.," described him as "a useful man" who became "a martyr in the sphere of his duty." "Philanthropy was his primary object, and many of the helpless Africans who have survived him will remember his goodness," A.B. declared. Despite the short notice, a substantial number of mourners, including "some of the most respectable citizens," turned out for the funeral. Wells left a large family "and thousands to lament his sudden death."[45] For decades thereafter, African

American families in Baltimore kept pictures of him on their walls and named their sons after him.[46]

Peter Hoffman Cruse's *Patriot* published Wells's obituary that had originally appeared in the *Republican and Commercial Advertiser*, but the editor privately denigrated the deceased African American doctor.[47] Cruse penned yet another letter to Kennedy on September 6, having taken a five-day break from his correspondence.[48] During that time, daily mortality counts in the city had fluctuated between twenty and thirty-five. "Its variations are incalculable," Cruse said of cholera, as the city took on a more abandoned appearance. "There have been two or three doubtful cases of cholera . . . among persons you know; but nothing fatal." Some enslaved servants belonging to a mutual acquaintance had died, but free people of color sustained the greatest losses.

Cruse described them in the vilest and most racist terms. They were "horrid wretches or apes," the editor privately declared, who "universally abandoned each other, sisters their sisters, and wives their husbands. Poor *Wells* that able rhetorician, the [bright light] of the Washington Med. College, died abandoned by his negro acquaintances." Wells, of course, had not been abandoned, but for the racist Cruse, who had kept his distance from the suffering that men like Monroe, Wells, and Jameson directly witnessed, free people of color were made to conform to the assumptions of white supremacy. They could not take care of themselves outside of the paternalistic care that enslavement supposedly provided. "You will have seen the blessings of *freedom* in the bills of mortality," Cruse confided to Kennedy.[49]

Those were among the last words the editor ever wrote. On September 7, the outbreak reached its peak in Baltimore, with a total of fifty-five deaths reported by the city's board of health. Peter Hoffman Cruse was one of them.

Grafton L. Dulany, a prominent lawyer in the city, filled Kennedy in on the details of their mutual friend's demise. "Notwithstanding the oft repeated injunction of Physicians to abstain from all green vegetables, & to eat sparing of rice & potatoes—poor Cruse habitually indulged himself in tomatoes, boiled onions &c.," Dulaney revealed. The editor had visited the lawyer in the latter's office on the early evening of the sixth. After "laughing & talking on indifferent subjects," Cruse had to excuse himself and remained indisposed for an unusually long time. When he came back, he told Dulaney that he "copiously vomited & purged" and "succeeded in getting rid of two peaches which he had eaten in the morning & felt much better." The lawyer "urged" him to go see his regular doctor, but the editor refused and returned to his room in seemingly good spirits. Dulaney went back to check on his friend later in the evening and found Cruse crying "out in a voice expressive of great agony." The editor's usual physician was nowhere to be found, and Dulany frantically searched for anyone to come and help. He finally found a doctor who bled him and tried a "great variety of remedies" through the night. It was to no avail. Cruse "quietly expired between 6 & 7 o'clock on Friday morning."[50]

Newspapers in Baltimore and in many other US cities noted Cruse's passing with both tributes and warnings.[51] "We are summoned, this morning, to the performance of a melancholy duty, in recording the death of PETER H. CRUSE, Esq.," his former colleagues at the *American* stated. "So far as we can learn, the immediate source of the attack was a slight, a very slight irregularity of diet." Even the "peach or two" he had consumed was enough to do in a man who was otherwise "temperate and prudent in all his habits and pursuits." The "moment's deviation, an imprudence scarce worth remembrance in ordinary times," ended a life of a man with "high hopes, a vigorous intellect, and a warm and generous heart." They added, "society grieves for the loss of one of her most rising and estimable members."[52] The *Patriot* reprinted the obituary from the *American* and prefaced it with praise of their own: "Baltimore has lost one of her most valuable citizens."[53]

The editor's death, along with the escalating mortality, shook elite Baltimoreans. "Such is the effect of a single blow of the Great Destroyer which is stalking through the land," the *American* opined. "Terrible indeed, and inscrutable is his march."[54] Even the most recalcitrant of the city's newspapers, the *Republican*, had to admit reality. "The destroying angel has fairly unsheathed his sword and is spreading desolation and destruction around us in a frightful and alarming manner," the editors exclaimed. "The bill of mortality... is appalling: and the inroads which have been made in the ranks of our fellow-citizens fill us with terror and dismay."[55]

After a peak of fifty-five deaths on the seventh, a daily average of twenty-two Baltimoreans perished over the next eight days. People of color continued to be overrepresented in the daily reports, but the numbers—a total of seventy-four white people and seventy-five black people—could not hide that cholera did not discriminate as much as advertised. "Consternation & dismay appear in almost every countenance," Monroe recorded after Cruse's death. One of his parishioners came down with the malady on the same day, and while she appeared to be recovering, he remained pessimistic. "I know so little of the nature of this disease that I cannot predict with any kind of confidence" whether she would survive, he confided to his diary. She died the next day.[56]

On the morning of the twelfth, Monroe visited Joshua Mummey, a member of his church who lay sick with cholera only two days after burying his wife. The reverend had to leave to administer a funeral and then returned to the Mummey home that evening and found Joshua "slumbering" and near death. He learned that Joshua's brother Thomas also had the disease, was not supposed to survive, and had also recently lost his wife. "Few would have thought that such respectable persons as these would have been called off by a pestilence which was supposed to visit principally the intemperate," Monroe bemoaned. "Here, however, its ravages for the last two weeks, have been among all ranks of citizens."[57] The next day, Monroe learned that both Joshua and Thomas had perished by the early morning. "Many have been the scenes of peculiar distress since the raging of this awful calamity in Baltimore—many families have been nearly exterminated—some entirely so."[58]

Editors seemed to no longer feel obligated to assign a reason for the death of respected white people. Jacob Steiner's passing, the *Gazette* mourned, "has contributed to deepen the gloom which the presence of the disease that proved fatal to him, is calculated to throw over our society."[59] The newspaper eulogized Jonathan Rogers as having "all the qualifications that constituted a useful citizen, an upright and honest man, and a pious Christian."[60] A couple of days later, the *Gazette* declared, "Death in making its ravages spares neither age, [n]or sex, not even the rich or the poor, the widow or the orphan, and in recording the decease of Mrs. *Elizabeth Sharkey*, the tear of sympathy may be shed... one of the best of Mothers, and a most exemplary woman." Sharkey was a widow who had raised six children, taught music, and had "but few superiors of her sex."[61] Cholera seemed to be convincing the Baltimore press that it would not abide by the rules that many, including editors in their own city, had imagined it would follow.

Vibrio took its time letting go of Baltimore. Daily mortality dropped substantially through the latter half of September and would remain in the single digits after September 20. City merchants took it upon themselves to declare an end to the emergency, and on the twenty-sixth, they issued a public address, inviting people from the countryside to come into the city and make their purchases. The merchants assured them that "the afflicting disease... only lingers feebly in... remote and unfrequented places."[62] Dr. Jameson concurred and reaffirmed his pre-existing belief in cholera's noncontagious nature. The board of health continued to record daily deaths and chastise residents for poor dietary choices, but on October 4, it ceased issuing reports because cholera had "entirely disappeared from Baltimore as an epidemic." Jameson had advised the board to do such and claimed that only "a few sporadic cases" were then occurring, all of which were "attributable to imprudence." The deadly bacteria lingered in Baltimore's water supply, however, and took an additional sixty-two lives before concluding with its last known victim on November 16.[63]

In his end-of-the-year assessment of the outbreak, Jameson struggled to make the event conform to the notion that the United States would fare exceptionally well with cholera's arrival, but he tried. The doctor had to revise the total mortality upward. By looking at interment records, he found that the board of health had not accounted for all deaths in its daily reporting. The total fatalities, according to Jameson, amounted to 853, with 502, or 59 percent, being white and 352, or 41 percent, being people of color. While he did not include the 133 who perished in the almshouse in his assessment, he did uphold the disease's reputation as a discriminate killer. Cholera had "excited the terrors of the people" and caused Baltimoreans "to lament the loss of a few of our most respectable citizens," but, he maintained, "the lower orders of our citizens, and the vicious" suffered the most.[64] "A very great majority of those who died were the most worthless," Jameson said of cholera's 1832 victims in his magnum opus treatise on cholera.[65]

Table 8.1 Reported Cholera Mortality in the Upper South, 1832

Location	Reported Deaths
Wilmington, DE	38
New Castle, DE	12
Baltimore, MD	853
Calverton Almshouse, MD	133
Hagerstown, MD	32
Williamsport, MD	34
Maryland, excluding above	76
Washington, DC	459
Alexandria, VA (then DC)	8
Georgetown, DC	9
Norfolk, VA	405
Smithfield, VA	25
Richmond, VA	478
Harpers Ferry, VA	14
Halltown, VA	16
Virginia, excluding above	239
Elizabeth City, NC	10
Total	2,841[a]

[a] Some C&O workers' deaths are represented in the tabulations for Williamsport, MD, and Harpers Ferry, VA, but most went uncounted, and the total necessarily falls short of the number who perished.

Frederick Douglass could have very easily been one of the 2,841 "worthless" victims who reportedly perished in outbreaks across the Upper South (table 8.1) and whom Jameson callously dismissed.[66] Somehow, the enslaved teenager managed to avoid ingesting a large enough dose of *Vibrio* from Baltimore's poisoned drinking supply. Somehow, he did not consume foods on which the deadly bacteria had proliferated due to being washed in contaminated water or handled with unclean hands. He survived, and in 1838, he seized the freedom that men like Cruse believed would only doom him to life of vice and degradation. Douglass escaped to the North, became one of the most famous and revered people in American history, and enjoyed a long life in freedom. In telling his life story, he transformed the cholera pandemic into the Lord's punishment for slavery. He gave the tragic event a divine purpose that countered what powerful public voices said about the scourge and its supposed intended victims.

9

What Happened in New Orleans

THE FIRST WAVE IN THE WEST

REVEREND THEODORE CLAPP did not try to hide cholera's terrors. In his 1857 autobiography, the Unitarian minister claimed to be among a crowd that gathered near the pandemic's first victims in New Orleans. Clapp recounted that on October 25, 1832, he saw a doctor ride up to two dying men abandoned at the levee and shout, "Those men have the Asiatic cholera!"[1] Word quickly spread, and many who could flee did so. The reverend recorded that even a hardened military veteran who fought under General Jackson at the Battle of New Orleans retreated. It was "no sign of cowardice, but common prudence," the veteran told Clapp. "But here is a foe that we cannot see, with his fatal scythe mowing down hundreds in a day."[2]

Clapp remained in the city for the duration of the terrifying outbreak. "A great many bodies, with bricks and stones tied to the feet, were thrown into the river," he described.[3] When he went to the graveyard to perform funerals, he discovered "a large pile of corpses without coffins, in horizontal layers, one above the other, like corded wood."[4] Grave diggers had no choice but to indiscriminately throw the deceased into large trenches. Staff abandoned a hospital, leaving bodies to rot, which later necessitated the mayor to have the corpses tossed into a bonfire.[5] Burning tar barrels and firing cannons into the air smothered the city with smoke as officials desperately tried to break up the pestilential atmosphere. These public health measures, Clapp decried, "conspired to add a sublimity and horror to the tremendous scene."[6]

Cholera, the minister emphasized, respected neither race nor class. "Many persons, even of fortune and popularity, died in their beds without aid, unnoticed and unknown, and lay there for days unburied," he maintained.[7] He performed a wedding of a young bride "possessed of the most extraordinary beauty" and a few hours later had to officiate her funeral. She was buried still wearing her wedding dress.[8] A next-door neighbor greeted the reverend one morning, and two hours later he had died. Ironically, the neighbor had proclaimed himself healthy but wondered that the reverend had not died yet, given his constant attention to his duties.

Clapp could not explain why he survived when so many did not. He could not abide by the prescribed diet even if he wanted to because of his irregular schedule and scarcity of food in the city. He even gulped down a glass of gin at one point and exposed himself to the most dangerous conditions. "My preservation has always seemed to me like a miracle," he intimated.[9] "Let the reader imagine a close[d] room, in which are lying half a dozen bodies in the process of decay," he asked, "and he may form a faint conception of the physical horrors in which I lived, moved, and had my being continually for two weeks."[10]

What happened in New Orleans, according to a mystified Clapp, escaped the attention of people outside of the Crescent City. He asserted that in just twelve days, cholera took six thousand of the thirty-five thousand people who had remained in residence after the fortunate got out. "This is the most appalling instance of mortality known to have happened in any part of the world, ancient or modern," he exclaimed. "Yet, in all the accounts of the ravages of this enemy... published in the northern cities and Europe, its desolations in New Orleans are not even noticed."[11]

Maybe the reverend exaggerated. If as severe as he characterized, the tragedy would seem unlikely to have escaped the attention of outsiders. But maybe he told the truth. After all, what he said happened in New Orleans did not fit the narrative that people wanted to maintain about the scourge.

Cholera spread into the West from the Northeast. During the first week of July, *Vibrio* crossed Lake Erie aboard steamboats filled with 950 US soldiers destined for Illinois. They intended to join forces already there to fight against the Sauks and Mesquakies (Foxes), whose leader, Black Hawk, conducted a daring yet unsuccessful attempt to avoid expulsion from their lands. Cholera began to dispatch the soldiers before they reached Detroit and continued to do so as they rounded the Great Lakes and arrived at their destination. About one-third of the troops from the East perished from the disease, and dozens of others already in the West fell to it after contracting it from the newcomers. An estimated four hundred men in all fell to cholera.[12] The Sauks and Mesquakies had been forced to surrender by the time the infected soldiers arrived, and no evidence suggests that they or their Indigenous neighbors contracted the deadly bacteria.[13]

American towns and villages along the Great Lakes did, however. Cleveland, Ohio, saw ten victims buried in July and then a sudden flare-up in October that killed fourteen more.[14] Detroit, with just a little over two thousand residents then, had widespread infections and mortality that began after infected soldiers passed through. Town officials stopped counting early on, but residents estimated that somewhere around eighty people had died.[15]

Eventually the pathogen reached Cincinnati. Known as "the Queen of the West," the city had doubled in population over the last ten years and reached around thirty thousand by 1832.[16] Numerous steamboats tied up at its wharves every day, and countless passengers stopped to rest and resupply before heading farther down the Ohio. The pandemic did not stop the traffic, but the pathogen stayed away from Cincinnati until late September.

In the interregnum, Cincinnati's *Gazette* published a series of Dr. Daniel Drake's essays to prepare residents. The University of Pennsylvania–trained physician—the first person born west of the Appalachians to receive an MD, founder of the University of Cincinnati, and perhaps the city's most famous resident—reiterated well-known beliefs about cholera: the disease was not directly transmitted from person to person; quarantines were useless; sanitation was the best preventative measure; and "Terror has every where been found to predispose to the disease."

In two aspects, though, the doctor deviated from the norm. First, Drake supported the unorthodox animalcular theory as the most plausible explanation for the disease's propagation. Small insects or animalcules, "too small to be seen by the naked eye," seemed to the doctor to be the most likely source of the infection. These beings could float in the atmosphere, attach themselves to travelers and cargo aboard ships, lay their eggs along rivers, circumvent quarantines and sanitary cordons, and deliver the cholera-causing poison into the bodies of people in a discriminating way. The "poor and filthy" rather than "those in more comfortable circumstances" would be the very people that these insects most infested. Second, he advised the intemperate to not immediately abstain from all alcohol. The shock of sobriety to a heavy drinker's system would make them more, not less, vulnerable to the disease.[17]

Drake had publicly advocated temperance before the pandemic and in no way called for the abstemious to start drinking with cholera's arrival, but his rivals rejected his apparent softness on alcohol.[18] One anonymous physician wrote the editors of the *Gazette*, claiming "the most prominent feature of [cholera's] mission is to rid society of drunkards." He warned drinkers that "you have no other rational alternative but to change sides immediately, so that cholera can have no legal demand on you." "Physicians may tell you that an entire abstinence will be fatal to you, but I tell you . . . that you may abstain with impunity," the letter ended, with a subtle jab at Drake.[19]

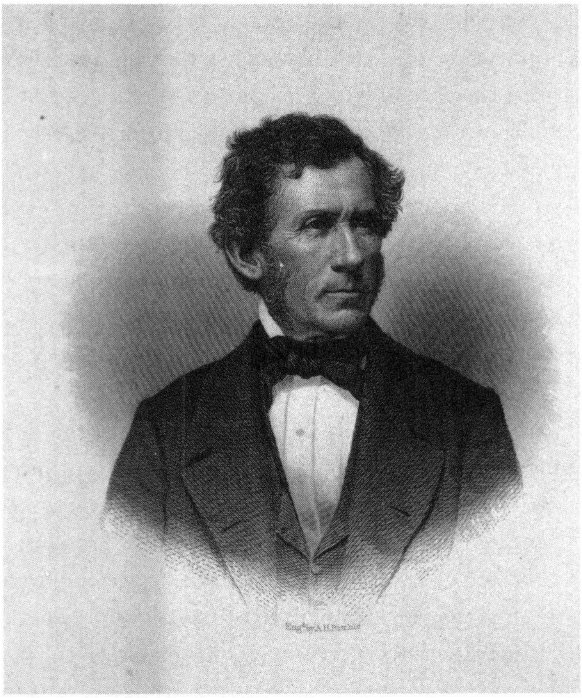

Dr. Daniel Drake. US National Library of Medicine, B07042.

As doctors argued about alcohol, *Vibrio* found its way into the Queen City. Sporadic infections started on September 30 and were followed by an explosion of cases during the second week of October.[20] Rain began to drench the city on October 6 and continued over the next four days, washing *Vibrio* from cesspools and outhouses down into the Ohio River, from which all residents of the city drew their water.[21] The official number of deaths reached its daily peak on October 19, when a reported forty-two Cincinnatians died.[22] Those deaths amounted to "an awful visitation," according to the *Cincinnati Journal*, which claimed (correctly) that per capita deaths in the city "has been much greater here... than it was during any week of its prevalence in New York."[23] "Cincinnati is filled with gloom," one resident privately bewailed. "The demon has reached us, and has let slip the dogs of death. Cholera, Cholera. The word is upon every tongue, its poison is in every constitution .... It has pervaded every section of the city."[24]

Editors of the city's newspapers tried to overcome cholera's apparent failure to discriminate.[25] "The disease has hitherto been confined to no class of our citizens," the *Journal* reported at the height of the outbreak, "although the intemperate, the careless, and the exposed have been the principal victims."

Causes of fatal cases, moreover, could be attributed to "great alarm," "an ignorance of the importance of guarding against the slightest symptoms," and "above all, the great excitement which accompanied the election."[26] Editors of the *Gazette* admitted that cholera's victims "have been selected indiscriminately from all classes" but qualified their observation that "the majority of those who have died with it here, as in other places, have been from the lower classes and many of them dissipated." They further lambasted municipal officials for not cracking down on "grog shops," decried the robust commerce in liquor, and condemned those who continued to drink.[27] The outbreak did not fizzle out until late November. At that time, the city clerk examined the available records and tallied 571 fatalities.[28]

Once *Vibrio* had become established in Cincinnati, the deadly bacteria infested steamboats traveling up and down the Ohio and infiltrated some adjacent communities in Kentucky. Louisville reported local spread and 122 fatalities, while another 36 deaths occurred in Maysville, Frankfort, Lexington, and Henderson before cold weather set in and arrested the first wave of the pandemic.[29] Among those unfortunate Kentuckians who Americans learned had perished was presidential candidate Senator Henry Clay.

Clay probably was the most shocked to learn the news. "You may hear that I am dead with the cholera," he quipped to his friend. "I assure you upon my honor it is not true."[30] He had been in Louisville to attend his son's wedding, and on his way back to Lexington, he experienced a minor illness. The Kentuckian's supporters charged Jacksonians with spreading the rumor of his demise to undermine his candidacy.[31] "You may probably hear that I caught the pestilence, and have been long since dead and buried," Clay joked to another friend. "You are authorized to contradict, most positively, such a report if you should hear it."[32]

Cholera was no laughing matter for residents along the banks of the Mississippi.[33] During the second half of October, the disease exploded in St. Louis, Missouri, a city of some 7,300 residents at the time.[34] "On the 25th and 26th," a Catholic nun decried, "our city presented nothing but a scene of dismal confusion and horror: people flying from the town, and many leaving their dearest friends to die quite alone, not daring to remain in the same house with them."[35] Editors of the *Republican* estimated that 140 St. Louisans fell to the disease by October 31 and that it had been a "consternation amongst all classes." *Vibrio* continued to infect people in the city well into November and pushed total mortality to a higher, unknown number.[36]

At the same time that St. Louis fell into the pandemic's grip, steamboats transported the pathogen to Memphis, Natchez, and Vicksburg.[37] The former two towns escaped local outbreaks, at least during this first wave, because cholera found it difficult to infiltrate their respective neighborhoods, which sat on bluffs high above the Mississippi; sewage usually drained away from the cities' wells that supplied the bulk of drinking water. Fatalities reported in both places were limited to travelers and local workers who went aboard the cholera-laden boats.[38] Several residents of Vicksburg, however, came down with the disease.[39] Residents were seen "flying from the dreadful scourge of nations" and leaving their town "almost deserted."[40] Nineteen total deaths were recorded as of November 8.[41]

As *Vibrio* wound its way down the nation's western waterways, Dr. Daniel Drake composed his analysis of what had happened. Cholera had persuaded him, perhaps more so than any other public figure, that it was not the selective predator as imagined. The Cincinnati physician concluded that cholera took fewer affluent victims in his home city because there were simply fewer of them to take: many prosperous people had left, so those in less privileged circumstances composed an even larger majority of the city's population during the outbreak.[42] Wage workers, he concluded, were not "more *predisposed* than the wealthy and more comfortable portions of the community." The survival of many people living in "filth and starvation," moreover, indicated that "this degraded class" was not particularly susceptible either. Most surprisingly, habitual consumption of alcohol appeared to have no bearing on an individual's fate. "I expect to be censured for *publishing* this fact," Drake declared. "But I am writing a *medical history*, not a *temperance address*."[43]

And the worst was yet to come. July and August passed in New Orleans without any unusual cases resembling cholera, although anxiety did not dissipate. Many believed that the pathogen's arrival was inevitable and that officials were not doing enough to prepare.[44] "It is a truly fearful calamity and the terror with which it inspires every one, is without parallel," the *Louisiana Courier*'s editors remarked about cholera's rampage through New York City. Meanwhile, the editors charged that New Orleans's streets "never were in a worse condition."[45] "We live in fear and trembling, our municipal authorities are under the influence of the most criminal apathy," one resident complained about the city's filth.[46] Residents were afraid that the foul air surrounding them made them sitting ducks for the approaching pestilential atmosphere.

It was their water that made New Orleanians so vulnerable. Natural springs did not exist in the city and were too distant to access. Wells were uncommon because the high-water table ensured that they would quickly fill with whatever ran off from the streets and yards. Some homeowners relied upon aboveground cisterns, but these were costly to build and maintain and mostly served the propertied classes. Cisterns also came with an unknown and deadly drawback. Their stagnant waters served as ideal breeding grounds for yellow fever–carrying mosquitoes, which made New Orleans especially deadly for newcomers.[47]

Most of the city's approximately fifty-seven thousand residents had little choice but to rely upon the Mississippi for hydration.[48] Public waterworks provided some of the city's drinking supply. The system involved a steam engine, which drew water by way of a pipe that extended along a pier into the river upstream from the city; the engine then pumped it into an elevated wooden reservoir in the center of the city and let gravity take it through wooden pipes to subscribers and to public hydrants on a few blocks. The water, however, thrilled no one. It supplied a silty brew that contained wastes discarded from steamboats and sewage that washed down from upstream communities.[49] Dr. Michel Halphen, a reputable physician among the city's French-speaking population, described the water as "full of organic material" and "unhealthy."[50]

If people did not get their supply from the city waterworks, they obtained it by other means. Vendors filled barrels with river water taken from the banks of the Mississippi, near where steamboats expelled their waste and where sewage trickled down from the wharves.[51] Those with the time and patience went to great lengths to try to render it into a form pleasant enough to drink. They filtered it through cloth, porous rocks, or peach pits, mixing it with alum and allowing it to settle in clay jars for hours before consumption.[52] Alum—a powder composed of aluminum salts—had some disinfecting qualities, but it was certainly not used in great enough quantities or by enough people to significantly lessen the pathogen load that New Orleanians consumed from their drinking supply. Enslaved and free laborers working in the hot and humid Louisiana weather especially did not have the time and luxury of transforming the liquid into a safer and more palatable form.

As September progressed, New Orleanians had reason to take their minds off cholera. Yellow fever cases escalated toward the end of September, reaching numbers not seen since a severe outbreak in 1822. The Crescent City's regular experience with this subtropical disease may have given some residents false confidence when considering the approach of the new pestilence. Yellow fever had regularly mowed down newcomers at an appalling rate, while leaving survivors with acquired immunity. These survivors understood that their "seasoning," or what historian Kathryn Olivarius calls "immunocapital," allowed them to stay in the pestilential city, take more risks, and accumulate more wealth from the speculative commercial world of cotton, human trafficking, and real estate. Enslaved people also went through the seasoning process, but the value of their immunity accrued to their captors, and, in the minds of white defenders of slavery, justified their perpetual bondage. Black people, it was believed, could work in the deadly environment, while whites could not. People of African descent did not have innate immunity to yellow fever, as imagined at the time and as medical scientists believed well into the twentieth century, but the perception that they did had become a key component of proslavery ideology by the 1830s.[53]

As fall advanced, then, residents who had lived in the city for years and the people they enslaved continued to go about their business, while newcomers were cautioned about pestilential dangers. "Strangers, perhaps, would act wisely," the *Courier* advised on September 29, "if they were to leave [the city] for a while."[54] Editors noted a week later, "There is not much said in the papers now about the Cholera, which seems to be on the decline every where, and appears to spread very slowly."[55] Yellow fever remained the obvious danger, and with cases continuing to be unusually high into mid-October, the *Courier* informed absentee readers that they ought to stay away a little longer.[56]

It was advice that had the fortunate, unintended consequence of lessening what would be cholera's frightful toll. The same steamboats that carried *Vibrio* to Memphis, Vicksburg, and Natchez began to arrive in New Orleans by October 21.[57] The deadly bacteria multiplied to dangerous levels around the wharf, where many people collected their daily drinking supply, and probably proliferated as well near the city waterworks' intake pipe. Infections and some deaths occurred but remained unnoticed for a couple of days. Suspicions mounted as the *Constitution* landed on the morning of October 24.[58] Word spread quickly that the vessel had lost passengers to the disease upriver, prompting the *Courier* to try to reassure a nervous public. The editors either believed the lie that the captain told or abetted it by printing his claim that only three people had died, whereas seven had, and by publishing his assertion that the deceased individuals "had not the slightest symptoms of the Cholera."[59]

On October 25, the novel malady became unmistakable and caused panic just as Reverend Clapp had indicated. One resident explained that two dying men had been thrown to the side of the street by a crowd "manifesting no feeling nor even offering to render any assistance to the dying."[60] Another observer described the dying as "two Spaniards who had lived for months in the most abject wretchedness."[61] Clapp claimed to have secured the services of two

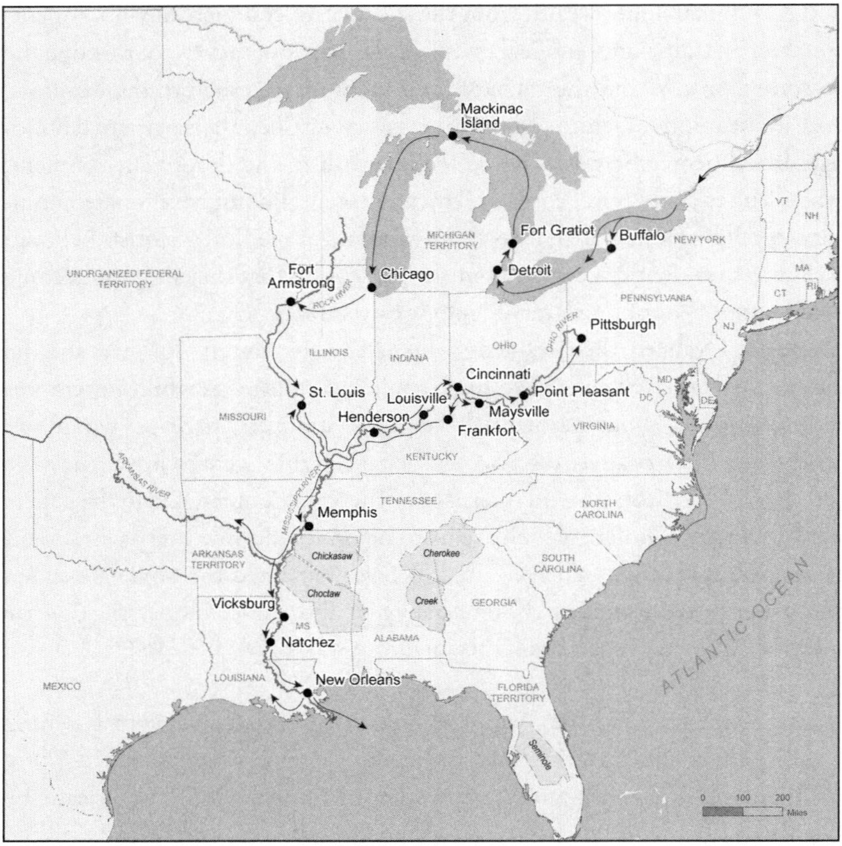

The Pandemic in the West, 1832. Map by Franchesca Rodriguez, Geospatial Center, Stony Brook University.

watchmen to cart the bodies away, not telling them that the dying men had cholera, because if they heard "that terrific word" they would have run off. The infected and discarded men passed by 11:00 a.m. that day. By the afternoon, the news had spread throughout the city.[62]

The following day, the outbreak became officially acknowledged. The board of health confirmed the disease's presence, drafted recommendations for treating the disease, called upon doctors to report cases, and requested inspections of "private hospitals in which the mayor may locate cholera patients."[63] The *Argus* was the first newspaper to deliver the bad news and did so with an indication that the disease had taken more than just a few people at the levee. "From the number of interments yesterday," the editors declared, "we are forced to conclude that the Cholera is raging with great fatality." The ongoing yellow fever outbreak had been taking an average of twenty-five lives a day since mid-September, but the one hundred burials on October 25 suggested an additional disease had entered New Orleans's notoriously deadly environment.[64]

The *Argus* as well as other newspapers broke the news with a mix of consternation, advice, and reassurance to affluent readers. "We are still induced to believe that this terrible pestilence is principally confined to the black population, and to the most exposed and imprudent classes of whites," the *Argus* explained. "We heard of but three or four cases among the better classes."[65] "Medicine, if instantly administered," the editors of the *Courier* remarked, "will in 19 cases out of 20, check the progress of the disease in people of temperate habits." More than anything, they charged, "*Fear* should not be allowed to exist. We do repeat it, banish FEAR, which is perhaps more to be dreaded than the disease itself, since it is sufficient to produce it."[66]

The *Emporium* gave a more mixed message. "The long expected scourge, the relentless ally of the king of terrors has, at length, landed and has commenced his ravages in our devoted city," the paper declared. Yet it qualified the horror with the usual description of those who should expect the worst: "We fear that our wretched blacks, whose filthy and irregular habits render them peculiarly liable to the assaults of this eccentric pest, as well as the still more culpable and reckless whites, will be sorely visited." They encouraged their readers to maintain "well regulated and systematic" habits as well "as near abstinence as possible from ardent spirits."[67]

The *Bee* proved more recalcitrant in acknowledging reality. The editors made no reference to cholera in their city until October 29, and in that day's issue, they only did so in the form of satirical suggestions. "Marvel makers and magnifiers of reports" should be locked in the graveyard; lawyers should be banished because "litigation discomposes the temper and irritates the nerves"; and "scolds, . . . speech making politicians, [and] disputatious physicians" should be confined in the insane asylum because "they promote one of the 'premonitory symptoms,' the buzzing in the ears!"[68] Finally on October 30, the editors took a somewhat serious tone, but they did so by expressing some doubt about the identity of the disease and disingenuously claiming the outbreak was coming under control.[69]

The *Bee*'s editors were hiding the terrible calamity already occurring in their city. Cases appeared in every part of New Orleans, and mortality escalated to astonishing levels within days of the *Constitution*'s landing.[70] "You cannot imagine, nor can I describe, the consternation, the terror, the agony which the pale-stricken countenance of our population betrayed," one resident wrote to a Virginia correspondent. "Such of our citizens as could afford it, left the city; some took passage up the river, some down; others fled across the lake Pontchartrain to seek consolation among the pine-groves."[71]

Dr. Halphen claimed "confusion set in" as the city became "gripped by horror."[72] "A universal panic prevailed, and business was entirely suspended," another resident reported.[73] Towns and villages along the opposite side of Lake Pontchartrain quickly overflowed with evacuees.[74]

Back in New Orleans, plans to deal with the long-awaited emergency never got off the ground. The board of health could not reach a quorum and failed to issue daily reports of cases and deaths as authorities did in other US cities.[75] Even if the body had managed to meet, physicians could not account for all of the cases and deaths and were in no position to give accurate statistics of cholera's horrible impact.[76] "We saw people from everywhere fall victim and die; there were not enough doctors to respond to all the calls," Halphen described. "Sick people were already completely filling the hospitals without any public buildings having been prepared to handle the overflow."[77]

Mayor Denis Prieur wanted advice and got none. His aldermen had either fled or were too ill or afraid to attend council meetings. His administration managed only to set tar barrels ablaze and shoot cannonballs into the air. "Perhaps there is something better to be done," he exasperatedly wrote to his council, "but I do not know what it may consist."[78] Halphen claimed, as Clapp retrospectively did, that this only made the situation worse: "Thick, black smoke darkened the dull, cloudy skies; night and day a reddish glow lit this theater of suffering, and the sight of all this shook the courage of the hardiest of people."[79]

Clapp was also correct about staff abandoning one of the hospitals, but even his recall of the event left out gory details. On November 6, citizens complained about an "insufferable odor emanating" from the hospital run by Dr. James S. McFarlane.[80] The following day, the mayor sent a committee to investigate, and they found a ghastly scene: corpses in a state of putrefaction after lying unattended for several days, survivors being left unfed and uncared for, and vessels overflowing with excrement. One man barely clung to life as he lay across the body a dead man; vermin or dogs had found one corpse, torn into its belly, and left entrails strewn along the floor; and in the hospital yard lay "the dead body of a negro, off which a fowl was picking worms." The committee declared to the mayor, "it is impossible for one to form an idea of what they have witnessed" and advised that the twelve to fourteen corpses be immediately burned.[81]

McFarlane responded to the committee's report defensively but did not deny what they had found. He had contracted the disease soon after it arrived, as did many of his thirteen "able bodied assistants." The physicians who took over for him could not find anyone to help at any cost. Meanwhile, the bodies poured in, and the only healthy people left were McFarlane's enslaved people.

They gave their lives in the care of others, but the doctor complained that he lost $5,000 worth of "property." The dead were stacked up in the hospital, McFarlane explained, because coffins were in short supply and the graveyards could not take any more corpses.[82]

The horror was not restricted to the hospital. Several New Orleanians described the scenes at the cemeteries in the same morbid terms that Clapp did.[83] "Cabinet makers & Carpenters cannot make the Coffins . . . fast enough for the demand," exclaimed M. M. Inskeep to his sister. Inskeep, writing just four days after the first cases were identified, reported that "dozens" of caskets stacked up and remained unburied for lack of graves. "It is awful my dear Sister and no one that has not been amidst such scenes can have any idea of it," he explained.[84] Thomas Overton Moore, later elected Louisiana's governor, commented that so many dead bodies piled up that workers used hooks to "drag them out and throw them in drays and tumble them in ditches prepared for their reception without either shroud or coffin." Overton added that "hundreds of bodies were buried so shallow that the first rain exposed them."[85] Dr. Halphen remarked the "chaos was so great that graves were dug anywhere and that often marked graves were dug up to make way for new bodies, and the old and new were reburied together."[86]

Many did not make it to formal burial grounds. Halphen observed corpses being thrown into the Mississippi, as did Clapp.[87] Jean Boze, an overseer who remained in the city to manage his employer's estate, remarked that "many Irish, Americans, and others have been buried in the cypress trees of the suburbs and in the courtyards, unable to find any cabriolet to transport them to the cemeteries."[88]

As Boze's comment indicated, Irish immigrants suffered high death tolls and unceremonious burials in New Orleans, just as they did in eastern cities and work zones. Hundreds worked on the New Basin Canal in 1832, and it was among them that Mayor Prieur identified the first cases.[89] Construction ground to a halt and did not resume until well into 1833 for lack of labor.[90] One citizen recalled many decades later that cholera "almost exterminated" the Irish workers and that along the canal "are buried hundreds, if not thousands, of the unfortunates."[91] At some point, the canal workers' tragic experience with *Vibrio* in 1832 and then during the next summer became memorialized in verse:

> Ten thousand Micks
> They Swung their picks
> To dig th' New Canawl, But the choleray was stroner'n they
> And twice it killed them awl.[92]

While barely acknowledged at the time, Irish fatalities have received more recent attention. In 1990, New Orleans's Irish Cultural Society erected a Celtic cross standing seven feet tall on Pontchartrain Boulevard, near the canal that had long since become obsolete and filled in. In 2023, with funds from the state of Louisiana, the Irish government, and other sources, the Louisiana Hibernian Charity dedicated a park around the cross.[93]

Cholera, of course, did not restrict itself to New Orleans's free and enslaved workers. The outbreak occurred so rapidly and so thoroughly in the city that a substantial number of affluent and well-known people perished.[94] Inskeep told his sister that yellow fever "has never been known so fatal as the Cholera" and that "a number of respectable persons have also fell victims in a few hours."[95] Catherine Dart originally thought it would just take "imprudent and intemperate" whites along with "poor blacks."[96] The novel malady made her change her mind. She and her husband stayed in a residence in which "people were dying around us...in our sight & hearing...day & night." "People of all ages, sex & condition fell, like grass in the meadow before the scythe," she described.[97] Carl Kohn stayed away from the city during the calamity, and upon returning, he found "that an unusual number of persons are in black, indeed every third Lady one meets in the streets is in mourning."[98]

Jean Boze found efforts to depict cholera as a discriminating killer insulting. "I assure you that an alarming scourge has brought trouble and desolation among the families of this city," he wrote to his absentee employer.[99] He consequently expressed his frustration with initial efforts by news editors to describe the many who passed away as filthy and dissolute. "Has anyone ever published anything more contrary to the truth," Boze privately complained. "Have we not lost many of our compatriots, of both sexes, who were all sick and still clean and proper?"[100]

After one week of trying to make the outbreak conform to expectations, the press generally gave up. "The eighth 'vial of the wrath of God' seems to have been poured over our ill-starred community," the *Emporium* proclaimed on November 1. The "appalling mortality," the paper told readers, "stands confessed in all its horrors"[101] The following day's *Courier* decried that cholera coming upon the heels of yellow fever constituted "a *compound of all the evils which hell may contain*." The scourge found "no obstacle to check its destructive course. The rich and the poor, the temperate and the intemperate, equally fall victims to its baneful influence."[102] The *Bee* eschewed such colorful language, but its editors no longer explained away the dead as the usual suspects and had to shift to a three-day-a-week publishing schedule because illness and death among their staff curtailed daily delivery.[103]

A number of shocking fatalities indeed occurred, just as Clapp suggested. Thomas Farrar McCaleb, Louisiana's thirty-five-year-old secretary of state, died in his bed unattended and was not found for a couple of days.[104] "His friends and society are by his untimely death deprived of an object of their dearest affection," his obituary proclaimed, "and his country mourns at his tomb the premature loss of talents and usefulness zealously devoted to her service." John Penrice, owner and editor of the *Louisiana Advertiser*, published in his paper a condemnation of the city's doctors for failing to turn in daily reports. He exclaimed, "there is not among the slave states a more scurvy set of white men than they are!" "Death has opened his 'workshop' amongst us; and the mortality has no ways decreased," he added.[105] The thirty-seven-year-old Penrice was then cut down by cholera at midnight.[106]

The *Emporium* made the most insistent case that the scourge did not follow the script, at least in the Crescent City. "We, most unqualifiedly, protest against the sweeping remark," the editors declared, "that 'the mortality has visited only the filthy and intemperate!' Hundreds of estimable members of society... have been consigned to the tomb." The editors had seen enough of the disease's power to not belittle it or dismiss the suffering of its victims. "Never was the general levelling of man's last enemy more signally illustrated than in the visit of the cholera at New Orleans," they remarked about death's universality. "May [cholera's] effect upon the hearts of survivors be salutary and lasting."[107]

As the *Emporium* called for its readers to not forget the calamity, city officials were trying to underscore an end to the outbreak. Civic leaders associated a decline in fatalities on November 8 with a cold front that came through that day, believing it had cleared the atmosphere of its disease-causing properties.[108] The *Courier* published an estimate of "no less than 2000 deaths" occurring since the outbreak began, giving the public the only somewhat official death toll.[109] By November 17, cases had declined enough for the board of health, finally in operation long after the peak of the calamity, to declare "that cholera, as an epidemic has ceased to prevail in this city."[110] Sporadic infection and mortality continued into December, however.

New Orleanians privately relayed messages that a historic tragedy had occurred. With countless corpses entombed in private yards, thrown into the river, and buried outside the municipality, survivors understood the magnitude of the calamity to be greater than the two thousand figure that the *Courier* published. William Worthington and John McDonogh each independently reported to their respective correspondents that five thousand people had perished.[111] The calamity had "no parallel in the history of our country," Worthington remarked, and was comparable to "the plague of the fourteenth century."[112] Nathan Morse and Eliza Noel Pintard Davidson each cited in their private correspondence a death toll of six thousand.[113] Davidson's father—John Pintard of New York—relayed the number to his correspondent with a comment that, compared to New Orleans, New York City's experience of losing 3,515 from its much large population had been "light."[114]

The Reverend Clapp's recollections thus do not appear to be exaggerations, but his autobiography did mislead in one unintentional way. People outside of the Crescent City knew more about the calamity than he realized. The *Emporium*'s piece characterizing the outbreak as the "eighth 'vial of the wrath of God'" as well as the *Courier*'s reference to the ordeal as a "*compound of all the evils which hell may contain*" found their way into newspapers across the country.[115] The shocking scene discovered at the hospital received mass attention; verbatim copies of the standing committee's report and Dr. McFarlane's response were reprinted widely.[116] Multiple editors chose to publish the *Emporium*'s protest against the idea that cholera only preyed on the "filthy and intemperate" as well as the notice of John Penrice's death.[117] In addition, a New Orleanian subscriber sent a letter to the New York *Journal of Commerce* that referenced mass burials, incinerated bodies, and other scenes "too horrible to relate." After publication in the New York press, the letter appeared in journals from Virginia to Vermont and from Ohio to England.[118]

Clapp's local vantage point made him unaware how widely information from his city had spread in 1832, but it is not difficult to understand why, looking back twenty-five years later, he thought his city's experience did not get noticed. Municipal officials never issued a final report. The *Courier*'s guess of some two thousand fatalities was what most people outside of the city read as a measure of the outbreak's magnitude. Dr. Michel Halphen, in his *Memoir Sur Le Cholera-Morbus de La Nouvelle-Orleans*, the only published medical account of the event, claimed, "Never, in any country, had cholera been so horrible." The doctor put forth an estimate of six thousand cholera fatalities occurring within just twenty days. Halphen's work, though, did not come out until the summer of 1833, was only published in French, and was ignored by the Anglo-American medical establishment (table 9.1).[119]

The news that did come out of New Orleans in 1832, moreover, reached the East Coast during an inopportune time to make an impact. By the end of November, cholera cases seemed to disappear from America's largest cities, and, except for Cincinnati's iconoclastic Dr. Drake, powerful public voices had loudly declared cholera to have taken only the expected victims. That the

Table 9.1 Reported Cholera Mortality in the West, 1832

Location	Reported Deaths
Cleveland, OH	24
US Troops Mobilized for Black Hawk War	400
Detroit, Michigan Territory	80
Cincinnati, OH	571
Louisville, KY	122
Kentucky, excluding Louisville	36
St. Louis, MO	140
Vicksburg, MS	19
New Orleans, LA	6,000
Total	7,392

new pathogen had the power to ravage places in the United States as severely as it had in Europe was unwelcome news. What happened in New Orleans ought to have challenged Americans to rethink their confidence, but preconceived beliefs about the disease proved implacable and would continue to be so as the scourge refused to leave the nation.

10

"They Just Covered It Up"

CHOLERA STRIKES CHOCTAWS ON THE TRAIL OF TEARS

GRADY JOHN KNEW the truth had been buried long ago. In the 1990s, he told an interviewer that President Andrew Jackson's agents had tricked his Choctaw ancestors into signing the Treaty of Dancing Rabbit Creek. The Choctaws, according to John, believed the 1830 document to be a "peace treaty," but it turned out to be a deadly instrument of dispossession. "All of them didn't make it," John explained. The deportation of his people that occurred over the next few years led to mass death. "Dehydrated," he described. "A lot of them just couldn't go. Died." Jackson's men just "buried them along [the route]—from Greenwood [MS] to Little Rock on to Oklahoma. If archaeologists looked for it, they could... find the Choctaw burial grounds somewhere..., but they just covered it up."[1]

Major Francis W. Armstrong was among the men to whom John referred but did not name. "No man but one who was present can form any idea of the difficulties that we have encountered owing to the cholera," he wrote to the War Department on December 2, 1832. "It is true, we have been obliged to keep every thing to ourselves, and to browbeat the idea of the disease." Armstrong served as a superintendent enforcing the Treaty of Dancing Rabbit Creek and witnessed the novel malady taking the lives of many Choctaws under his direction. "Death was hourly among us," he confessed at Little Rock, "and the road lined with the sick." He had hired extra wagons to haul the incapacitated and kept those healthy enough to travel by foot moving forward, callously declaring, "fortunately they are people that will walk to the last, or I do not know how we could get on."[2]

That cholera had already taken thousands of American lives was no secret, but that Choctaws were among the fatalities was not something that Armstrong wanted known. Deaths of deported Indigenous peoples would generate bad publicity for the president's controversial Indian Removal policy.[3] Jackson had campaigned back in 1828 on the promise to allow states to extend their jurisdictions over Indigenous lands and to commit the federal government to removing Indigenous inhabitants. He advocated the plan as "not only liberal, but generous": the federal government would pay Indigenous peoples for their land, finance and organize their relocation to western territories, and protect them there from further white interference.[4]

Indigenous leaders and their white allies saw through the faux humanitarian rhetoric. Jackon's policy, they declared, sanctioned the unconstitutional actions of state governments to abrogate treaties and to nullify federal laws that obligated the national government to protect Indigenous peoples. Indigenous peoples would have no choice but to leave as they saw their sovereignty disappear and themselves becoming second-class citizens with few, if any, rights.[5] Opponents also condemned the policy as a dangerous experiment with human lives that would have dire consequences. "The constrained migration of 60,000 souls ... must be attended with much suffering," Jeremiah Evarts, a Congregationalist minister opposed to Jackson, warned in an anti-removal essay. He added that "much exposure, sickness, hunger, nakedness, either on the journey, or soon after their arrival" would necessarily result from the policy.[6]

Congress nonetheless passed and Andrew Jackson signed the Indian Removal Act in the spring of 1830. States had the green light to oppress Indigenous peoples, and Jackson's agents were empowered to pressure Indigenous leaders to sign treaties in which they gave up their land and agreed to move. The Choctaws predicted calamity, telling a Methodist missionary that immediate enactment of the policy would "force them off to suffer and to die."[7]

They were right, but Jackson never let up. As cholera swirled through North America, he continued to push Indigenous peoples to leave their homelands and tried to hide the reality they faced on what the Choctaws and other deported Indigenous nations called the Trail of Tears.[8]

In 1830, the Choctaws, a nation of 19,954 farmers and ranchers, held ten million acres that the states of Alabama and Mississippi claimed. The cotton boom drove the thirst for land, and the president sent Secretary of War John Eaton and trusted friend John Coffee to get it. According to a white trader who observed events at Dancing Rabbit Creek, Eaton and Coffee told Choctaws that "evils ... would speedily befall them" when they became "subjected to the operation of the state laws." They would have to pay taxes, serve in the state militia, and labor on public works. He further warned them, "white men . . . would come among them like flocks of blackbirds and swarms of locusts; that they and their children would become paupers and beggars; that they would be broken up and utterly destroyed as a nation." Jackson, his commissioners threatened, would do nothing to stop this. A treaty giving them land in the West in exchange for theirs in the East was the final and last offer. If they did not take it, the western land that had been promised to them would be given to other tribes. Panicked, many Choctaws signed the treaty, and the commissioners hastily left without giving them copies.[9]

The Choctaws did not know what was in store for them. The US Senate ratified the treaty on February 24, 1831. It stipulated that Choctaws who stayed could receive an allotment of land, on the condition that they become citizens of the state of Mississippi. Those who chose to leave would have to sign up for removal before the end of 1833. The treaty lightly mentioned any logistical detail, only stipulating that the federal government would secure transportation aboard wagons and "with steamboats as may be found necessary" and provide one year of subsistence in Indian Territory. The journey would also occur "under the care of discreet and careful persons, who will be kind and brotherly to them."[10] Choctaws were shocked about both the contents of the treaty and the fact that it had been ratified.[11]

White people were determined to take away the option of staying. Many Choctaw families had hoped to accept an allotment and remain, but the corrupt US agent, William Ward, refused to assign them their plots of land. Speculators filled the agent's pockets with bribes, and he opened up the yet to be evacuated property for purchase.[12]

The land rush led to the first deportation being a disaster. George Gaines, superintendent of Choctaw removal in 1831, was completely unprepared for the nearly four thousand Choctaws who wandered into Memphis and Vicksburg in the early fall to await transportation to the West. They had lost their lands, had planted no crops, had seen their livestock disappear due to forced sales or thefts, and arrived destitute. Gaines had to spend more money than he was authorized and even used his own funds to ameliorate the calamity. Still, he could not immediately find enough boats, leaving thousands of hungry and cold Choctaws stranded well into November.

The steamboats that Gaines eventually managed to hire were in wretched condition. One removal agent, Captain William Colquhoun, found the vessels "disgusting" because "human beings under no control or regularity" had to relieve themselves wherever they could.[13] Many sickened aboard the vessels, and some died. The water levels of the Arkansas and Red Rivers were not high enough for the boats to reach Indian Territory, and roads had not been constructed to get them there. Food was scarce along the way, a particularly severe winter set in, and dozens perished from exposure, pneumonia, and malnourishment. When they arrived at their destinations, federal agents did not have food available, and when they did acquire it, it quickly ran out. By June 1832, the US agent at Fort Gibson offered to satiate their hunger with spoiled and condemned barrels of pork. Malaria and typhoid also began to set in as the newcomers struggled to find well-drained spots to build homes and healthy drinking sources. The first removal's total fatalities cannot be known.[14]

The deadly fiasco did not lead to any apparent second thoughts on the part of Jackson and his administration. The president pressed his agents to make treaties with all Indigenous nations who remained in the East, including the Choctaw's northern neighbors, the Chickasaws. "I hope the Chickasaws, will be provided for west...," he privately remarked to one of his supporters, "we will get clear of all Indians in Mississippi, and have a white population in their stead."[15] Meanwhile, Jackson's new secretary of war, Lewis Cass, and the army's commissary general for subsistence, George Gibson, who oversaw removal operations, implemented a set of regulations to control costs and expedite departures. To this end, Cass and Gibson dismissed the supposedly spendthrift civilian agent Gaines and appointed Jacksonian loyalists to superintend. Captain William Armstrong was to oversee operations on the east side of the Mississippi, and his brother Major Francis Armstrong was in charge on the west side.[16]

Choctaw leader Peter Pitchlynn tried to have some say in how the planned removal for fall 1832 would occur. He had escorted a party of his people to the West during the previous winter and had seen the deadly consequences of packing too many people aboard steamboats and then forcing survivors to walk the final leg of the journey.[17] "At the time the treaty was made our understanding... was that we should be removed to our new country in the same comfortable manner as the whites do in moving from one country to another," Pitchlynn wrote to Lewis Cass. "There are many amongst us who are young and many who are old and infirm, none of whom can walk, and they have no horses." Pitchlynn reminded Cass that the United States and not the Choctaws benefited from the deportations. "The privation of a whole nation... are all calculated to imbitter the human heart," he declared. "These can be softened by a generous fulfilment of the Treaty."[18]

The Jackson administration gave the Choctaws no indication that removal would be conducted on more generous terms. The War Department responded to Pitchlynn's letter curtly in late July. The Choctaw leader was

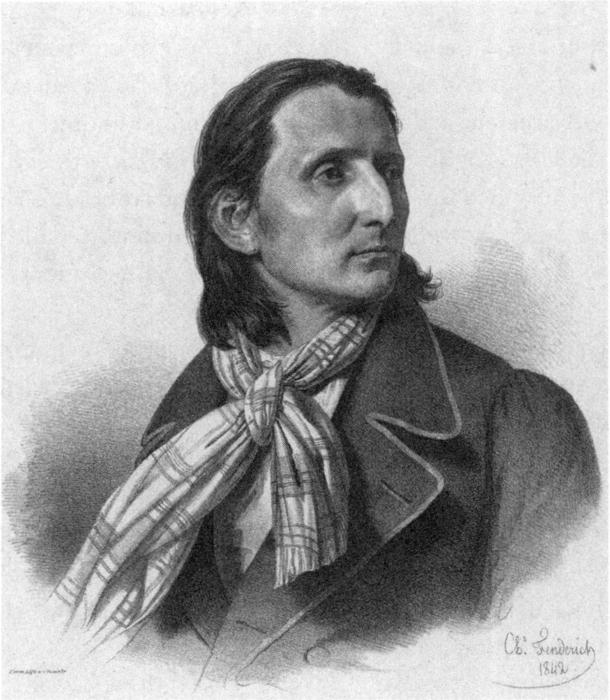

Peter Pitchlynn. Lithograph by Charles Fenderich, 1842. National Portrait Gallery, Smithsonian Institution, NPG.72.64.

informed that the Armstrongs would be in charge and that they "will together carry into effect all the provisions of the treaty in a spirit of kindness and liberality."[19]

The brothers arrived in Mississippi late in the summer, knowing that they were racing against a deadly disease. "We are making every effort to cross the Mississippi as early as possible," William Armstrong informed Gibson. "If the cholera should reach the western country, doubtless it will be at Memphis and Vicksburg."[20]

They planned for several thousand Choctaws to be on the move in October. Indigenous peoples who preferred to make their own arrangements and travel without direct government supervision could do so, but they would only get a commutation payment of thirteen dollars after they arrived in their new homeland.[21] The Armstrongs discouraged commutation and thought only the wealthiest would take this option—the few Choctaws who enslaved African Americans and had substantial numbers of horses, oxen, and wagons to use.[22] Around one thousand people would set out on their own that fall, however, exceeding their expectations.[23]

The vast majority of Choctaws did not have the means to go it alone. The Armstrongs planned on followers of Chief David Folsom to gather at Memphis and followers of chiefs Joel Nail, Nitakechi, and Greenwood LeFlore to meet up at Vicksburg.[24] Folsom's people would have the option of being ferried across the Mississippi and traveling by land to a place on the White River known as Rock Roe, or they could take steamboats down the Mississippi and then ascend the White all the way to the rendezvous point. The Vicksburg groups would have to board steamboats and ascend the Mississippi and White rivers to the staging location. From Rock Roe, Choctaws would be sent overland in staggered parties of about one thousand each, with eight provisioning stations established over the more than two hundred miles to Indian Territory.[25] If all went well, the Choctaws would arrive in Indian Territory by early December.

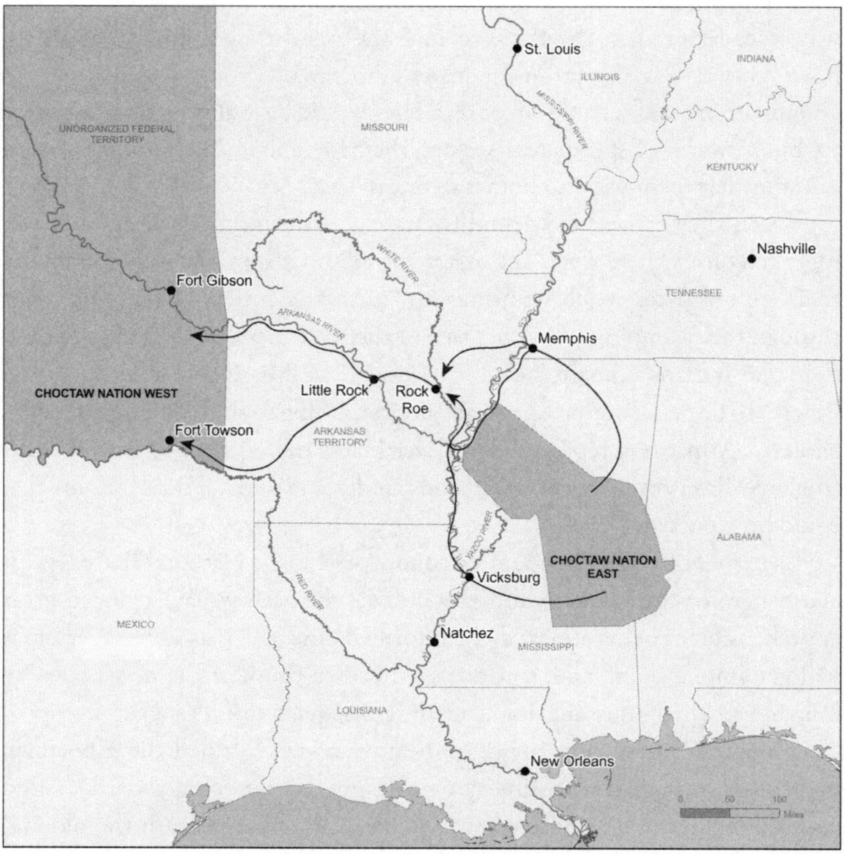

Choctaw Removals, 1832. Map by Franchesca Rodriguez, Geospatial Center, Stony Brook University.

All did not go well. *Vibrio*-infested steamboats began arriving in Memphis and Vicksburg and dropping off corpses and infected passengers before the Choctaws got there. "It now becomes my duty to apprize you of what we have a right to expect," Francis Armstrong informed Gibson. "Should we escape all will be well, but I confess I fear that we are to encounter the cholera with our Indians." He ominously added, "Nothing but the cholera will prevent our giving a satisfactory account to the department of the duties we are engaged in."[26]

Choctaw departures from Memphis began under the worst of circumstances. On October 23, Folsom's people were within eighty-two miles of the Mississippi River. "The Indians have understood the cholera is in Memphis and are much alarmed," William Armstrong reported. "I hope it is not so, for I fear it would nearly disperse the Indians."[27] The news likely contributed to many turning back and refusing to go; the 2,700 of Folsom's people on their way were fewer than the three to four thousand they estimated. Staying, however, was not an option for many Choctaws. Given a viable choice to remain during that terrible fall of 1832, they would have almost certainly done so, but a swarm of speculators seeking their fortune in the booming cotton economy left them with no homes to return to.

When they arrived in Memphis, Francis Armstrong met them and was eager to convey them west. The major vowed to Gibson that his brother and their subordinates would continue to "push the Indians from this point through the swamp" on the other side of the river and send "the baggage and the lame Indians" aboard steamboats down the Mississippi for the White River. "To be plain, our prospects are gloomy, owing to the breaking out of the cholera," Armstrong reported. He nevertheless touted his and his brother's frugality. "Everything goes on well and rapidly, and with all the economy that could be expected."[28]

Lieutenant J. A. Phillips painted a more pessimistic picture. "There is great alarm here of the cholera; and the Indians themselves have evinced great apprehension of being attacked," he informed Gibson. "I am almost certain it will get among them, and, if it does, I dread to think of the destruction of human life which must inevitably be the consequence of its appearance."[29]

Climbing aboard notoriously unhealthy vessels terrified the Choctaws, even more so with the possibility of a deadly disease being aboard. "I find much difficulty in getting even the women and children, with the old and infirm, to take the steamboat," William Armstrong observed.[30] In the end, Armstrong let the Choctaws decide for themselves, later explaining, "in these *cholera times*, I felt unwilling to coerce them, but left it to their own choice."[31] Those who made the "choice" to stick with water travel were those least able to travel on foot: children, the sick, and the elderly. Armstrong estimated that about one thousand chose the water route, with a group embarking on the *Reindeer* on November 2 and another leaving soon after aboard the *Archimedes*. Some 1,700 crossed over the Mississippi and took their chances traveling through the rain-swollen swamps of eastern Arkansas.[32]

The *Reindeer* carried cholera to the White River. Major A. S. Langham, the assistant superintendent in charge at Rock Roe, greeted the vessel on the fifth and interviewed Dr. Fulton and Dr. Rayburn, whom Armstrong hired to attend the travelers. They reported that a terrible illness struck on the second day of the voyage and continued until they arrived. Two Choctaws perished during the three-day period. Fulton did not believe the culprit to be cholera, but Rayburn thought it was. Circumstances over the next three days after the *Reindeer*'s arrival convinced Langham that Rayburn was right. Fifty-three cases and eight deaths occurred among the Choctaws encamped at Rock Roe.

Major Langham had an emergency on his hand. "The disease has caused so great and so general a panic," he proclaimed, "that the consequences cannot be calculated." Seventeen teamsters employed to transport Indigenous peoples across Arkansas fled, taking three of the wagons with them. Waggoneers who were supposed to arrive refused to come. Unable to stop the departures, the major agreed that the drivers could evacuate to nearby neighborhoods until the situation improved. "Until this calamity," he lamented, "the agents of Government had cause to congratulate themselves that their arrangements had been fortunate as well as judicious."[33]

Folsom's Choctaws who traveled by land would not escape the scourge. After pushing the deportees through swamps and mud for several days, William Armstrong stopped on November 10 some fifty miles from Rock Roe to update Gibson. "We have . . . had seven deaths since we left Memphis, which is in part pronounced cholera," he informed his superior. He refused to believe that they had a case of genuine cholera among them and instead blamed "severe exposure" because they had traveled for thirty miles in water "from knee to waist deep."[34] The captain, of course, could have been correct; it is not hard to imagine that the hardships of traveling took a toll without any assistance from *Vibrio*. Still, he knew that cholera stood in their way. Travelers informed him that the scourge raged at Rock Roe. "I fear we are to have a serious time in getting on if we escape here," he informed Gibson.[35]

Captain Armstrong was correct. Four days later, the land travelers began to arrive. If they did not have cholera with them as they traveled, they certainly picked it up at the rendezvous. One removal agent, who crossed paths with the party, said flatly, "they suffered dreadfully with the Cholera."[36] Francis Armstrong described the overland deportees from Memphis as being "sorely handled with sickness" and experiencing "very many deaths."[37]

Choctaws collecting at Vicksburg also faced an epidemiological nightmare. White residents fleeing the Mississippi town crossed paths with deportees from Chief LeFlore's district. Lieutenant W. R. Montgomery and Captain Samuel T. Cross steered the party to a destination two miles above the cholera-ridden place, warned Choctaws to stay out of city, and requested residents to stay away from the Indigenous peoples. "These precautions were not, however, sufficient to prevent communications," Montgomery admitted. Forty or fifty Choctaws developed symptoms, with the first person attacked dying. The lieutenant hired a local doctor, bought medicines, and constructed a tent to serve as a hospital.[38]

Francis Armstrong, who had been in Memphis until October 28, arrived in Vicksburg on October 31 and found his plans in trouble. LeFlore's Choctaws were supposed to number some 2,500, but Montgomery only had 617. Major Armstrong blamed Indigenous leaders for holding back their people, insinuating that they did so to skim off some of the commutation money that the federal government would pay individuals to remove themselves. He gave little thought to the possibility that Choctaws wanted to protect themselves from what was unfolding before his very eyes. "The cholera is actually in our camp," Major Armstrong informed Gibson, "and all through the country, at all the landings and towns even in the rear of this." He fretted, "we must go ahead, for in this matter we cannot stop to *look around*."[39]

Armstrong rushed the cholera-infected Choctaws aboard the *Heliopolis* and *Tom Yeatman*. He and Lieutenant Montgomery traveled along with the deportees to the mouth of the White River, where they disembarked and headed back to Vicksburg to oversee further operations. They left Captain Cross in charge, and as they churned up the White River, cholera became more widespread and deadly on the steamboats. Montgomery, in his report to Gibson, attributed this to "a sudden change in the weather," although everyone involved in the sordid process knew that the Choctaws had been packed on vessels under the worst of hygienic conditions. Rock Roe offered no respite. Illness and mortality continued as they encamped there before making their way west.[40]

Choctaws from Nail's and Nitakechi's districts remained out of the cholera cauldron, at least until the second week of November. Captain William

Colquhoun and Lieutenant J. P. Simonton had a difficult time gathering up 1,908 people and getting them across the Pearl River.[41] Soon after, they learned that "the Cholera was raging with its usual violence in Vicksburg and its vicinity." Colquhoun consequently steered the people in the direction of a low bluff on the Yazoo River above the city to avoid the disease. Simonton thought the decision foolish because the new location did not have food ready for the people and steamboats could not reach them there.[42]

The decision did not sit well with Francis Armstrong. He thought Nail's and Nitakechi's Choctaws should have been at the pickup location on the Mississippi by October 31. When he did not find them there, he ordered Colquhoun to make haste and get them to the river landing. The captain complied, but Armstrong stewed with anger because the delay of several days added more expenses.[43] Along the way, 109 Choctaws disappeared, presumably running away in fear of a deadly disease that awaited them.

They were right to be afraid. Francis Armstrong had the same cholera-ridden steamboats waiting for them that had done the morbid work of Indian Removal over the previous two weeks. On the twelfth and thirteenth of November, Armstrong sent the remaining 1,799 Choctaws up the Mississippi.[44] The deported certainly faced horrors that exceeded the federal agents' vague and cryptic references. "On the way up the Mississippi, the cholera broke out among these Indians," Lieutenant Montgomery wrote.[45] "I hope our difficulties are nearly over," Armstrong reported to Gibson after the final boat arrived on November 21, "and, although we have suffered from the cholera, the mortality in this party has not been great, and I now consider them as healthy." The major did complain of expenses being too high, "owing to the influence of cholera" and consequent reluctance of residents along the shores of the Mississippi and White rivers to sell them supplies. He admitted that local residents "had cause of alarm" because steamboats, in general, had been landing and burying deceased passengers.[46]

The stressful situation of seeing such misery and death under Armstrong's command got the better of Captain Colquhoun. He constantly argued with Francis Armstrong and eventually fired a pistol at him. The bullet grazed the major's skull, but he remained fit enough to serve out his removal duties.

Circumstances are not entirely clear, but even in his own account, Major Armstrong did not come across as an agent of a humane policy. Colquhoun, according to Armstrong's report to Cass, prevailed upon Chief Nitakechi "to insist" that the government disperse blankets to his people aboard the steamboats for Rock Roe. Armstrong claimed he could only make the distribution once they completed their journey to Indian Territory. Yet as the steamboats advanced toward their destination, and with "the cholera then pressing hard on us with difficulty," Colquhoun approached Armstrong aboard the *Heliopolis* and demanded that the Choctaws get their blankets. The allegedly drunk captain charged the major "with being a tyrant & cruel" and fired the glancing shot. Armstrong condemned Colquhoun's actions as "a cold blooded attempt to murder" and "outrageous in favor of the *poor Indians*."[47]

Colquhoun did not make much of a coherent defense, but he did include in his journal a charge that nobody seemed to deny. When the steamboats stopped to get wood, Armstrong "kept a fellow to beat [the Choctaws] back from the shore where propriety & necessity urged them to repair."[48] In other words, the major kept cholera's presence hidden by forcing Choctaws who hoped to relieve themselves in a more private manner to remain on the boats with their common and disgusting toilets. In the end, the War Department kept the affair quiet. No trial was held, and both Colquhoun and Armstrong remained employed in Indian Removal.

Choctaws continued to battle the dreaded disease as federal agents pushed them out of Rock Roe and across Arkansas. Captain J. A. Phillips, for example, left the White River rendezvous on November 13 with eight hundred from David Folsom's district and did not shake the scourge for another eleven days.[49] Six children, two elderly persons, and a woman—the very people who Jackson's opponents warned would be sacrificed by the Indian Removal policy—died before they reached their destination.[50] Captain Samuel T. Cross pushed LeFlore's people west only two days after arriving at the White River rendezvous and recorded fifteen more fatalities among them before they reached their new homeland.[51] J. P. Simonton departed Rock Roe on November 22 with some 1,800 of Nail's and Nitikechi's people. "The Cholera which had been raging in our own camp for some time past, now raged with increased violence," he recorded two days out, adding, "the woods are filled with the graves of its victims."[52]

Mourning Choctaws arrived in Indian Territory after experiencing unimaginable trauma, yet removal agents revealed an astonishing level of callousness and self-congratulation in the records they produced. When Folsom's people arrived and met friends and kinsmen who had been deported the previous year, Phillips could only remark to Gibson, "It was a night of great joy & rejoicing."[53] Cross said nothing about the terrible voyage from Vicksburg, bragged about his management, and sugarcoated the entire experience. The Choctaws, he claimed, "did not lose one day the whole route, performing their daily march with much cheerfulness, and arrived in their new country in good spirits."[54] Simonton chastised the Choctaws for being lazy. "So perfectly inefficient are they," he recorded, "that on one occasion my assistant Mr. Oury, and myself were obliged to get off our horses and put a man into a cart, who was in the last stage of the Cholera." He wrote that fifty Choctaws stood by and would not assist. "Having received assistance once, they would not bury their own dead afterward without asking for help," he complained.[55]

That Choctaws lost hundreds of lives during the fall 1832 removal and that cholera caused the bulk of those deaths cannot be denied. Just how many fatalities occurred cannot be known, however. One missionary claimed that altogether cholera "cut off about 200 of them" but that "some accounts say more."[56] A higher count was probably correct. Federal agents had enrolled 5,317 Choctaws in the East and approximately another 1,000 took the commutation option and moved themselves. Of these 6,317 deportees, federal agents counted only 5,538 arriving.[57] The difference of 779, to be sure, cannot be entirely attributed to fatalities on the trail. Some Choctaws turned back after learning cholera was in Memphis and Vicksburg. Deaths from causes other than cholera also occurred. Nevertheless, it seems safe to conclude that the scourge took around seven hundred Choctaws, or 11 percent of those being deported, a higher proportional loss than what New York, Philadelphia, and Baltimore experienced.

The Choctaws need not have had any experience with the disease. They would have been safe had they been allowed to stay in their homeland. Roughly six thousand of their kinsmen escaped cholera because they remained in the East, biding their time until Jackson's agents would try again to force them to leave during the next year's removals.

Indigenous deaths did not remain as much of a secret as Francis Armstrong wanted them to be, but he had help from powerful people covering up the full scope of the tragedy. Editors of Little Rock's two newspapers, the *Weekly Gazette* and *Times and Advocate*, for example, treated the first whiff that something terrible was happening at Rock Roe as rumors.[58] After Little Rock's Dr. Bushrod Lee investigated and confirmed that Choctaws suffered from the novel malady, both papers reassured readers that it had not afflicted any white people. Dr. Lee's public letter dated November 16 from Rock Roe, moreover, reassured Arkansans that Choctaws suffered because they "indulged in . . . fruits, vegetables, &c" and had irritated their bowels by drinking the Mississippi's water. Even though Lee lost a patient after subjecting him to Dr. Chapman's famous treatment, he claimed "a large majority of the deaths occurred with those who from ignorance or obstinacy, refused medical aid."[59]

After Major Armstrong pushed the last groups from Rock Roe, Little Rock's papers curiously became mum about cholera's presence among the Choctaws. The *Weekly Arkansas Gazette*'s editors, likely "brow-beat" by the major, informed their readers on November 28 that they had nothing to fear. "Some alarm was excited previous to the arrival of the Emigrating Indians," they said of cholera, "but since a large portion of them have passed through, without spreading the disease, it has entirely subsided, and many now doubt whether it has ever prevailed among them to any thing like the extent that was reported."[60] One week later, the *Gazette* reported that Armstrong left the Little Rock area on December 2, after getting the last deportees across the river. "There had been considerable sickness among them, previous to reaching this place, and 19 had died since leaving Rock Roe," the editors admitted without referring to cholera. They added the previously ill were recovering "and the general health of the several parties very much improved."[61] The *Times and Advocate* merely informed its readers that the last Choctaw groups had crossed the Arkansas River.[62]

The most powerful man in the United States did his part as well to cover up the Choctaw tragedy and falsely represented cholera as having a mild impact on the nation as predicted. On December 4, 1832, Andrew Jackson delivered his Fourth Annual Address, and he could not avoid mentioning the pandemic; it had impacted the lives of too many Americans to be ignored. Yet as thousands of his fellow citizens died and as hundreds of Choctaws were marched right into the scourge's path, Old Hickory pronounced that cholera was operating just as it was expected to. "It has pleased Almighty God," he stated about cholera, "to mitigate its severity and lessen the number of its victims compared with those who have fallen in most other countries over which it has spread its terrors." Witnesses to outbreaks that took more than eighteen thousand American lives over the course of the year (table 10.1) certainly thought otherwise, especially the Choctaws. The president, however, wiped out their suffering in one sentence: "I am happy to inform you that the wise and humane policy of transferring from the eastern to the western side of the Mississippi the remnants of our aboriginal tribes, with their own consent and upon just terms, has been steadily pursued, and is approaching, I trust, its consummation."[63]

Ezekial Roebuck, his family, and their descendants knew the policy as anything but "wise and humane." Roebuck, according to family history passed down to his great-granddaughter Josephine Usray Lattimore, farmed about

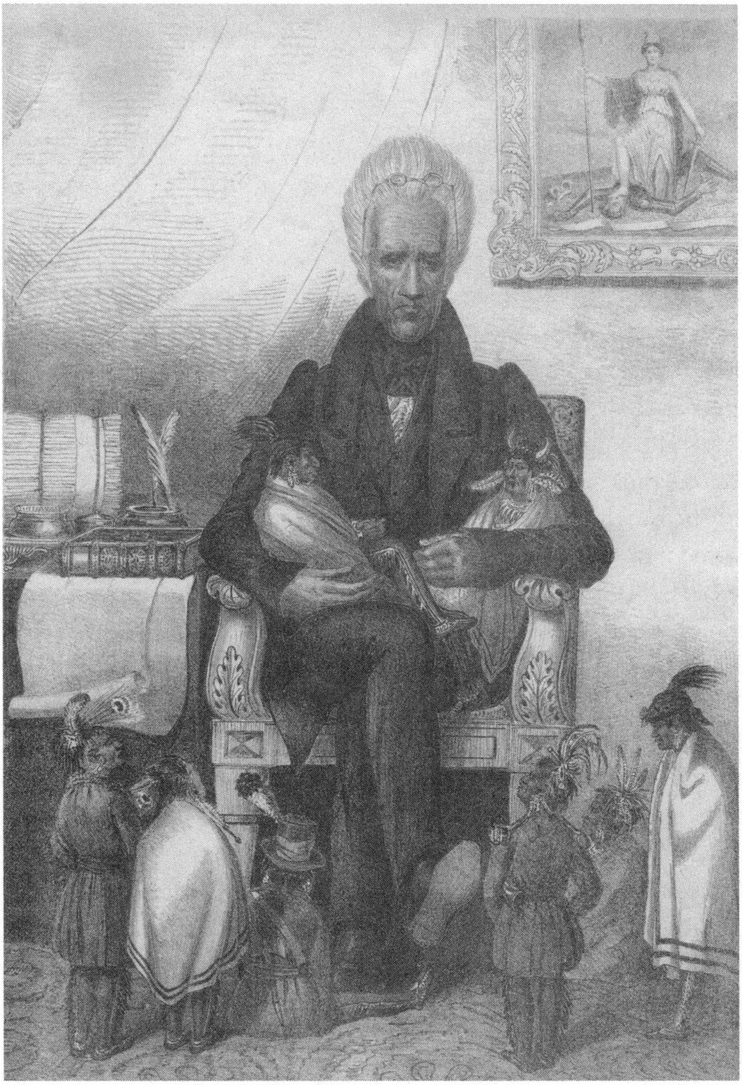

Andrew Jackson as the Great Father. Jackson is pictured here in a satirical broadside mocking his claim to care for his "Indian children." William L. Clements Library Image Bank. William L. Clements Library, University of Michigan Library.

eighteen acres in the Pearl River Valley, earned respectable income with his apiary, and earned the nickname "Honey King." In fall of 1832, he, his wife Elsie, their twelve- and ten-year-old sons, and an infant daughter were forced from their prosperous Mississippi home, gathered at Memphis, and boarded one of the steamboats that the Armstrongs had contracted for use. They sang a farewell song to "Nunialchwayah," or the "land we love so dear," as they

Table 10.1 First Wave, 1832

Location	Reported Deaths
The Northeast US from table 5.1	7,081
The Upper South from table 8.1	2,841
The West from table 9.1	7,392
Choctaws	700
Total	18,014

departed.[64] Rain, cold temperatures, and illness plagued their journey across Arkansas. "Many were weak and broken-hearted, and as night came there were new graves dug beside the way," Lattimore learned.[65]

Among those who suffered were Lattimore's ancestors. While encamped, waiting before the Ouachita River crossing, her great-grandfather became ill and could not stand. A wagon driver said, "I will have to stop and put him out as we can't afford to have any one with the Cholera along." Elsie refused to abandon her husband, and the family stayed behind.[66] She "begged" the driver not to leave them without supplies, and he "grudgingly" gave them four blankets and one day's worth of food before he left.[67] They then spent an anxious night in which they feared wolves or panthers might attack them. The next morning, Roebuck continued to deteriorate but prayed "that his little family might be spared from the dreaded disease."[68] He passed at sunset. The boys and their mother dug a deep grave, packed rocks atop of it, and marked the trees around the site so they could find it when they wished to visit.

The Roebucks still had a long journey ahead of them. The day after her great-grandfather's passing, Lattimore learned, "the brave mother with her three children bade farewell to the Honey King's grave, by the roadside of the Trail of Tears."[69] They swam across the Ouachita, walked the entire way to Indian Territory, and subsisted on honey, flour, and whatever roots and berries they could find along their route. "The Honey King's prayers were answered," his great-granddaughter recited: "not a one of them took the cholera." In their new homeland, relatives fetched them from a trading post on the Red River and helped them recover from the traumatic ordeal.[70] Today, Roebuck descendants are counted among some 220,000 members of the sovereign Choctaw Nation of Oklahoma.

If Andrew Jackson had had his way, Lattimore's story of the Trail of Tears would not represent how Indian Removal would be remembered. "The experiment which has been recently made has so far proved successful," the president boasted in his annual message of 1833. "The emigrants generally are represented to be prosperous and contented."[71] When his agents tried to remove the remaining Choctaws that year, however, few agreed to go on the dangerous journey to a place that the Pitchlynn family called "a Land of Death."[72] The rest fled into "the swamps & the settlements."[73]

Grady John's ancestors were among them. Today, their descendants compose the Mississippi Band of Choctaws, a sovereign Indigenous nation of some ten thousand members. The Choctaws' story—one that John correctly knew to be shaped by a deadly disease and injustice—could not be covered up, not even by the most powerful voice in the United States.

11

Isaac Franklin's Dark Deeds

TRAFFICKING ENSLAVED PEOPLE INTO THE HOT ZONE

ISAAC FRANKLIN SPECULATED in Black lives. He had been purchasing enslaved people in the Upper South since the early 1800s, trafficking them to the Lower Mississippi Valley, and selling them to labor-hungry white planters. With every shipment, he gambled. He hoped that proceeds from his sales would more than cover his purchase costs as well as food, clothing, and transportation expenses. Franklin won his bets more often than not. By 1832, he, along with his partners John Armfield and Rice Ballard, oversaw the nation's most extensive slave-dealing firm.

Risks were always part of Franklin, Armfield, and Co.'s sordid business. By the time their human cargo reached its destination, demand might have fallen due to a momentary downturn in cotton prices, and their sales might not cover expenses. Captives also could be so ill or injured during the grueling journey that would-be buyers refused to pay the marked-up prices, or an occasional death of one or more trafficked people might wipe out hundreds of dollars of profits. The company factored these risks into its business model and routinely reaped substantially more gains than losses from commodified bodies.

Human trafficking from the Upper to the Lower South was, in fact, one of the United States' largest commercial enterprises in the 1830s. Enslavers moved an average of more than thirty thousand Black people across state lines per year. On average, every three and a half minutes, a human being was sold somewhere in the nation. A young enslaved person in the Upper South, according to historian Joshua Rothman, "faced a roughly one-in-three chance of being taken into the slave trade." Professional dealers dominated the business, being responsible for 60 to 70 percent of interstate trafficking.[1]

Even cholera did not deter Franklin, Armfield, and Co. from gambling the lives it robbed from Black people. As the pandemic swept the Upper South, ravaged the Lower Mississippi Valley, and resurged in 1833, Armfield and Ballard bought hundreds of captives from enslavers in Virginia, Maryland, and the District of Columbia and sent them by both land and sea to Isaac Franklin's trading house in Natchez, Mississippi.

Cholera posed a threat to enslaved people at every stage of their horrifying journeys. African Americans were ripped from friends and family members; they were forced to travel along routes that *Vibrio* increasingly saturated; and they arrived in the Lower Mississippi Valley as it became the hottest of the disease's hot zones. Isaac Franklin, nonetheless, continued in the morbid yet highly profitable enterprise during the deadly times and resorted to clandestine and scandalous activities to hide his role in enhancing the pandemic's terrible impact.

By the time cholera arrived, Black people had long lived in constant fear, especially of being sold and sent far away. John Boggs, for example, witnessed the day-to-day trauma that trafficking produced. Born enslaved in Maryland in 1803, Boggs believed that his disfigurement from a severe reaction to poison oak and the loss of one of his fingers kept him from being sent to the Deep South. "I would have been in a cotton-field forty years ago if it hadn't been for that," he recalled after escaping to freedom in the 1850s. "That is what our people dread the most.... When a man goes out in the morning, he may have a wife and a parcel of children, and maybe when he comes back at night, he will find nobody who will tell him anything about them." Women who came in from the fields may have found their children sold off, and if they complained, they "would be whipped or knocked and slashed about." Boggs's first master, William Merrick, impregnated slave women he raped and even sold his own children, a practice that Isaac Franklin and many other enslavers engaged in as well.[2]

J. W. Lindsay conveyed an account similar to Boggs's. Born a free person of color in the District of Columbia, Lindsay was kidnapped as a child and wound up in Louisville. Before he ultimately ran away, he saw steamboats arrive with dealers picking up captives for transportation to the Deep South. "Sometimes a young girl would come, looking like she might be 16 or 17, with a little bundle, & tears streaming, or a young man, about the same age," he recalled. "Old gray-headed fathers & mothers had come there to bid their children a long and last farewell." He remembered, "One man ran up the wheel house, and put his head into a window, to see his wife, perhaps, and one of the keepers took him by the shoulders and flung them back." Lindsay claimed the experience was "the most horrible scene I ever saw in my life.

Such sighing, such groaning, such lamentation! Well, they groaned with groanings that cannot be uttered."[3]

The trauma continued aboard filthy steamboats that provided ideal breeding grounds for germs. William Wells Brown, after escaping enslavement, recalled his experience working for his master aboard a vessel that plied the Mississippi with captives for sale. Dealers knew that the frequent stops that the steamboats made for wood and water provided opportunities to flee, and they tried to minimize those opportunities. "There was on the boat a large room on the lower deck, in which the slaves were kept, men and women, promiscuously—all chained two and two, and a strict watch kept that they did not get loose," Brown recalled. "It was almost impossible to keep that part of the boat clean." During Brown's experience only one captive was ever lost. An unchained woman "who had been taken from her husband and children, and having no desire to live without them, in the agony of her soul jumped overboard, and drowned herself."[4]

Traveling overland also subjected captives to terrible epidemiological conditions. Drivers tied dozens of men, women, and children closely together with ropes and bounded men even more securely with iron shackles around their wrists. The cheapest food available was provided to the captives in just enough quantities to keep them alive and moving forward. Streams along the route, which had served as receptacles of the excreta from all groups of migrants, served as the most convenient source of water for captives, whose thirst grew insatiable as the marching continued for days on end. Sanitation was not an issue for traffickers. Captives were forced to eat, sleep, relieve themselves, and march in close proximity to each other during the length of the trip.[5]

At the outset of their forced journeys, many enslaved people understood their destination to be a place of misery and death. "The trader was all around, the slave-pens . . . ," the escapee Lewis Hayden told an interviewer, adding, "we did not know what time any of us might be in it." If they did end up there, they knew they would be sent to a faraway rice, sugar, or cotton plantation. "We had had them held before us as terrors, by our masters and mistresses, all our lives," Hayden recounted. "We knew about them all; and when a friend was carried off, why, it was the same as death, for we could not write or hear, and never expected to see them again." He lost his first wife and one of their sons to the traders, losses that scarred him more than the death of another son who remained near him. "I have one child who is buried in Kentucky, and that grave is pleasant to think of," he told his interviewer. "I've got another that is sold nobody knows where, and that I never can bear to think of."[6]

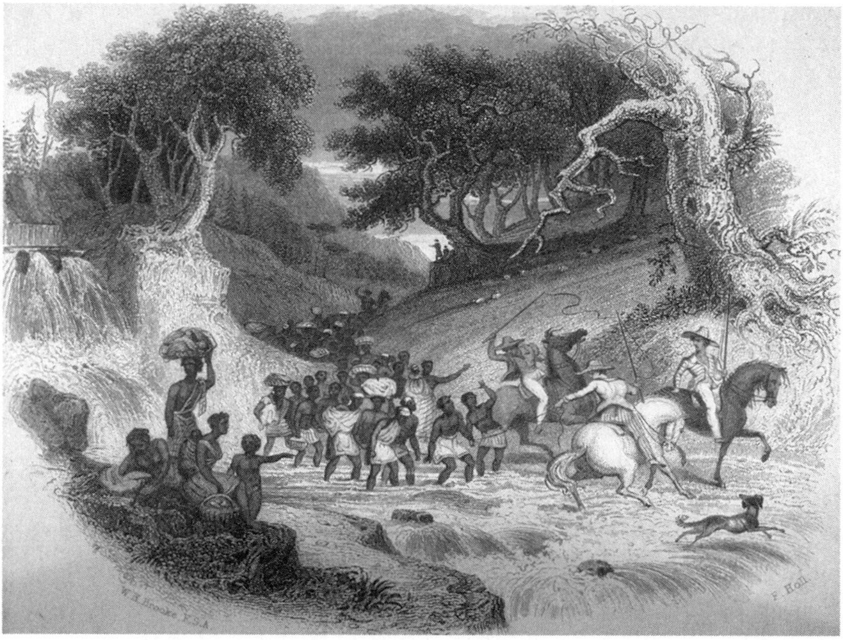

Slave Coffle, Virginia, 1839, in James Buckingham, *The Slave System of America* (London, 1842), Vol. 2, facing p. 553. Special Collections Department, University of Virginia Library, NW0250.

Captives whom Franklin, Armfield, and Co. assembled in July 1832 experienced all the horrors of being trafficked and then some. Early in the month, an illness broke out in Armfield's Alexandria jail. It could not have been cholera, given that the pandemic had not yet reached Virginia, but several prisoners became very ill, and a man, valued at $400, perished.[7] The death essentially amounted to "spoilage," the expectation that businesses have that some products they intend to sell will be ruined before they can be sold in the market.

Armfield, of course, wanted to limit the damage. He cleared his jail of healthy prisoners and sent them to Richmond, where Rice Ballard combined them with captives he had bought for export. James Franklin—Isaac's nephew and a junior partner in the company—arrived at Ballard's, organized a large coffle, and set off with it in August on the thousand-mile march to Natchez.[8] The exact size of the coffle is uncertain. A rival trader put the total number at 230, but it was probably a little more than half of what he understood it to be.[9]

James Franklin got the enslaved group out of Richmond before cholera struck the city, but he raced against the deadly disease as he forced the captives on their westward journey. The coffle may have intersected with the deadly pathogen somewhere between the Blue Ridge and the middle of

Tennessee as two children and "a boy" died during a brief rest at Isaac Franklin's Fairvue plantation, about twenty-five miles northeast of Nashville. Four or five remained too ill to travel any further when James Franklin, accompanied by his uncle, departed Fairvue in early October.[10]

If the coffle had not encountered cholera in western Virginia or in Tennessee, it would have in Mississippi. On October 31, Isaac and James Franklin pushed their captives as far west as Port Gibson, Mississippi, some thirty miles south of Vicksburg and some fifty miles north of Natchez. They likely crossed paths with Choctaws being deported and certainly encountered pandemic refugees from the Mississippi Valley. Isaac Franklin found the latter "so much alarmed that they would not purchase" people from him.[11] They had good reason to shun him. White evacuees, according to the Indian Removal agent Captain William Colquhoun, blamed "the negroes belonging to traders" for spreading the disease.[12]

Franklin, Armfield, and Co. bore responsibility for trafficking humans amid a cholera pandemic, and those they trafficked paid a dear price for their gamble. It took two weeks for the coffle to complete the remaining fifty miles of their march to Natchez. Cholera slowed them down and led to the deaths of several more people. "We have buried since the negroes left Alexandria [Virginia] 9 negroes and 6 or 7 children," Isaac Franklin informed Ballard.

Isaac Franklin took an extreme and wicked measure to hide the fact that he brought infected people to sell. He had deceased captives secretly buried after sunset. "The way we send out dead negroes at night and keep dark is a sin," he confessed to Ballard. "No person in this country knows that we ever have had a case of Cholera."[13] Survivors certainly did know, however. Tired, abused, and already traumatized from being ripped from friends and family, enslaved people had to witness a gruesome disease take lives from among them and wonder if they would be next.

For his part, Isaac Franklin breathed a sigh of relief as cholera disappeared among the coffle but worried about future shipments. On November 22, after keeping their people camped in the woods for a little over a week, the company entered Natchez and quickly sold all but fifty of their enslaved people. "The cholera has nearly subsided...," James Franklin informed Ballard. "I have no fears about the negros we have in this place but entertain great fears about those shipped."[14]

As Isaac Franklin peddled bodies in the West, his partners in the East went about their business with even more vigor than they had in years past.

The company's standard advertisement, offering "Cash for Negroes," ran in District of Columbia newspapers as cholera ravaged the Upper South. Armfield claimed to have enough funds to buy "one hundred and fifty likely Negroes, of both sexes, from 12 to 25 years of age" and that he would "give a higher price for slaves than any purchasers who are or may hereafter be in this market." Interested sellers could meet with him at his Duke Street property in Alexandria.[15] In October, Armfield changed the company's advertisement for the first time in about two and a half years by increasing the number wanted for purchase to two hundred.[16]

The company also continued to expand into Maryland. Austin Woolfolk had dominated in trafficking enslaved people from Baltimore to New Orleans for years, but political affairs disrupted his business. Residents of the Deep South grew concerned that Virginia planters were sending them rebellious captives in the wake of Turner's Revolt, and early in 1832, Louisiana's legislature banned traders from importing enslaved people for resale within the state's boundaries. This moved the center of the business to Natchez, where Isaac Franklin held the competitive edge.

Around the same time, Franklin, Armfield, and Co. sent James Purvis to oversee its Baltimore operations. He rented a property northeast of the city and advertised that he would buy up to 350 people. The ad ran from May 1832 through the end of the year, not only in the Baltimore *Republican* but also in newspapers published on Maryland's eastern shore. Purvis busily purchased people, shackled them into coffles, and marched them through the District of Columbia to Armfield's Alexandria jail.[17]

Woolfolk did not give up. During the pandemic, he continued to run his usual ad in Maryland, Virginia, and the District of Columbia. As newspapers reported grisly statistics of cholera's power, Woolfolk announced his desire to buy up to four hundred enslaved people and his willingness to offer "the HIGHEST Prices" to sellers and "Liberal commissions" to any middleman who arranged transactions.[18]

Then, much to his surprise, Woolfolk learned of his own death and had to change his advertisement. "A. Woolfolk wishes to inform the owners of Negroes in Maryland, Virginia and North Carolina," his revised ad of October 1 announced, "that he is not dead as has been artfully represented by his opponents, but that he still lives to give them cash, and the highest prices for their Negroes." Woolfolk requested all papers that he advertised in use the revised one, which let the public know that the rumors of his death were exaggerated and that he would "give them CASH and the *highest prices* for their Negroes."[19] Franklin, Armfield, and Co.'s agents may have been behind the rumor.

They certainly were attempting to drive him out of the business and take over his territory, which they would eventually do over the next few years.[20]

If Woolfolk, or for that matter all slave dealers, had died, a female African American captive being marched to the auction block would have believed they had gotten what they deserved. She belonged to a "negro trader" who stopped with his captives at an inn near Fredericksburg and had a conversation with a local white man that a witness overheard. The man obliviously asked the unnamed enslaved woman, "If she was willing to go?" The woman unsurprisingly responded, "No, I am not, 'willing.'" She then said, "Master, do you know why God has sent this cholera among the people?" When the man asked her why, she pointed to the twenty men in the coffle, who were "handcuffed, two and two, [with] a chain passing between them." The enslaved woman held the same beliefs as Frederick Douglass and many other African Americans at the time. The scourge "was a judgement from the All mighty" for the sin of slavery.[21]

The coffle that she was in may have been one of several that were headed toward John Armfield's jail. Traumatized by what they had already endured, captives arrived in Alexandria terrified of being sent away forever. James Wilson avoided this fate, at least temporarily. He escaped from Armfield's clutches on October 30, leading the company to advertise a ten-dollar reward for his capture and return.[22] If Armfield successfully retrieved the twenty-five-year-old man, he did not do so before November 2, when the *Tribune*, a brig that the company had constructed a year earlier, set sail for New Orleans. James Wilson did not appear on the ship's manifest listing the names of ninety-six captives consigned to Isaac Franklin or the names of another eleven consigned to another enslaver who contracted with Armfield to transport his human cargo.[23]

A gauntlet of cholera awaited those who could not escape. The disease persisted in New Orleans after the devastating outbreak in late October and early November; steamboat passengers continued to sicken and die aboard the filthy vessels; and *Vibrio* spilled into several plantations.[24] "There has been more sickness in this country within three months than ever was known before in the same space of time," William Trowbridge observed after arriving in the fall at the Deslondes plantation about thirty miles upriver from New Orleans. "Cholera set in . . . and made a general sweep through the country," he learned, adding, "some planters have lost from 30 to 50 negroes by the cholera alone." The Deslondes family had twelve to fifteen cases among their enslaved people, with three dying within ten hours of first becoming sick.[25]

Henry McCall lost so many enslaved people to "the great Cholera epidemic of 1832" that he sold off one of his plantations, bought more slaves, and concentrated his workforce on his Evan Hall Plantation in Ascension Parish.[26]

The scourge also visited the Labranche family's sugar plantation in St. Charles Parish. Mary Austin Holley, the governess of the Labranche children, observed that cholera broke out among enslaved field workers in early November and within a couple of weeks had killed several hands whom the Labranches valued at $10,000.[27] After seeming to disappear from the distant slave quarters, cholera invaded the plantation household. Holley saw the house servants John, Patience, and Louisa die within hours of being attacked. "Instead of the habitual *bon jour* so gaily pronounced, we met in tears & dismay, not knowing where the pestilence would end," she informed her daughter before detailing her own ordeal with the disease. "I felt the circulation arrested & a coldness fast spreading over me like the chill of death, with a terrible distress at my stomach," she described. The Labranches' doctor came to her aid and fortunately did not follow a toxic regimen of bleeding, calomel, and laudanum. He administered ether, peppermint, and hot brandy toddy while keeping her warm and rubbing out her cramps. She "had such terror of another attack" that she could not sleep, but the mild treatment her doctor administered helped her body heal. Others were not so fortunate, however. A total of sixteen enslaved people died on the Labranche plantation.[28]

The continuing pandemic led Franklin, Armfield, and Co. to have mixed thoughts about cholera's impact on their business prospects. Ballard, on the one hand, seemed resigned to the possibility that the disease endangered the lives of his colleagues and threatened the company's bottom line. "I hope for the *Best*...," Ballard wrote to Isaac Franklin, "[and] if it please *God* that the Negroes should get it I hope you will be careful of yourselves. We had better lose all and begin again than lose ourselves." On the other hand, he came to the heartless conclusion that cholera's ravages could be good for business. He advised his partner to resist the temptation to sell captives at a low price before the disease had a chance to take them away. The novel malady appeared to be depleting the Lower Mississippi of its labor supply, and the company could reap the rewards of being patient. "My opinion is that we had best hold on," Ballard told Franklin, as "the more negros lost in that country the more will be wanting."[29]

Rice Ballard was not the only peddler of human bodies seeking to profit from a morbid situation. Paul Pascal set sail from Norfolk aboard the *Ajax* with fifteen of his enslaved people on October 16.[30] They arrived in New

Orleans on November 9 and managed to reach Natchez without contracting cholera. The disease, and particularly its association with traffickers, continued to keep buyers away. Pascal lamented the state of the market but saw an upside to the fatalities. "I think that the slowdown in commerce could seriously hamper the trade in negroes," he informed his partner, "but I think [planters] will be forced to buy because of the losses they have just experienced."[31]

Isaac Franklin was making the same calculations, although on a grander scale as he had a large shipment aboard the *Tribune* arriving in New Orleans on November 26. Before it got there, he sent a message back to Virginia expressing his "uneasiness" and informing company agents to suspend all purchases "until further orders." He also detailed his plan to intercept the ship before it reached New Orleans, take the captives across the lakes below the city, and conduct them overland "to avoid the pestilence."[32]

Franklin did not completely succeed in his plan. He got the entire cohort to Natchez without losing anyone along the way, but a few days later, tragedy struck. "Yesterday to my Great Mortification had one case of the great Asiatic Cholera," he wrote to Ballard on December 8, "and it killed a first rate man in 8 hours." Seven or eight captives remained severely ill at the time he composed his letter. Franklin described the situation as "the most trying times that ever sailed in my high seas" and confessed to Ballard that the deceased man would be buried secretly at night, just as he had done with the corpses of other people he trafficked into the pandemic's hot zone.[33]

Undeterred, Franklin, Armfield, and Co. sought to cash in on what became a seller's market. They steadily sold off their inventory through December and January. James Franklin bragged to an eastern associate that "good men" sold for $650 to $700 and women for $450 to $500.[34] He followed up a month later, claiming demand for slaves to be at an all-time high.[35] Isaac Franklin lamented that they could have made more money had cholera not interfered, but he planned for a more prosperous future. "For the losses we met with last summer & fall by deaths," he remarked to Ballard, "we would have made a better business this season than we ever have in proportion." He advised his East Coast partners to "go on and buy all of the right kind you can get at a fair price" and assured them that the company would "be sure to realize a profit."[36]

They would have to outlay more capital, though. The residual impact of the pandemic led to inflated prices in Virginia. "We have never known of Negroes selling or hiring at such high prices as they do at present," editors of Richmond's *Compiler* remarked in their January 12, 1833, issue. "We have heard of a carpenter selling at $1200—of boys of 14 selling at more than

$400." The editors speculated that the increased costs could be due to booming demand from tobacco factories, internal improvement projects, farmers seeking to profit from increased produce prices, and settlers building new farms in the West. Yet they also cited a labor shortage. Could the increased cost be "for slaves to supply the want of those who have died with the cholera?" they asked.[37]

Franklin, Armfield, and Co. knew the answer to be yes, and they had the capital to give them the competitive edge in buying and reselling people. The company's finances depended on complicated arrangements, making it difficult for Isaac Franklin to transform profits made in the West into cash that his eastern associates could use to make purchases. That changed with a $50,000 loan that Franklin secured from the newly chartered Union Bank of Louisiana, which was itself capitalized by the Baring Brothers of London.[38] As 1833 approached, Armfield had ample funds on hand to do "all sorts of purchasing."[39] The company also changed its standard advertisement on January 15 to indicate that it would not limit the number of enslaved people it would buy. "We will pay cash and the highest prices for any number of Likely Negroes, of both sexes," the new notice read.[40]

For the remainder of the winter and into the early spring, the company outcompeted all others in marketing human bodies. Armfield packed eighty-three enslaved people aboard the *Lafayette*, which set sail on January 16, 1833.[41] Six days later, he sent another shipment aboard the *Tribune*, which departed with an unknown number of captives from the Alexandria jail, stopped at Norfolk, and picked up thirty-eight that Ballard had sent down from Richmond.[42] One month later, the company sent another group of captives to New Orleans aboard the brig *Ariel*.[43] More cash and encouragement arrived in March from the Franklins. "We are selling fast at present," Isaac and James Franklin wrote to Ballard.[44] The *Tribune* had returned to Alexandria in mid-March, took aboard another load of captives, and then arrived back in New Orleans on April 9.[45] Altogether, Isaac Franklin collected around three hundred captives from the four shipments.[46]

Their ambitions got ahead of them, however. Some thirty-one individuals and slave-trading partnerships had set up shop in the Natchez market, flooding it with hundreds of captives.[47] Sales started to become "dull" in early March.[48] Isaac Franklin still had seventy captives on hand at the end of March and knew another shipment would arrive aboard the *Tribune* in early April.[49]

Franklin had more to worry about than dull sales. Cholera had never disappeared from the Gulf South. After sweeping away countless enslaved people along the Lower Mississippi in the fall of 1832, the pathogen made its way west and circulated among coastal estates into the early spring of 1833. An untold number of captives continued to perish, with plantations around the town of Franklin, Louisiana, experiencing especially severe outbreaks.[50] Cholera not only lurked to the west of New Orleans, but it erupted frightfully in Cuba. *Vibrio* made it to Havana by mid-February, escalated to a peak within a couple of weeks, and abated by April 6. US newspapers relayed reports of hundreds dying per day and a death toll reaching five thousand in the Spanish colonial city of some one hundred thousand people by the end of March. Among the dead was William Shaler, US Consul to Havana.[51]

The ongoing pandemic, along with the warming weather, led the editors of Natchez's *Mississippi Free Trader* to worry. "The Cholera is raging with extraordinary violence in Havana, near a thousand persons it is reported have died there in a day," they informed their readers on April 19. They emphasized the widely held belief that cholera often returned to places it had previously visited and referenced its suspected reappearance in New Orleans. There, city officials denied the actual presence of the scourge, but the mayor did acknowledge that one ship arrived from Havana on April 5 after a man died onboard with a disease suspected of being cholera. That ship, along with others that were then on their way, were ordered to anchor on the opposite side of the river until inspected and cleared. The *Free Trader*'s editors recommended their own city's officials enact protections and pointed to the influx of "an unusual number of slaves for sale" as a reason not to be cavalier about the scourge.[52]

The editors were right to be alarmed. On April 9, the *Tribune* arrived in New Orleans for the third time during the pandemic. Franklin collected the approximately one hundred enslaved people, put them on a steamboat, and brought them to his slave pen. On their arrival, many began to sicken, and more than a dozen had died by April 19. Franklin had five buried in the public graveyard, but to hide the extent of infections at his trading house, he resorted to his old trick of clandestinely burying the deceased.[53]

This time he got caught. A "slight rain" fell on Saturday, April 20 and exposed a recently deceased woman who had been tumbled into a gully and covered with a thin layer of dirt.[54] The washed-out grave drew the attention of residents, who reported it to city officials. The next day, more hastily disposed bodies were discovered. Most were in such a decayed state that no one would touch them for fear of contracting a deadly disease. The coroner and his jury of inquest exhumed and examined three of the most recently discarded corpses. They were identified as African Americans: a fifteen- to twenty-year-old woman, a forty-five-year-old woman, and an eight-month-old child. The jury determined that none of the three died from violence and that whoever buried them did so in violation of city ordinances requiring notification of the town's sexton and interment in coffins at a proper depth below ground. The jury was particularly indignant about the treatment of the infant, who was "put into a hole, washed out by the rain as it run into the bayou, with its head downwards, and which was only hid from view by a few shovels of dirt." That the deceased had belonged to one or more traders was obvious since one of them wore the same type of clothing as the Franklins' enslaved people.[55]

News of the clandestine burials traveled fast and incited outrage within the Natchez citizenry. A gathering of people, described by the editors of the *Courier* as "the largest, that we remember ever to have witnessed in this city," occurred on Monday, April 22. Calls for the slave traders to be expelled had mass support.[56] One petition, bearing eighty-four signatures, condemned "the horrible and inhuman practice of throwing the Bodies of their Dead Negroes into the Bayous." Yet opposition revolved around issues of public health and not disdain for the buying and selling of other human beings. The exposed corpses, the petition complained, would add "noxious exhalations" into the atmosphere "at a time when the *cholera*, that King of Scourges is lurking in our neighborhood."[57]

City officials called traders to publicly testify. Representatives of eight outfits swore oaths declaring that they had nothing to do with the crime. Five enslaved people belonging to those who came forward had perished, they claimed, but none from cholera, and all the deceased had been properly buried.[58] Isaac Franklin was conveniently out of town, and none of the company's employees testified. Dr. Samuel Guastain, the city's health officer, nonetheless examined all the slave pens and found that Franklin had lost five captives over the last week, one from an unknown cause and four from cholera. The notorious traffickers also had three prisoners recovering from the disease. Guastain could only identify one case of cholera as having been among other traders.[59]

A citizen committee investigated further on Tuesday, April 23 and delivered a finding of facts that evening. The preamble to their report verified that the "clandestine burial of several negroes" had occurred and that the deceased were "supposed to have died of the cholera." They consequently delivered what the citizens wanted to hear. Because the "large numbers of negroes" brought into their town was "a great nuisance . . . calculated to create disease," the city council should outlaw the slave trade from city limits. Ten traders preemptively signed a public declaration that they would voluntarily leave.[60]

Isaac Franklin was not among the signers, but the city gave him no choice. On April 24, the council passed an ordinance giving all traffickers three days to move their businesses beyond city limits.[61] "We shall have to take the woods in haste," James Franklin informed Ballard after the measure passed.[62] One of their employees would not go with them, however. Samuel Jacobs, a driver, died of cholera and was properly buried in the Natchez cemetery. Evidently, the Franklins scapegoated their employee for dark deeds that they had orchestrated. Notice of his death in the *Courier* claimed he "was supposed to have had the principal hand in putting the bodies of the negroes, reported last week, into the bayou."[63]

The company took the scourge with them to their new location at the Forks in the Road, a place just outside Natchez's boundary where a major avenue split into two routes heading into Mississippi's interior. "We are not selling any [slaves] at present," James Franklin informed Ballard. "In fact my partner is alarmed & not without a cause for I do assure you it is dreadful. We have 4 or 5 down at present and it takes all the well negroes to attend to the sick." He closed his letter abruptly, explaining that he had to attend "another sick negroe."[64]

Still, Isaac Franklin reaped profits, as he had the year before and would in the two years to come. The monetary value of enslaved people continued to rise throughout 1833 and into 1835 as cotton prices surged and as cholera continued to deplete plantations in the Lower Mississippi Valley of their captive workforce. Isaac Franklin made the Forks in the Road the preeminent slave market in the United States, and his profits continued to far exceed the losses that cholera caused. He retired from the trafficking business in 1835 a rich man. He used his fortune to develop his Fairvue operation in Tennessee, purchase new plantations in Louisiana, and accumulate wealth through the forced labor of more than six hundred people he enslaved. At the time of his death in 1846, according to historian Joshua Rothman, Isaac Franklin possessed "the modern equivalent of more than $435 million," making him one of the richest men in the country prior to the Civil War.[65]

Isaac Franklin sacrificed numerous people along the way, especially during the deadly cholera years of 1832 and 1833. One of those who paid the ultimate price for the risks that trafficking entailed was Betty. She was dragged away from loved ones—possibly a mother, father, siblings—and confined in Ballard's Richmond jail. She was then sent to Natchez and experienced wretched conditions and treatment along the way. By the end of her journey,

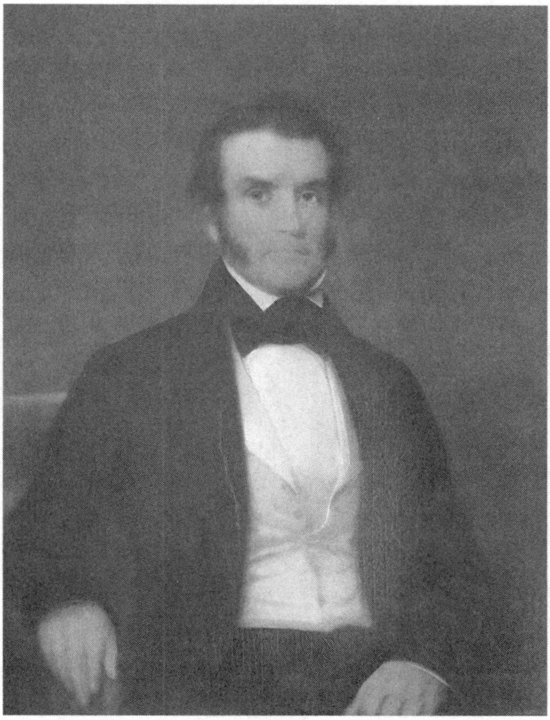

Isaac Franklin. Courtesy of the Belmont Mansion Association, 2016.13.01.

her body could no longer endure the disease-filled ordeal that her enslavers put her through. "Girl Betty who died" is recorded in a company ledger on January 3, 1833, with her market value listed at $350.[66] Not just a financial loss on a balance sheet, she was a human being exposed to cholera's terror when her traffickers risked her life for their own profit.

Phillip Willis was another tragic victim of Franklin, Armfield, and Co.'s speculative enterprise. He was the "first rate man" that Isaac Franklin lamented losing in early December and had secretly buried. Armfield had packed the five feet and five-and-a-half-inch-tall eighteen-year-old aboard the *Tribune*, which set sail on November 2, 1832. Like Betty, he left behind heartbroken family members who feared they would never see him again. He had to endure nearly three weeks on a ship, most of it chained below decks, breathing foul air, consuming the scant food and water that his captors gave him to keep him alive, and feeling seasick as waves rocked the vessel. Near the end of his long journey, he met his deadliest obstacle, one that he might have escaped back in Virginia. In Franklin's Natchez pen, *Vibrio* replicated rapidly in his

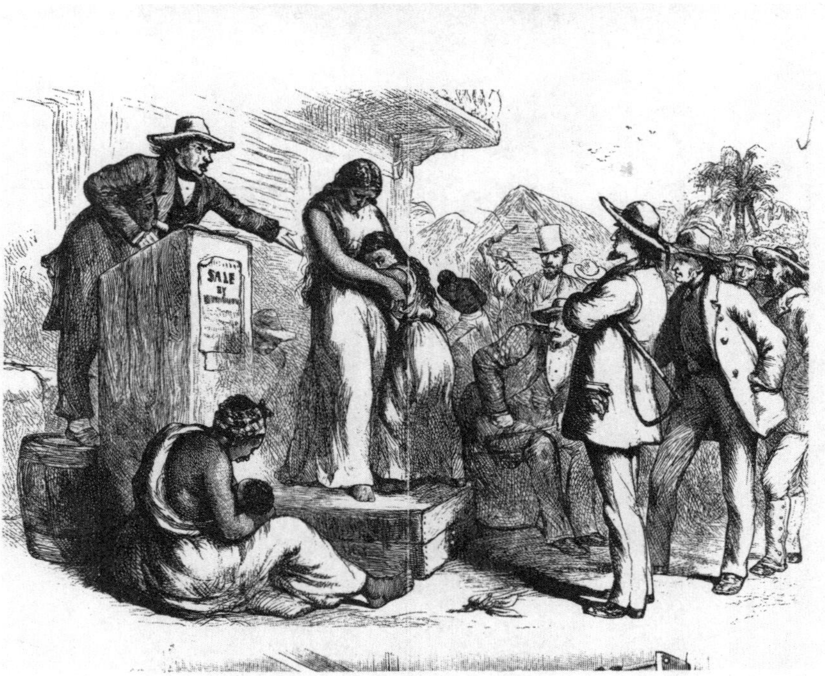

Woman and Child on Auction Block. Franklin and Armfield would have acquired Betty in an auction like the one depicted here. Schomburg Center for Research in Black Culture, Photographs and Prints Division, The New York Public Library, 1710249.

body and caused excruciating symptoms. As his consciousness faded in and out, was he thinking about people back where he came from—people who valued him as a loved one or friend instead of a commodity? Probably. To Franklin, Armfield, and Co., though, he went from a living asset to a dead liability, and they covered up his agonizing death to protect their bottom line.[67]

12

Noise over Troubled Waters

THE DEAFENING CONSEQUENCES OF TEMPERANCE

ON FEBRUARY 26, 1833, the First Presbyterian Church of Charleston held a "Temperance Celebration."[1] The star of the evening was Thomas Grimké, a Yale-educated lawyer, the president of South Carolina's main anti-alcohol organization, and a rising public intellectual whose reputation extended well beyond his home state. He was an enslaver but a firm unionist, who spoke out against his state government's failed attempt to nullify federal tariffs, which had brought the nation to brink of a civil war during Jackson's first term.[2] He also committed himself to promoting peace, diffusing knowledge through public education, and upholding Protestant Christian morality as the key to his nation's progress.

Grimké gave his listeners a lot to think about that night. His remarks, when published, consisted of thirty-five pages that hammered home the message that drunkenness and the social disorder associated with it posed a grave threat to the individual enjoyment of life, liberty, and property. Ending intoxication thus was "*the cause of* PATRIOTISM."[3]

The pandemic served as a useful rhetorical weapon in his efforts. The South Carolina reformer had read French physician F. J. V. Broussais's *Le choléra-morbus épidémique: Observé et traité selon la méthode physiologique* in its original language, and he translated passages for his audience confirming that cholera had preyed upon Paris's brandy drinkers. He used evidence from a study of Albany, New York, suggesting that only two members of temperance societies in that city succumbed to the scourge and that the vast majority of deaths fell on those who habitually drank. "In a word," he declared, "the vice of Intemperance, is the prolific parent of disease in every age and condition of life, and in every state of society, whether civilized or barbarous." Giving up alcohol and encouraging others to do so, thus, were acts of "GENUINE PATRIOTISM" because they would "deliver every community from . . . loathsome, excruciating and obstinate disease."[4]

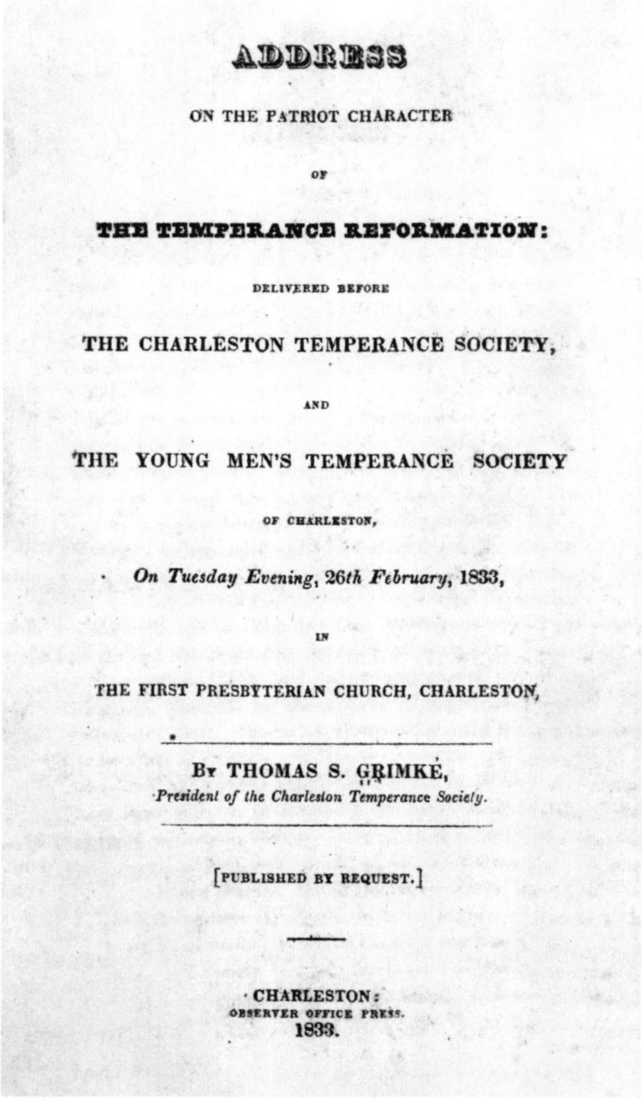

ADDRESS

ON THE PATRIOT CHARACTER

OF

THE TEMPERANCE REFORMATION:

DELIVERED BEFORE

THE CHARLESTON TEMPERANCE SOCIETY,

AND

THE YOUNG MEN'S TEMPERANCE SOCIETY

OF CHARLESTON,

On Tuesday Evening, 26th February, 1833,

IN

THE FIRST PRESBYTERIAN CHURCH, CHARLESTON,

BY THOMAS S. GRIMKÉ,

President of the Charleston Temperance Society.

[PUBLISHED BY REQUEST.]

CHARLESTON:
OBSERVER OFFICE PRESS.
1833.

Address on the Patriot Character of the Temperance Reformation by Thomas Grimké (Observer Office, 1833). Throughout the pandemic, temperance advocates lectured listeners and flooded the reading public with addresses that employed cholera in their war against inebriation.

Charlestonians were not the only Americans to have a temperance celebration on the day Grimké spoke. Back in September 1832, the American Temperance Society proposed February 26, 1833, as the time for organizations devoted to the anti-alcohol crusade to make their voices heard in unison. The reasons for it were manifold, but the mass disease mortality occurring when they announced it provided a major justification for their cause. With inebriation's disappearance, the society declared, "the cholera, that scourge of the nations, which has spread sackcloth round the globe and threatens to cover our land with mourning, would be nearly if not altogether unknown."[5] In every state in the Union and in the largest cities and the smallest towns, simultaneous events called on Americans to champion sobriety and thus keep their nation safe from cholera's full onslaught.

If attendees did not have the disease on their mind when they flocked to churches on the appointed day, they would have as they heard speeches similar to that of Thomas Grimké. Alvan Stewart told a crowd assembled in Utica's First Presbyterian Church that the disease preyed on drunks in "Paris, Montreal, New-York, and New-Orleans" and "has been preaching to the nations of the earth, from the burning plains of India to the arctic snows, . . . 'The intemperate are my chosen victims.'"[6] Reverend William Jackson showed young men in New York City a certificate with two sets of images, one with "Poverty, Disgrace, and Ruin" inscribed alongside liquor bottles and the other with "Health, Wealth, and Happiness" inscribed underneath a water well and bucket. If any of the men turned to alcohol during times of cholera, the reverend warned, they would be throwing themselves "into the paws of a raging bear that knows no pity!"[7] In Norwalk, Connecticut, the Congregational Pastor Edwin Hall said of the disease, "Go where it will, there it seems to scent out the breath of those who have tasted the poison" of liquor.[8] Reverend Thomas H. Stockton emphatically told a gathering at the Methodist Episcopal Church in Easton, Maryland, that "THE CHOLERA THIRSTS FOR THE BLOOD OF THE DRUNKARD."[9]

Loud jubilation for temperance reverberated through the nation in the wake of the pandemic's first wave. Celebrating sobriety seemed the best way to make sense of what had happened during the previous summer and fall and to prepare for the scourge's potential return. The moralistic noise that reformers produced had tragic consequences, however. The voices of Americans who proposed that the global killer lurked in their waters were stifled.

On August 1, 1832, Baltimore's *Gazette and Daily Journal* brought renewed attention to "telluric theory," which posited that subterranean gases infused underground water with harmful toxins. A story from a Leipsic, Germany, newspaper published in late 1831 originally brought this idea to wide attention and even suggested that ordinary people were not merely superstitious in claiming that their drinking supplies had been poisoned. The story also gave plebians credit for treating their water before swallowing it. "Many persons drink boiled water, as they consider this as a preservative against the disease," the article concluded. The Leipsic piece appeared in American newspapers in February and March of 1832, but thereafter editors forgot about it until the pandemic gripped the United States.[10] After Baltimore's *Gazette and Daily Journal* reprinted it, newspapers shared it with readers across the country.

None did so with enthusiasm. Many simply published the piece with no commentary, while others included the postscript added by the editors of Baltimore's *Gazette and Daily Journal*: "There is certainly no end to the various theories which the Cholera seems likely to engender—it might be a gratification to see any two of them assimilate."[11] A few papers reprinted the piece from the Camden, South Carolina, *Journal* with its dismissive preface: "These theories amuse, but prove nothing, except absolute ignorance which prevails."[12]

Charles King, editor of New York's *American*, had been encouraged to give drinking water more attention by his famous friend, novelist Washington Irving. While on a retreat at Saratoga Springs in August, Irving privately complained to King, "the cholera is proving so powerful an ally of the temperance society" that the liquor trade was in ruins. "I wish you would endeavor to interest it in the cause of good water," he quipped about the disease to the editor, "by intimating how much of the virulence of this malady and the prevalence of other maladies in our city may be owing to the nature of the water we drink." Irving further lamented that "so rich and luxurious a city which lavishes countless thousands upon curious wines, cannot afford itself wholesome water."[13]

Charles King kept private any thoughts on the matter. His paper ignored the Leipsic piece and did not include any suggestions that the disease may have come from drinking water.

The press in Cincinnati, however, did give the idea of cholera's presence in water some consideration. On October 15, a reader, simply identified by the initial "P," composed a letter to the *Daily National Republican*'s editors supporting "telluric" theory. "Among the means of preserving health, at his fearful period, pure water may not be considered the least," declared the writer. P's method of purifying water involved pouring water into an upright cask, affixing a faucet near the bottom and another six inches above, adding an eighth of an ounce of alum per gallon, stirring the mixture, and allowing to set for twenty-four hours so the sediment would settle at the bottom. P, of course, was not the first to practice this method of clarifying water, but at a crucial time this explanation pointed people in the right direction of discovering cholera's route of transmission and teaching them an effective means of making drinking water safer. The process, according to P, rid the liquid of "animal or vegetable poisons."[14] Modern studies verify that alum mixed into untreated water can significantly reduce *Vibrio* levels within one to two hours.[15]

Henry Boyd, a free African American resident of Cincinnati, also suspected an aqueous origin to the novel malady. Boyd, then in his late twenties, had been born enslaved, bought his freedom at age eighteen, moved to Ohio, and earned enough money to buy the freedom of his brother and sister. As cholera exploded in his city, he correctly identified the vector of the disease and offered even clearer directions to avoid illness. "It is an old saying that in every emergency 'even the weak may give some help,'" the *Gazette*'s editors paternalistically remarked. "Mr. Henry Boyd, a man of color, has suggested that the source of cholera is in the water, and that it may be removed by boiling all the water we use and letting it cool again before used." Hoping to keep trade flowing, the editors added that "our country friends of the market may boil and bottle their water, before they come to the city, and if the theory be well, bring it with them and incur no risk."[16] Boyd's advice unfortunately appeared to be confined to Cincinnati, where few seemed to take it.

Even the iconoclastic Dr. Daniel Drake could not believe that water delivered cholera. He gave Boyd no notice in his own analysis in late 1832, and in an 1833 essay, he referenced the "theory of [cholera's] aqueous origin" only to dismiss it as "equally unsatisfactory" as all other proposals. He had even given up on animalcular theory and did not believe any true knowledge of what caused the pandemic had been produced.[17] Part of what vexed Drake about water was that in some plagued cities, such as Cincinnati, rivers quenched thirst, whereas in other afflicted places, local wells provided the bulk of what people drank.

Albany, New York, was one of those places where wells served a large portion of the population, and one resident pointed to those as sources of the scourge. James P. Goold, a well-to-do carriage and railroad car manufacturer, remained in the city during the outbreak in the summer of 1832, served on a relief committee to provide for workers and orphans the pandemic had left destitute, and paid close attention to the daily mortality reports. Between August 6 and 19, he counted that among the 103 nonhospital deaths, 83 were of individuals living in neighborhoods not served by the Albany Water Works Company. This company piped a supply from Maezlandt Kill, a creek northwest of the city, into an elevated reservoir and then through wooden and cast-iron pipes to some, but not all, homes and businesses.[18] On August 23, Goold drummed up the courage to reveal his discovery, although remaining anonymous as he did so. Under the pseudonym "Common Good," Goold informed the editors of the *Evening Journal* of his conclusion: "From these facts, I am led to believe that, from some (to me) unknown cause, the water of our wells must be unhealthy."[19]

Editors of the *Evening Journal* published the letter with additional statistics he supplied in a short piece titled "How is this?" Over the previous four days (August 20–23), twenty-nine of the thirty-two cholera victims who had perished relied on well water, and over the previous twenty-four hours, only one of the fourteen recorded deaths had occurred where the city's water lines reached. The editors identified their informant only as a "friend who is always alive to the interests of the city" and called for an official investigation. "It is remarkable that most of the cases, since the disease appeared, has been in neighborhoods not supplied by the Water Works," they wondered.[20]

If Goold had fears of being accused as a purveyor of superstitious beliefs, they were realized just three days after his statistics were published. The rival newspaper, the *Argus*, published a letter from "A. PHYSICIAN" ridiculing the buzz that had been created. "I trust we are not returning to the madness of the populace of Paris, who supposed their water to be poisoned." He referred to the suggestion as a "mare's nest," or a discovery that turns out to be a hoax, and then dismissed it, as the scourge's complex origin was self-evident. "A disease which has ravaged Asia and is now ravaging Europe and the Americas," the anonymous doctor declared, "can hardly owe its origin or progress to 'well water,' even if it be somewhat impurer [*sic*] than spring water."[21]

The unnamed physician's letter led Goold to reveal his identity and defend his findings, although with some equivocation. The manufacturer responded that he did not believe "the disease was produced by the water" but that "its existence is prolonged among us by the use of water from wells." Or, in other words, the causative agent or agents probably lay elsewhere but drinking poor water made one more vulnerable to those agents. Goold provided further "facts" that cast suspicion on wells. Of the forty-six cholera deaths over the most recent week-long period, thirty-eight were of people who "lived in the vicinity of wells and used the water." Meanwhile, a surprising absence of the malady occurred in an area served by the waterworks but had all the ingredients associated with cholera: poverty, open sewers, poorly ventilated homes, and pools of stagnant water.[22]

The debate led the mayor to order an investigation. He called upon Dr. Theodore Romeyne Beck, an Albany medical professor and author of America's first significant treatise on forensic medicine, to examine samples collected from the suspected wells. Beck found that the samples smelled and appeared normal and dismissed the idea that cholera came from drinking it. Residents, to be sure, should use their "common sense" and avoid rancid and turbid liquid and refrain from guzzling cold water when overheated. He then dismissed the controversy as making the situation worse by enhancing cholera's most important predisposing cause. "Fear or dread of the element which forms one of the principal sources of our animal nutriment, must concur in hurrying on that state of the system which lays it open to the attack of our fearful visitor," he warned. "If the mind becomes diseased with apprehensions, bodily illness will sooner or later follow."[23]

Few people outside of Albany paid attention to the statistics that pointed toward cholera's true vector. Some newspapers reprinted the *Evening Journal*'s "How is this?" piece, but only Baltimore's *Gazette and Daily Advertiser* did so with commentary.[24] "The facts set forth may furnish a hint for the investigation of the same subject here," the *Gazette*'s editors noted, "and we are inclined to the impression that much sickness is produced by the use of the water from pumps, which is so often deficient in that purity essential to the promotion of health."[25] As the outbreak abated, the Baltimore brewer Samuel Lucas referred readers of the *Gazette* to the issue of contaminated water. Lucas noted observations made in France, England, and the United States that consumers of malt beverages fared much better than the general population, citing "the Albany papers" as evidence that alcohol was not to blame. People instead got cholera "by drinking cold spring and well water."[26]

Neither Baltimore nor any other American city carried out an investigation along the lines that Goold did in Albany. Complaints about municipal water supplies, to be sure, grew louder during and immediately following the pandemic's first wave, and city officials in New York, Baltimore, and New Orleans were increasingly pressured to enact plans to tap purer and more ample supplies. The Fairmount Water Works were held up as a model for other cities and heralded as a reason for Philadelphia's low per capita mortality rate. Nevertheless, public support for improvements did not include what Henry Boyd had suggested—the possibility that a deadly agent that caused cholera had infiltrated drinking water. Instead, political pressure stemmed from the belief that municipalities needed better water to cleanse the streets, gutters, and alleys of miasmatic-causing filth.[27]

Troubled waters were of little concern to reform-minded Americans who had long since made up their minds that alcohol above all other factors made one predisposed to cholera. Conversely, they promoted membership in a temperance organization as a way to increase one's chances of survival. Months before Richmond's *Southern Religious Telegraph* bragged that only one of their city's 1,000 members belonging to anti-alcohol organizations had died, a report circulated that cholera had taken only one life among the 350 temperance members in Montreal during the pandemic's first few weeks.[28] On July 4, 1832, the Reverend George Duffield cited the statistic to warn the young men of Carlisle, Pennsylvania, that God "is giving an awful admonition to the world at present" that habitual drinking would lead to being swept "off the face of the Earth." Their membership in a temperance society was "patriotic" and a "guard against such a dreadful scourge of human existence."[29]

As the first wave abated, Albany's *Temperance Recorder* published the study that seemed to demonstrate what Duffield preached and that Grimké would later utilize. Commissioned by the New York State Temperance Society (NYSTS), "An Authentic Record of Deaths in the City of Albany" was the product of an unnamed "gentleman of intelligence, of integrity, and of warm benevolence," who investigated all cholera deaths of people aged sixteen and older in the city. He compiled a list of 336 deceased people, identified by their gender, age, ethnicity or race ("native," Irish, German, or "coloured"), social standing ("low character" or "respectable"), drinking habits, and any dietary imprudence immediately before their demise. Since the dead could not speak for themselves, however, one wonders how the gentleman learned all the details that he recorded.

In any event, the findings revealed that all but ten of the deceased were moderate to heavy drinkers. The "facts speak for themselves" the committee declared. "Cholera has an affinity, close and intimate with ardent spirits." To add weight to the findings, nine of the eleven members of the board of health's medical staff signed the report and recommended its publication. The two who did not sign, Dr. McNaughton and Dr. March, were out of town.[30] Albany's *Recorder* published the NYSTS's "Authentic Record" on November 6, and abridged forms of the findings found their way into numerous newspapers in many different states in November and December.[31]

The *Recorder* provided reformers with additional, useful information in its next issue. The editors not only pointed out what Grimké had told his audience—that just two people out of the five thousand members of Albany's multiple anti-alcohol organizations had fallen to cholera—but also that sobriety protected all people regardless of race, class, or ethnicity. Not one of the 123 members of the Irish Catholic Hibernian Temperance Society and not one of the 192 members of the African Temperance Society had died, they touted.[32]

Thomas Grimké was not the only crusader to bolster his speech with evidence from the *Recorder*. The NYSTS's "Authentic Report" presented "not solitary facts," Dr. Thomas Sewall told fellow attendees at the American Congressional Temperance Society's inaugural meeting, held two days prior to the appointed celebration day. "Over whatever region this disease has passed, it has singled out the intemperate for its victims in a marked and extraordinary manner," proclaimed the doctor, who had attended patients during the pandemic's sweep through the District of Columbia.[33] Cholera's discriminating nature was perhaps the only thing Sewall's audience could agree upon. Partisanship, sectionalism, and bitter policy differences over the National Bank, Indian Removal, and tariffs did not stop Democrats and Whigs, northerners and southerners, and easterners and westerners from collectively attending the inaugural event and uniting to condemn ardent spirits.

"And who were the victims of the pestilence," Bellamy Storer asked his Cincinnati audience on the temperance celebration day. The lawyer and reformer did not rely on Drake's analysis. Instead, he named the NYSTS's "Authentic Report" to proclaim "that a very large proportion of the deaths in the United States, from cholera, were of those who were habitually addicted to the use of ardent spirits." His published remarks included a footnote citing an unnamed French medical authority that "persons given to drinking, have been swept away like flies" and the New York City physician Dr. John R. Rhinelander, who observed the scourge "invariably" cutting down the inebriated in Montreal.[34] Editors of the *National Intelligencer* found Storer's speech so persuasive that they published it in full.[35]

New York's highest judicial officer, Chancellor Reuben H. Walworth, was instrumental in the production of Albany's "Authentic Report" and utilized it forcefully in his celebration day address. He admitted to his audience that during the pandemic's first wave, he and his fellow members of the executive committee of the NYSTS could not "stay the suicidal hands of those who were addicted to the daily use of ardent spirits."[36] He spoke with pride that the statistics they published in the *Recorder* would demonstrate "the results which may ever be expected from such madness and infatuation." He personified cholera as "a preacher of temperance" that would likely return and warned that even "self-styled temperate drinkers" should be wary.[37]

The chancellor then attempted to do what other crusaders dared not try. He explained why "Some few indeed, of the most regular and temperate habits, have fallen its victims." He mentioned the passing of Justice Ewing as well as an unnamed "devoted sister of charity" as examples and claimed these losses were the fault of the drunkards who infested the land. The deaths were, he claimed, "the natural consequence" of the intoxicated masses who polluted "the atmosphere" until it became "so impure as to render it deleterious to human life." Ewing and the unfortunate Catholic nun were still exceptions. Even doctors, nurses, and others who cared for the ill and had close contact with the dying survived. Walworth called upon his audience to think about those "fearless men" and "devoted" women "and then say is not the dreaded Cholera disarmed of nearly all of its terrors...for those who are strictly temperate in all things, and who rely upon the Almighty to sustain them in the faithful discharge of duty."[38]

Loud condemnations of alcohol found support in a steady stream of medical writings published in the interregnum between the pandemic's first and second wave. Only Drake's account of the Cincinnati outbreak bucked the consensus view. Dr. Hunting Sherrill of Poughkeepsie, for example, recorded that, in the fully formed cases he and his peers treated, only one in twenty resulted in death. "The fatal cases," he claimed, "were all of intemperate habits, or very unfavourable ones." He further explained that the mild heroic treatments were enough to cure temperate patients, but physicians had to resort to larger bloodlettings and "liberal doses of calomel and opium" for "those of intemperate habits and impaired constitutions."[39]

Thomas Spencer of Utica and Samuel Jackson of Philadelphia offered more detailed explanations for the differential outcomes between the intoxicated and the sober. Spencer found that for prudent and healthy people coming down with the disease, "a few grains of calomel" and induction of vomiting would "in a great measure disarm [cholera] of its terrors."[40] Drunkards stood little chance. They had become inured to the frequent diarrhea that accompanied their inebriation and thus remained unaware when the more serious disease set in. If physicians came to their rescue, it was often too late. In the hospital that Jackson oversaw, sixty-nine patients received treatment. Twenty of them died, with fourteen of the deaths occurring within a day after arrival.[41] The Philadelphia doctor explained that these patients were "from the very lowest portion of society" who were "scarcely conscious of the first approach of disease."[42] Predisposing factors, especially "gross intemperance," caused them to advance very rapidly to the final stage of the disease, in which heroic interventions were futile. "No one can boast of more than few and scattered triumphs," he admitted.[43] Meanwhile, Jackson attended fifty-five patients in their homes. Because they were "of perfectly temperate habits, of easy circumstances, and regular lives," medicines had "their desired effects" and all but one individual survived.[44]

Dr. David Meredith Reese of New York City made the most explicit indictment of alcohol. Reese had reason to believe himself to be an expert on cholera. During the summer of 1832, he attended to ill patients, took case histories, and observed autopsies on the pandemic's victims. He tracked the disease as newspapers reported on its movements across the United States, and he analyzed the writings of his peers that proliferated in the wake of the scourge's first wave. As he did, he prepared his own massively titled book, *A Plain and Practical Treatise on the Epidemic Cholera, as it Prevailed in the City of New York, in the Summer of 1832, Including its Nature, Causes, Treatment, and Prevention. Designed for Popular Instruction. To Which Is Added, by Way of Appendix, A Brief Essay on the Medical Use of Ardent Spirits; Being an Attempt to Show That Alcohol Is as Unnecessary and Mischievous in Sickness as in Health.*[45] Released in May 1833, Reese's work was advertised for sale by booksellers in multiple cities and towns throughout the nation. The New York *Spectator* praised the work, explaining to potential readers that it would show that cholera "is entirely manageable, and will therefore tend to diminish the terrors of those who may experience its attacks."[46]

Reese left no doubt about the key step for robbing cholera of its frightening power. Even to the general public, he declared, the connection "between Rum and Cholera became so apparent in the course of the disease in this city and elsewhere, that it needs not the testimony of the faculty in any place to declare and maintain it."[47] Fear, poor diets, and filth, to be sure, allowed the noncontagious disease to take hold of individuals. But even those in comfortable circumstances made themselves vulnerable by imbibing even small amounts of alcohol. "In some melancholy instances," the doctor supposedly observed, "a little crackers and cheese, with a glass of beer or wine, taken before retiring at night, has developed the disease in a fatal form before morning, and in persons who were not previously sensibly indisposed."[48] Reese warned that if authorities continued "to sanction the sale and use of spiritous liquors" amid cholera's return, then "we may expect a repetition of the calamitous results which spread such a gloom over our city and country during the last summer."[49]

Reese emphatically claimed that in no instances did liquor promote health, not even as an additive to New York City's notoriously bad water. Whatever was in the city's water, the doctor stated, was not as bad as alcohol, and consumers who added ardent spirits to it further jeopardized their health. This flew in the face of what many New Yorkers, especially thirsty laborers, observed. Many cholera victims were described as dropping dead soon after drinking municipal water. Alcoholic beverages seemed a safer alternative, and if city-supplied water had to be used, then it was best to mix some rum into it.[50] Reese decried what he thought were casual and lazy observations. Those who died after drinking the supposedly "villainous pump water," he claimed, were "intemperate foreigners" and native-born drunks who already had bellies full of booze. Their bodies could not stand the shock of cooling liquid ingested into their already weakened systems. "Among the hundreds of thousands who practice total abstinence from all intoxicating drinks, there cannot be an instance produced of death from drinking cold water," he boldly asserted.[51]

The temperance movement also found support from practitioners outside of the medical establishment, most notably Samuel Thomson and his followers. Thomson, a non-university-trained healer, frequently accused physicians of lining their pockets by purposely prolonging their patients' sicknesses with bloodletting and toxic drugs. Tapping into the anti-elitism of Jacksonian America, he marketed a system that ordinary people could use themselves. Steam baths to produce perspiration and plant-based substances to serve as purgatives or laxatives, he maintained, were best at restoring the body's natural balance.[52] As cholera spread across the nation, the pages of the *Thomsonian Recorder* were filled with testimonials about how botanicals and steam saved lives while calomel and laudanum accelerated death.[53] Thomson himself attributed the mass mortality to the medical establishment promoting fear, driving patients into their care, and then accelerating their deaths with their dangerous practices.[54]

Still, Thomsonians did not step far out of the mainstream in their thinking about cholera. Subscribers to the journal found no suggestions that the disease might be lurking in drinking water and instead read the common refrain that it was atmospheric in nature, preyed on the inebriated, and shunned people with "regular habits."[55] John Thomson, Samuel's son and a practitioner in Albany, to be sure, took issue with the NYSTS's "Authentic Report" signed by his city's medical staff. "My object is not to injure the temperance cause, for I believe it to be a good one," he explained when publicly criticizing his mainstream peers. He wondered, though, why his name was listed as providing medical care for twenty-two of the deceased individuals listed in the report while other doctors who lost patients were not identified. As many as five thousand Albanians may have taken his treatment, he claimed, boasting that his methods must have had a much higher success rate than those of his professionally trained peers. He also pointed out that the deceased who used his medicine were moderate to heavy drinkers, a class of people that no doctors, whether using botanicals or mercury, had success treating.[56]

Thomsonians continued their praise for the anti-alcohol movement throughout the first half of 1833. "Temperance societies have our best wishes for their ultimate success and triumph," the *Recorder*'s editors opined in April, "we mean ever to co-operate with them in bearing an uniform testimony against intemperance of every description."[57] Later, as the second wave of the pandemic rapidly accelerated, the editors reminded their readers that Samuel Thomson was an early advocate of the cause and "always pointed a nervous and determined veto against the drunkard and the dram-drinker." They added that the inebriated "have lost that dignified sense of moral propriety which give impulse and direction to ingenuous, honorable, rightminded men."[58]

The anti-alcohol crusade created a lot of noise and rapidly gained adherents. In 1831, a total of 170,000 Americans belonged to 2,200 individual temperance societies. In 1833, approximately one million Americans belonged to some six thousand distinct temperance organizations.[59] Missing from the clatter were serious reflections on the deaths of Judith Roosevelt, Peter Hoffman Cruse, Charles Ewing, and other elites who were not "supposed" to die from cholera. Ignored were the large numbers of Choctaws and enslaved people who perished not because of their own moral choices but because of those of their oppressors. Overlooked were Drake's insights that the impoverished died in larger proportions because of the fact that the affluent quickly fled when the scourge approached or erupted. Dismissed were the cries from New Orleans that cholera did not discriminate as advertised. And drowned out were ideas that pointed to cholera's true conduit in drinking water. Instead, most, if not all, temperance enthusiasts reinforced their preconceived notion that the scourge was a predator that could be avoided by laying off the booze.

One of those who took this message to heart was Angelina Grimké, Thomas's younger sister. Angelina developed strong anti-slavery views and moved from her family's home in Charleston in 1829 to join her sister Sarah in Philadelphia.[60] There, Angelina experienced heartbreak on October 10, 1832, when her suitor, Edward Bettle, died. His obituary did not indicate whether he had cholera, only indicating he "been seized with the attack of illness," held on for a couple of weeks, and then perished one day after he consented to "a remedy... of rather a painful character."[61] "Death has snatched from me one whom I had fondly hoped would my friend & counsellor, my help mate in best things," she recorded in her diary, "but my Heavenly Father

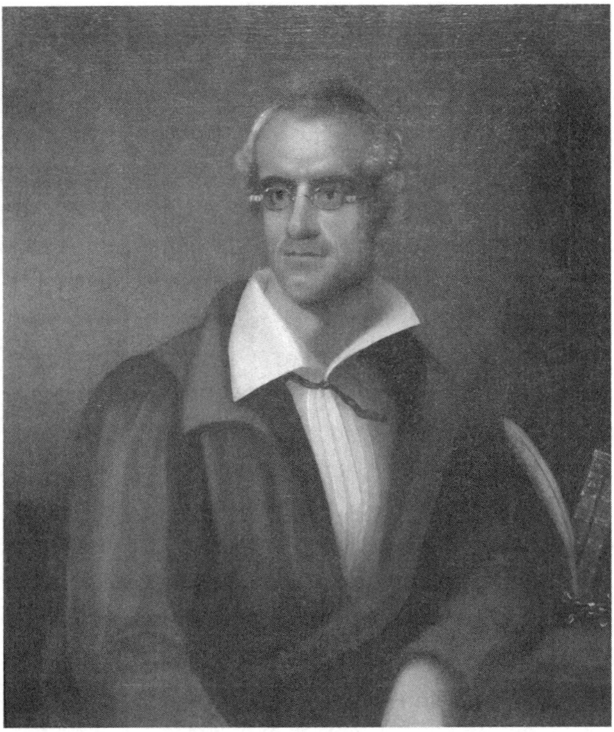

Portrait of Thomas Smith Grimké, 1834, by Abraham G. D. Tuthill. At the time when Thomas collaborated with his sisters Angelina and Sarah in getting his anti-alcohol tract edited and published, cholera was far from over and would inflict pain on many more American families, including their own. Image courtesy of Richard and Carole Cocks Art Museum at Miami University.

whom I love more than ever has in his wisdom & mercy left me to look up to him alone as my head & husband."[62]

Her brother helped her through this difficult time.[63] Angelina and Sarah edited Thomas's works, offered feedback, and arranged for their distribution in Philadelphia and beyond. He responded to Angelina's lengthy letters in which she offered her thoughts and asked theological questions. Despite their differences over slavery, they shared a perfectionist millennialism, one in which moral reform movements were leading individuals to abandon sin and gradually preparing the world for Christ's reign on earth. "I have no doubt that this is the brightest era the Church has yet seen," she effused to her brother after receiving his published temperance address. The 1830s was not a period of widespread persecution and execution that early Protestants suffered, she admitted, but it was a time in which "hundreds, perhaps thousands, who carry the spirit of martyrs about them & are now preparing the way for the universal reign of Truth & Righteousness in the earth."[64]

Cholera would continue to test Angelina's faith, as it would for thousands of other reform-minded Americans. As she wrote those lines, the second wave was exploding in the Lower Mississippi Valley and heading northward. It would wash over people who were enthusiastically celebrating temperance and basking in self-confidence that sobriety offered the best protection.

13

The Lessons of Lexington

THE SECOND WAVE, 1833

HENRY DUMESNIL LIVED long and eventually prospered. Born in Lexington, Kentucky, in 1820, he worked aboard steamboats as a clerk as a young adult, married Mary Ormsby (a member of one of Louisville's most prominent families) in 1846, had a series of ups and downs in his mercantile businesses in the Mississippi Valley, and settled permanently in Louisville after the Civil War. There, he invested in railroads and real estate and became wealthy. He even had a street named after him. Henry and Mary had seven children—one of whom became president of the Hydraulic Brick Company—and many grandchildren. Upon his death at the age of eighty-five, the Louisville *Herald* hailed him as "one of the oldest and most prominent citizens." The editors lauded him as "always going around doing good for suffering humanity."[1]

Dumesnil knew something about suffering. Just shy of thirteen years of age, he had escaped the 1833 Lexington cholera outbreak, but his father, Anthony, and mother, Molly, had not. "When the first case was announced, it looked to me like the town was to be deserted," Henry recounted in 1905 in his unpublished autobiography. "All around [us, people] were packing and crowding into carriages, wagons, etc. and fleeing to the country." [2] His family did not leave and paid a dear price; his sixty-one-year-old father, a prosperous silversmith, and fifty-four-year-old mother died within six hours of each other on June 11. It was "almost impossible to procure even boxes in which to bury the dead," Henry described. He and his sisters, Adelaide and Sarah, however, managed to obtain caskets, secure "a common cart" to transport them to the graveyard, and persuade six friends to attend the burial.[3]

Deprivation accompanied the heartache. Henry, Adelaide, and Sarah followed dietary advice and abstained from eating fruits and vegetables they grew in their garden, but they could not find enough bread and meat to purchase. They stood in long lines at the local bakery, which had to curtail production amid the calamity, and appreciated the small bundles of crackers that their Louisville relatives sent with a stage driver. Henry rode his horse into the country to buy provisions from farmers, who "seemed almost afraid to talk to me even at a distance of several hundred feet." He stopped at one farm that offered food for sale but had to leave the money at the gate, gallop off some distance, and return later to avoid human contact. After the outbreak subsided, he and his sisters were sent to live with relatives in Louisville.[4]

The Dumesnils were just one family among many to directly experience cholera's indiscriminate power during an explosive resurgence of the disease in 1833. As the weather grew warmer, *Vibrio* mushroomed again in New Orleans, swarmed up the Mississippi Valley, simultaneously branched both east and west, and covered a vast swath of the nation's western states and territories. Wherever it went, cholera presented clear evidence that it could produce unimagined mass mortality and could take Americans from all walks of life, even in Lexington, widely regarded as one of the healthiest cities in the nation. The Kentucky city's experience provided powerful lessons for Americans grappling with an invisible and mysterious global killer for a second year.

Vibrio again ravaged New Orleans. "On some days there have been upwards of a hundred deaths," Mary Bryan Harford exclaimed from the Crescent City on June 11, 1833. "The panic is excessive," she described, guessing that some would not stay even if offered "thousands" of dollars.[5] On June 12, hospitals filled up with patients and would not accept any more unless the city agreed to pay the expenses.[6] Letters from New Orleans painted a scene that was "truly awful." Refugees who escaped upriver said of cholera, "they cannot describe its horrors."[7] City officials again proved unable to assess the extent of the damage, but one reputable resident estimated that about one thousand people had died of cholera by early summer.[8]

Several New Orleanians believed the malady to be even less discriminating than it had been during the previous outbreak.[9] "This cholera is the darndest thing I ever did see," John Striker scrawled on June 21, 1833. "It has killed a number for us here of all kinds and all classes."[10] Dr. Michel Halphen thought he knew why cholera acted even less selectively during its resurgence. Back in the fall, the disease had struck when many departed their homes due to the prevailing yellow fever epidemic. The scourge's return in the spring, he claimed, occurred "when nobody was thinking of leaving."[11]

With New Orleans again a hot zone, *Vibrio* struck Louisiana plantations particularly hard. Edward Rawle recorded the deaths of nine enslaved workers—Litty, Old Bacchus, Toby, John, Elizabeth, Maria, Luke, Anna, and Tom—on an estate he managed nine miles above the city.[12] Rawles knew of another 220 enslaved people who had died on four different plantations near him.[13] One of those, owned by Colonel Proctor, was the horrific scene of 83 out of 150 captives being swept away within a seven-day period. "When it commenced there, it broke out so suddenly that the [white] family became so alarmed that they came directly to [New Orleans]," one Louisianan learned. "The negroes were left to themselves and some went to the lake [and] some ran into the woods, and having no one there to do anything for them in that horrible situation, many of them died."[14] Plantation records and newspapers recorded that another 262 enslaved people along with 40 white people died in Ascension, Iberville, West Feliciana, and Carrol parishes.[15] Cholera also spread west up the Red River and through Rapides Parish, causing a significant yet unrecorded number of losses among the enslaved population.[16] The pathogen continued to find new victims west of New Orleans along the Gulf Coast as well, where at least 343 deaths were reported by the fall.[17]

The number of deaths among Louisiana's enslaved population had reached catastrophic levels. The total since the beginning of the pandemic, according to one newspaper, was "estimated at not less than *ten thousand*; or about eight percent of the entire slave population of that state."[18] Editors of the New York *American* relayed the figures to a broader reading public and did the morbid math: "Valuing each slave at $400, which is not an exaggerated average, this would make the pecuniary loss alone of Louisiana *four millions*."[19]

The domestic commerce in human bodies in fact escalated because of the pandemic. Its first and second waves had taken so many enslaved lives that Louisiana planters successfully clamored for their state to rescind its ban on the interstate slave trade.[20] Franklin, Armfield, and Co. capitalized on the turn of events. The company again lost several captives to cholera during the second wave yet had even more buyers to bid up prices and offset their losses.[21]

The pandemic's resurgence also created widespread devastation in Mississippi. In Natchez, local infections began to pick up after the council expelled slave traders from the city. The sexton counted the burials of seventy-four cholera victims from April 17 to July 2.[22] At the outbreak's peak, the hospital refused to take cholera patients, fearing the disease would spread to their regular patients, leaving infected "indigent boatmen and paupers" stricken, with no place to go but the poorhouse. Most well-to-do residents fled the city.[23] Dozens more people died in Port Gibson, Vicksburg, and Amsterdam (now Edwards).[24] *Vibrio* penetrated the interior, where it slew Governor Abram Scott at his home in Jackson, along with an untold number of other individuals.[25] The enslaved population of the state sustained the most casualties. Editors of Natchez's *Mississippi Journal* guessed that as of mid-July, the number of captives who had perished in their state "cannot exceed one thousand" since cholera had arrived back in the fall.[26]

Cholera veered west from Mississippi and up the Arkansas Valley. Nine total passengers died aboard the *Reindeer* before it reached Fort Gibson, Indian Territory.[27] There the vessel's captain, David Miller, succumbed to the disease, and then eleven soldiers fell as well.[28] An unreported number of Cherokees who had voluntarily left their nation over the years and lived near Fort Gibson also sustained some losses.[29]

The extent to which the disease spread among Choctaws who had settled in Indian Territory is not clear. Many survivors of the 1832 fiasco had been immunized, and the disease likely did not find ideal conditions to spread among their new, scattered homesteads as it had when they were confined on the boats and encampments during their Trail of Tears. They suffered immensely from the deportation and resettlement process from causes other than, or in addition to, cholera. Approximately 20 percent of the Choctaws who had relocated to Indian Territory over the previous two years reportedly perished before the end of 1833.[30]

Back in the Mississippi Valley, cholera entered Memphis with some success. With its location on a bluff, Memphis did not appear to have local infections during the first wave. The high volume of traffic as the weather grew warmer in 1833, however, made it easier for the pathogen to stay in the city and spread among residents.[31] By July 26, the sexton had buried thirty-two cholera victims in a town that probably had a population of around one thousand people at the time.[32]

On the Missouri side of the river, on the single day of June 6, cholera killed nine people in Jackson, a small town near Cape Girardeau. The fatalities included United States Senator Alexander Buckner and his wife.[33] The senator, the press reported, did not receive medical care in time to survive, while his exhausted wife nursed him as best she could and then collapsed and died.[34] About fifty miles upriver, the pathogen invaded Ste. Genevieve, where it took forty people before burning out by the end of August.[35]

St. Louisans again saw cholera casualties in their midst. Colonel William McRee fell to the disease in the city in May and "was buried with military honors." He was widely regarded as a hero for his exploits in the War of 1812 and served as surveyor general of public lands in Missouri and Illinois at the time of his death.[36] The bulk of the fatalities occurred among newcomers, especially German immigrants who were arriving by the thousands.[37] City officials never counted cases, and a mass exodus did not happen this time.

It was a different story just to the west, in the Missouri River town of St. Charles. Sixty-two fatalities occurred there in rapid succession.[38] One resident expressed his dismay that the pestilence preyed on the "temperate, cleanly and excellent," whereas the "intemperate have scarce been touched." It became so bad, he moaned, that "you may literally smell death in the streets."[39]

Steamboats took *Vibrio* farther up the Missouri Valley. In early July, it hitched a ride on the *Yellowstone*, infected many of the crew along the way, and forced the vessel to stop at the mouth of the Kansas River. Residents there refused to allow the boat to stay and threatened to torch it if the captain did not steer it further upstream.[40] Nearby, the Reverend Isaac McCoy planned on conducting a baptismal ceremony for recently converted Lenapes, but they became so alarmed at the arrival of cholera that they "removed their ferry boat to prevent travelers from crossing to them."[41] Kickapoos, who had been removed to the area years earlier, refused to go into Fort Leavenworth to negotiate with the federal government for fear of the disease, which had incapacitated a number of soldiers there.[42]

Cholera traveled even further up the Missouri River. It struck the Bellevue Indian Agency, about fifteen miles south of present-day Omaha, where it debilitated federal agent John Dougherty and killed a number of employees, settlers, and traders congregated near the post. The farthest it was known to reach was a federal outpost, commanded by Major Joshua Pilcher, some fifteen miles north of Omaha. Except for an Indigenous Omaha man who worked at the Bellevue agency as a blacksmith and interpreter, no confirmation of cholera's presence in Indigenous villages in or near the Missouri Valley existed.[43]

As *Vibrio* branched into the west, it simultaneously moved north of St. Louis on both sides of the Mississippi. In Belleville, Illinois, the disease put Ninian Edwards in his grave. Edwards, Illinois's former governor, stayed in his hometown as the scourge approached and supposedly cared for others until he became too weakened to fight off the disease.[44] The total number of fatalities in Belleville went unrecorded. Carrollton, Illinois, lost thirty-three of its residents, and Quincy, Illinois, lost fifty.[45] Cholera extended its reach as high as Galena, Illinois, where it took sixteen lives within a thirty-hour period at the beginning of the summer.[46] Some thirty to forty people, mostly workers in the lead mines there, had perished by the time the outbreak ran its course (table 13.1).[47]

Palmyra, Missouri, suffered the most of any Mississippi Valley town. On June 3, nine or ten residents suddenly died in the recently incorporated town of seven hundred residents, and dozens succumbed over the next few days. Those who could escape the town did so.[48] By mid-June, cholera found no

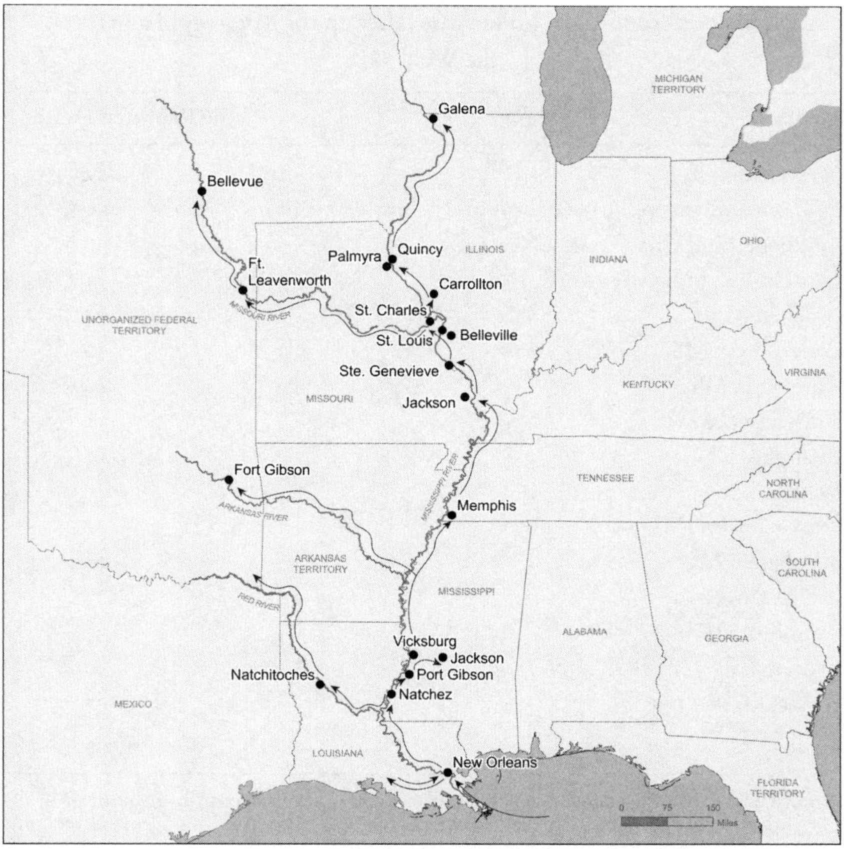

Resurgence in 1833: Up the Mississippi and into the West. Map by Franchesca Rodriguez, Geospatial Center, Stony Brook University.

more victims. The Palmyra *Courier* published a list of 104 deceased, which included the names of several prosperous men and women. "Whatever elsewhere, may have been its course, here at least its ravages have been indiscriminate," the editors said of the novel malady. "The virtuous and the vicious, the temperate and the intemperate, have alike been prostrated in its desolating march."[49]

Before *Vibrio* reached St. Louis, it had forked east, traveled on the Cumberland River, and made a violent foray into the heart of Tennessee. On April 19, the *Tobacco Plant* arrived in Nashville from New Orleans after eight people had died on its passage up the Mississippi. Alexander Porter, a wealthy Nashville real estate magnate, stock investor, and enslaver, got off the boat and proceeded overland. He only made it thirty miles before he, too,

Table 13.1 Reported Cholera Mortality up the Mississippi and into the West, 1833

Location	Reported Deaths
New Orleans, LA	1,000
Louisiana, Mississippi Valley, above and below New Orleans	531[a]
Louisiana, Gulf Coast west of New Orleans	343[a]
Fort Gibson, Indian Territory	21
Natchez, MS	74
Port Gibson, MS	10
Vicksburg, MS	44
Amsterdam, MS	10
Memphis, TN	32
Jackson, MO	6
Ste. Genevieve, MO	40
St. Charles, MO	62
Palmyra, MO	104
Carrollton, IL	33
Quincy, IL	50
Galena, IL	35
Total	2,395

[a] Most fatalities among enslaved people on plantations did not appear in the press or in the available records. These numbers, which are derived from the sources used in this chapter, necessarily fall far short of the total.

died of the disease.[50] The ill-fated vessel's arrival spurred rumors that cholera had taken hold of the city.[51] Still, only sporadic cases were reported through late May.

Cholera's flirtation with Nashville might have lolled its officials into complacency. An eruption of twenty cases, with seven terminating in death, occurred over the course of a day on May 28. The city's board of health did not convene, and the *National Banner* reported that with the continued prudence of its citizenry, the outbreak would quickly pass.[52]

It did not. Thirty-one deaths occurred between May 31 and June 3. Among the dead was Josiah Nichol, president of the Nashville branch of the United States Bank.[53] While he had "the temperance of his habits," which ought to have protected him from the scourge, he supposedly neglected premonitory symptoms and died on June 1.[54] Francis Porterfield, a wealthy merchant, died two days later. The *National Banner* described him as "one of our most enterprising, upright, liberal, and useful citizens" and could not find a reason to explain away his death. "In no instance since its appearance among us, has the cholera made a more sudden and rapid blow, than in the death of this worthy man," the editors explained.[55] "A general gloom pervades our town," Colonel Andrew Hynes informed an associate, adding that "the stillness of death pervades a great many of our business places."[56]

Nashville's outbreak may never have been as explosive as in other communities, but the steady toll that cholera took added up. Nineteen inmates fell to the disease in the state's penitentiary, which housed eighty total prisoners within the city's limits.[57] With those added to the number of residents who perished, a total of ninety-two people died from early May to June 20.[58] Again, what proved most shocking was not how many died but who died. As the outbreak began to abate, Thomas Yeatman, one of the richest men in the South, who had amassed a fortune as a cotton and tobacco merchant, iron foundry owner, transportation entrepreneur, and banker, climbed aboard a steamboat and would never return. Cholera took his life when he was two days away from the city.[59]

From Tennessee's capital, *Vibrio* devastated at least two small towns. Pulaski, a community of some one thousand people, lost sixty-nine, including a Presbyterian minister and a physician.[60] Forty people fell to the disease in Shelbyville between June 29 and July 1, including a doctor and his wife.[61] One resident explained that cholera "has been fatal to nearly all those who have been attacked" and that nobody had a cure for "the dreadful epidemic."[62] A mass exodus occurred, but many did not make it out in time before *Vibrio* found its way into their bodies. More than 109 of the town's 600 residents succumbed.[63] People could not find help burying their family members, and corpses were "rudely placed" in "exceedingly shallow" graves.[64]

While Tennessee suffered, *Vibrio* saturated the Ohio Valley. Steamboats dropped off sick and dying passengers in Louisville and Cincinnati into the summer. Immediate escalation, though, did not occur in either of these cities, because the previous year's scourge had immunized substantial portions of their respective populations.[65] The Louisville Board of Health did not do any daily reporting, while an uptick in mortality in Cincinnati during the week of July 16 led its health authorities to monitor and count cases and deaths for a short while.[66] Dr. Daniel Drake examined his city's sexton reports and counted a total of 370 burials of cholera victims from April through September.[67]

An almost imperceptible return of the scourge was not the case in Maysville, a Kentucky city of around three thousand on the Ohio River. When only three cases occurred there during a seven-day period before May 25, local authorities thought they would get off lightly, as they had the year before.[68] During a twenty-four hour period from May 29 to May 30, however, twenty cases suddenly erupted, with twelve terminating in death, including two respectable merchants.[69] Cholera's rapid escalation put people to flight in "terror," as one Kentuckian observed.[70] By the time the disease had run its course, sixty-seven residents had died.[71] "The disease has made no discrimination in its ravages . . . the prudent and the imprudent, the vigorous and the feeble," one resident described, "have fallen before the pestilence as the leaf is shaken by the wind."[72]

Vibrio forked from the Ohio into the Kanawha Valley. A Charleston, Virginia (now West Virginia), physician indicated that fifty cases occurred between May 26 and June 8 in the town of one thousand, with twelve of the cases terminating fatally.[73] People were "dying around us every day more or less with that fatal Epidemic, the Cholera," Dr. John Cabell remarked from his home some seven miles upriver.[74] One family left devastated was that of Charleston's postmaster, James Lewis, and his wife, Prudentia. On July 8, their six-year-old daughter, Wilhemina, died within six hours of being attacked by the illness, and the next day their eldest daughter, Letticia, followed her sister to the grave. While Letticia struggled for life, an express rider arrived at the Lewis home with a message that the scourge had just taken the life of Prudentia's sister Margaret. James and Prudentia packed themselves and their three remaining children, fled into the mountains, and remained there until they believed they could safely return.[75]

Further up the Ohio River, Wheeling received a severe blow. Sporadic cases occurred over the last half of May, and then suddenly the disease raged. Twenty people died during a twenty-four-hour period that ended on June 1.[76] "The old and young, the rich and the poor, are alike its victims," one correspondent declared after observing three days of heavy losses.[77] The city of about 3,500 people lost 153.[78] Eleven individuals died suddenly just across the river in Bridgeport, Ohio. All but fifty residents reportedly fled from the town, leaving unburied corpses behind them.[79]

With one exception, *Vibrio*'s eastward advance stopped at Pittsburgh, where only fifty-two deaths were recorded in that city of thirteen thousand people.[80] Pittsburgh had a five-year-old central waterworks that pumped water upstream from the city from the Allegheny and was thus largely free of the sewage that residents produced.[81] The scourge managed to make it over the mountains to the south and into the headwaters of the Potomac. Fifteen to twenty workers on the Chesapeake and Ohio Canal near Williamsport, Maryland, lost their lives to the disease in late June and early July.[82]

As cholera circulated up and down the Ohio, it branched away from the river and made its way to interior communities. Lexington, Kentucky, was its most surprising target. The city of approximately six thousand people had a reputation as one of the healthiest spots in North America.[83] Its boosters bragged that its elevated location kept it well drained and provided its residents with the freshest of air. Some cholera cases occurred in November 1832, and deaths happened to only a few transients.[84] The brief and relatively painless visitation seemed to confirm the belief that, if any place stood a chance against the scourge, it was Lexington.

Lexingtonians thus were caught off guard with a sudden explosion of cases during the first week of June 1833. Rumors of the disease percolated on the first day of the month, followed by a few confirmed cases over the next few days, and then twenty-seven fatalities occurring on the single day of June 6. The disease subsequently erupted throughout the town, and mortality grew to more than fifty on the ninth, surpassing the yearly average number of deaths in a single day.[85] Heavy daily losses occurred through the middle of the month.

Lexington proved more vulnerable than people thought because of its location atop the particularly porous surface that the city sat upon. Throughout the city, sinkholes existed, which ordinarily kept the city well drained by funneling surface water into caverns within a limestone base. Lexingtonians tapped these caverns to supply the numerous public and private wells that satisfied the population's needs. Rainfall was noted as particularly heavy during May and early June, leading Elkhorn Creek—the town's main form of drainage—to overflow and flush much of the waste it carried into the sinkholes. *Vibrio*-laden sewage thus made it into the city's drinking supply as the weather warmed, bacteria replicated to dangerous levels, and the deadly germs caused widespread infections.[86]

The number of highly respectable people who fell at the outset proved most startling. The deceased included Thomas Skillman, editor of the Presbyterian journal the *Western Luminary*; General Thomas Bodley, clerk of the district court; William Smith, clerk of the US Branch Bank and secretary of the local temperance society; Joseph Towler, cashier of the US Branch Bank; Joseph Ficklin, postmaster; Captain John Postlethwait, owner and manager of the city's main hotel; George Boswell, a prominent merchant; and three doctors—Drs. Boswell, Challen, and Steele.[87] The "city is all most depopulated by deaths and persons leaving," Sarah A. Bell observed on June 13. Her friend Miss Jane Anderson, sister of Captain William Anderson, had just succumbed to the disease, and Bell saw little hope that the outbreak would abate anytime soon. "There has been death all around us but through the mercy of our heavenly father our lives are still spared," she prayed to her sister.[88]

By June 20, the outbreak had subsided to the point where businesses began to reopen. The Kentucky *Gazette* resumed its operations, and its June 22 issue published what it morbidly titled a "Catalogue of Deaths." "Mr.," "Mrs.," or "Miss" preceded several of the names of white people, denoting their perceived respectability. Also on the list were two ministers, four doctors, and three men with military titles. Free people of color were not accorded titles of respectability, but their full names were given. Enslaved people had their first name listed before that of their owner. Inmates in the Lunatic Asylum, where the disease spread rapidly and thoroughly, were also named. Perhaps most surprising was that only one person—"Mr. Thompson"—had the term "stranger" next to his name. Altogether 381 names were listed, but the editors believed that the true number of deaths to be "about 400" as several people likely died soon after leaving town.[89]

Some smaller communities in Kentucky's interior suffered proportionally higher losses. In Flemingsburg, a town of about seven hundred people, sixty-three fell to the disease.[90] John Rogers, an itinerant preacher in the nearby village of Carlisle, recorded that twenty perished near him in June. His family escaped infection but not fear. "To say I felt no alarm, during its prevalence, would be a vain boast, as well as false," he admitted.[91] In nearby Paris, the postmaster's wife, children of a local doctor, and General Roger Williams were among the first to fall.[92] By July 5, a total of 133 people had perished in and around the Kentucky town of 1,300. Nine died in the nearby village of Millersburg, nineteen at Flat Run, and twenty at Centerville.[93]

Vibrio infested Georgetown. It killed thirty-two in the town before the end of June and then spread to the nearby Choctaw Academy, an Indian boarding school on US Senator Richard M. Johnson's property.[94] Twenty-four of the two hundred people associated with the school perished, including one Miami, two Seminole, and six Choctaw students; a white employee; and fourteen enslaved people, including Julia Chinn, the mother of Senator Johnson's two biracial daughters.[95]

In Harrodsburg, the pathogen took thirty to forty people within a matter of two days.[96] Among those who died was a member of the Corlis family. Back in July 1832, John Corlis had received a letter from his friend Otis Ammidon of Philadelphia. "It is a remarkable fact that in almost every instance it attacks the Intemperate & the filthy," Ammidon recited as the first wave began. "The finger of God is directing it to sweep from the face of the earth the dissolute & abominable."[97] At the time, John's son Joseph was a Presbyterian teacher in Harrodsburg and eager to work as a missionary among Indigenous peoples. He would never get that chance. A year later, John Corlis wrote back to Ammidon, informing him that the supposedly discriminating scourge had taken Joseph. His son, according to his father, had stayed in Harrodsburg, "where he believed it was his duty to remain nursing the sick."[98] Ammidon wrote back—this time with no reference to cholera's predilection for dirty drunks—and expressed his belief in Joseph's salvation. He told his Harrodsburg friend that Joseph "was leaving a World of Sin & trouble for a world of eternal happiness beyond the Grave."[99]

The deadly bacteria reaped another harvest of victims in Danville. The first cases in the town of 850 people occurred among enslaved people who, according to the local resident Joseph Huber, "had a clandestine party," feasted "on forbidden trash," and refused to reveal their symptoms "for fear of having to take medicine."[100] Soon thereafter, Sidney Clay, a friend in Paris, Kentucky, wrote to Huber to tell him that the Clay family had stayed at home and fortunately escaped cholera's ravages. "I cannot say the same of mine," Huber responded to his correspondent. His wife died after exhausting herself "visiting & administering help or comfort to the sick."[101] The Reverend Kerr, principal of the Kentucky Asylum for the Tuition of the Deaf and Dumb, and his wife also perished.[102] Fortunately, none of the pupils were reported as victims, but fifty people in Danville ended up in graves.[103]

Lancaster, a town of 570 people, had the most tragic death toll. Thirty-two people, including "the most esteemed members of society," fell to the disease between June 19 and 22.[104] "In one instance, the entire family deserted their house, leaving its head dead & unburied," Senator Henry Clay learned from a constituent.[105] "It seemed to baffle all medical aid, and . . . no case was cured," a resident exclaimed. "I believe that greater mortality has not attended it any where in the United States."[106] The resident may have been correct. Cholera took the lives of 116 from the town, a loss of more than 20 percent.[107]

Springfield was the scene of similar horror.[108] "We have attempted to account for the death of many persons, who seemed to have the promise of longer days than some of the survivors," a subscriber to the *Western Luminary* lamented. "But most of such efforts were in vain. Death has moved over us like a despot king, giving and leaving no reasons for his mysterious havoc." Many of the deceased went without funerals. The Presbyterian church lost twelve members. Eighty people died up to July 13, which represented 14 percent of the town's population of 650.[109]

Cholera penetrated as far into the interior of the Bluegrass State as Greensburg.[110] Hector Green entered the town in early July, passed by the graveyard, and observed multiple burials taking place. "There was not a house of business open," he described, adding "the inhabitants all looked as if they expected the next moment would be their last."[111] Forty-one total fatalities occurred in the town of around 669 people.[112]

Although not as widespread as to the south, *Vibrio* found its way into some communities north of the Ohio River. A total of ninety-two fatalities, including eleven in the state penitentiary, were recorded in Columbus, Ohio, before the board declared an end to the outbreak on September 29.[113] A resident privately claimed that cholera had only "somewhat abated" and that city officials undercounted the number of deaths, which he believed reached close to 150 by October 7.[114]

Salem, Indiana, a town of eight hundred to one thousand people, suffered even greater per capita losses. Sixty-two residents died in rapid succession in early July, and twenty-three died while in flight from the town.[115] At the beginning of the outbreak, Salem resident James McCoy wrote to his brother Rice, expressing "a fearful foreboding" but giving no indication that his large family would leave. Rice lamented that his brother chose to stay and attend to the sick. Cholera took James, his wife, Nancy, and their son Milton to their graves, leaving the surviving children to be divided up and sent to live among family members in Indiana and Kansas. Rice McCoy summed up the experience as one in which "good citizens were generally taken." He made no reference to intemperance or imprudence.[116]

A severe episode occurred in Jacksonville, Illinois, as well. The Reverend John M. Ellis was absent from the town in mid-July when cases began, and when he returned home, he entered his church and heard one of his parishioners praying for him. The content of the prayer made him fall to "the floor as if he had been struck by a butcher's ax." He learned that his wife Frances, son John, and daughter Frances had been quickly taken to their graves.[117] A professor at the local college heard nothing but cries for help. "The doctor! The doctor! For Heavan's sake, sir, can't you tell me where is the doctor," he remembered hearing. "My father is dying, my wife is dead, and my children are dying."[118] Fifty-three people died in the town up to August 14, and many more were suspected of perishing during their flight from the town (table 13.2).[119] A doctor from another town observed the outbreak and stuck to the standard line that "moral causes" led to cholera's devastation.

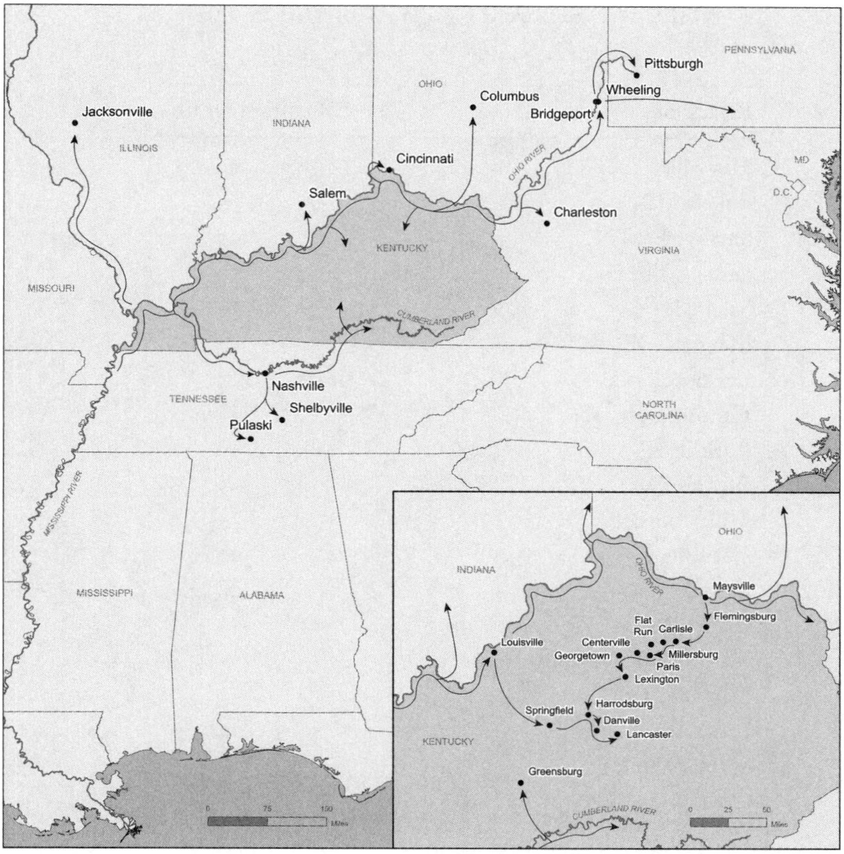

Resurgence in 1833: Up the Tennessee and Ohio. Map by Franchesca Rodriguez, Geospatial Center, Stony Brook University.

A Jacksonville paper retorted, "The timid and the bold, the temperate and the intemperate, the moral and the vicious, none, none, can claim exemption from this liability."[120]

Cholera's dramatic resurgence in 1833, particularly its rampage through Kentucky, shocked some Americans. "It is like the returns of the killed after a dreadful battle," editors of the Washington *Globe* commented after reading the widely circulated list of Lexington's dead. "Among those who have fallen, we recognize many of the most respectable citizens of the place—many young and healthy persons of both sexes—many of the most robust constitutions and temperate habits." The *Globe* suggested that "the general law of the disease, which confined it in a great degree to the poorer classes, has been inverted."

Table 13.2 Reported Cholera Mortality up the Tennessee and Ohio Valleys, 1833

Location	Reported Deaths
Nashville, TN	92
Pulaski, TN	69
Shelbyville, TN	109
Jacksonville, IL	53
Salem, IN	85
Maysville, KY	67
Lexington, KY	489
Flemingsburg, KY	63
Carlisle, KY	20
Paris, KY	133
Millersburg, KY	9
Flat Run, KY	19
Centerville, KY	20
Georgetown, KY	56
Harrodsburg, KY	35
Danville, KY	50
Lancaster, KY	116
Springfield, KY	83
Greensburg, KY	41
Cincinnati, OH	370
Columbus, OH	92
Bridgeport, OH	11
Charleston, VA (now WV)	12
Wheeling, VA (now WV)	153
Pittsburgh, PA	52
Williamsport, MD	18
Total	2,317

Included in this supposedly "new peculiarity in the history of the disease," the editors pointed out, was the fact that more white people perished than people of color. Only seven fatalities occurred among the numerous enslaved workers at the bag and rope factories, which seemed perplexing given "the multitudes" of laborers crowded into these plants.[121]

To counter suggestions of his city's deviation, Dr. Lunsford Yandell immediately and publicly wrote Lexington's experience into the pandemic's preconceived narrative. Yandell, a local physician and professor who received his MD from the University of Maryland, finished his essay by July 18 and rushed it into the delayed spring issue of the *Transylvania Journal of Medicine*, which he edited. It read much like the reports that had come out of New York, Philadelphia, and Baltimore the year before. The professor parsed the list of 381 official fatalities that occurred up to June 22 and pointed out that 25 were "lunatics" in the asylum. "It is unnecessary to speak of the liability of the . . . class to attacks of cholera," he dismissively wrote of them, adding vaguely, "there is every thing in their situation to predispose to it." He castigated the 168 people of color who fell to the disease as "filthy and careless, poor and ignorant" people who "nearly always live in low, damp, or ill ventilated houses." They neglected their symptoms and "inevitably" perished.[122] Yandell conversely used the observation of cholera's comparative absence from the rope and bagging factories to support his claim that people of color could not take care of themselves. At these plants, enslavers and overseers intervened at an early stage with heroic treatments that supposedly kept the disease at bay.[123]

The higher number of white people on the list of the dead posed the more perplexing problem. He solved it, however, with the same worn-out explanations, which clearly did not rest on any research. Some white people lived "in squalid wretchedness," and their vulnerability was obvious, while respectable victims consisted of those who had the usual predisposing causes: advanced age, prior illnesses, or intemperance "in the use of ardent spirits, or guilty of some excess, in eating, exercise, &c." Without giving any specific examples, he chalked up the deaths of the "few robust young persons" to "some indiscretion."[124]

Yandell's attempt to have Lexington teach the predictable lesson did not correspond with his and his wife Susan's personal experience. On June 11, the doctor himself came down with cholera, became bedridden, and started treatment from one of his colleagues.[125] Susan informed her father, David Wendel, about the turn of events but tried to reassure him that Lunsford was on the mend and that, so far, people whom she knew who had died had predisposing conditions or acted with great imprudence.[126]

It was a useful fiction to assuage the anxiety of her geographically distant father. Cholera had not discriminated in her city, and Lunsford was, in fact, much sicker than she let on. For twelve days, she could not pick up the pen to write to her father again. She had to run the household during a stressful time in which she observed her husband enduring painful spasms. He seemed to be at death's door, and she pondered what would become of her and their children and prayed continuously for his recovery.[127]

On June 24, 1833, she again wrote to her father and started with a cryptic apology for tardiness, explaining that "various things" had occupied her time. She did not reveal how sick Lunsford really was, other than to say that he "mends slowly" and had only within the last two days been able to resume his work. While glossing over details of her husband's ordeal, she was franker when discussing the horror that Lexingtonians had endured. Newspaper accounts, she admitted, had not been exaggerated, and among the list of the dead were respectable people. Many names did not even appear on the list, and she "confidently" estimated "that not fewer than 500 have fallen." "Such mortality has not been known on this continent," she declared. "In some cases, three were buried in one grave & numbers were put into any kind of a box that could be nailed together." She made no effort to explain away deaths as the result of underlying health problems or poor decisions.[128]

The disease had also persuaded Yandell's colleague Charles Wilkins Short that it was like nothing imagined before. Cholera, "that awful scourge of the human race," Short privately wrote to his Philadelphia uncle on June 16, "has proved more malignant, fatal, and indiscriminate in the selection of its victims in Lexington, than in any other town of the Union—perhaps the world." He acknowledged that Lexingtonians "rested in supposed security" because of the city's reputed "general healthfulness." The malady, however, acted "as if to mock the calculations of men." He knew many "respectable, sober, and useful citizens" who succumbed to the disease, including his neighbor Mr. Gratz and almost all members of his family. Meanwhile, he had "not heard of the death of one solitary drunkard!" He tracked cholera's course to Kentucky "with fearful apprehensions," he admitted, and confessed "that its horrors have surpassed my most horrific conceptions, and its mortality has baffled the best concerted and most boldly executed practice."[129]

Short wrote his uncle again one week later. He, too, believed that more than five hundred residents had perished. "Does not this go far to confute the reasonings of those who contend that Cholera is alone the product of malarious situations," he asked rhetorically, "and confined in its usages to the dirty hovels of wretchedness and want?"[130] Short observed sporadic cases of cholera occur through July and then disappear by the end of the month. The city council updated the previous list to give a final and official death toll. The scourge took the lives of 489 residents, comprising 229 white people, thirty-three white inmates in the Lunatic Asylum, 182 enslaved people, and forty-five free people of color. Lexington lost over 8 percent of its population.[131] Short believed even this was an undercount. He concluded that six hundred had perished, although it would be five more years before he publicly stated that figure and revealed to the reading public the lessons he learned about cholera during that terrible summer of 1833.[132]

Henry Dumesnil kept the lessons he learned for a lifetime. Memories of losing his parents in the Lexington outbreak remained vivid to him seventy-two years after the tragic event. In his autobiography, he demonstrated his gratitude to his sister Catherine and her husband, Bowes Reed McIlvaine, for welcoming him, Adalaide, and Sarah into their "happy home." Mr. McIlvaine, who passed in 1866, Dumesnil recorded appreciatively, "should ever be remembered and his memory cherished for his kindness to the orphan children."[133] When he left the McIlvaine home in 1837 to work on the notoriously dangerous steamboats, Dumesnil recalled his sister saying, "Henry I am afraid this is the last of you." Those words, Dumesnil wrote, "have rung in my ears ever since."[134] He survived steamboat accidents, yellow fever, another round of cholera in the 1850s, and business failures. He knew how arbitrary life could be and wondered why he, of all people, survived so long. "But why should I, yes even I, have been so . . . blest," he wrote, "and so many good and righteous people should be condemned to extreme suffering in this world." [135]

14

Back to Charleston

THE PANDEMIC ENDS, 1834, 1835, AND 1836

CHARLESTON'S THOMAS GRIMKÉ departed from home in the summer of 1834. His publications on temperance, pacifism, and education had earned him invitations to speak to audiences both near and distant, including the Erodelphian Society of Miami University in Oxford, Ohio.[1] That he could visit his brother Frederick in Columbus almost certainly influenced his decision to accept the invitation.

His journey began near the midpoint of the pandemic. A third wave engulfed a wide swath of territory in 1834. The disease branched from the Mississippi in the spring and scourged communities into the summer from the farthest reaches of the Ohio River to the western prairies of Kansas. It also recrossed the Atlantic from Europe, traveling westward along the Great Lakes and popping up on the Eastern Seaboard from Massachusetts to Georgia. In 1835, *Vibrio* traveled its familiar routes along western waterways, revisited some places it had been before, and found new paths into some previously unscathed communities. Yet it remained west of the Appalachians and fizzled out before summer ended. All seemed quiet through most of 1836, giving the nation hope that the pandemic had come to an end. But then cholera exploded in late August for one grand finale. Grimké's home city, which had up to that point escaped, became cholera's final counter to the delusive narrative constructed about it.

Like others with powerful voices, Grimké had not publicly expressed any doubt that cholera stuck to its preconceived script. Back in February 1833, he had echoed confidence that sobriety ensured safety. Cholera preyed on the inebriated and debauched, he assured his audience at Charleston's temperance celebration. His subsequently published address became noticed throughout the United States as the pandemic's second wave and its nondiscriminatory rampage swept the Trans-Appalachian West. When delivering his annual speech as president of the Charleston Temperance Society in February 1834, he did not specifically mention cholera, but he made the connection between alcohol and illness quite clear. "Intemperance," he declared, was "the great fountain of disease," and abstinence would rescue from death "tens of thousands of our fellow men!"[2]

As he made his way to Ohio, however, Grimké privately expressed some personal concern about cholera. He twice wrote Dr. Daniel Drake of Cincinnati, asking him if it was safe to continue with his travels, given the scourge's presence in Ohio.[3] He must have also worried about his wife, Sarah, and their six children in Charleston. He publicly professed that abstemious values protected people like him and his family, but he clearly had doubts.

As the weather of 1834 turned warm, *Vibrio* reascended the Mississippi Valley and its tributaries. Dozens of steamboat passengers perished from the disease before reaching their destinations, while plantation residents along the river found themselves under renewed threat.[4] The pathogen found some previously unscathed towns in Mississippi, Tennessee, Kentucky, and Illinois and inflicted the devastating damage it had repeatedly shown itself capable of producing.[5]

The pandemic also intersected once more with the deportations of Indigenous peoples, which had continued to be relentlessly conducted despite the process's obvious hazards. Lieutenant John Harris escorted a party of 550 Cherokees from Georgia during the spring, but more than eighty did not make it. Measles, whooping cough, and dysentery began to take a toll soon after the party departed, and then cholera killed around fifty of them just west of Little Rock, including a white doctor from Little Rock.[6] "I advised [the Cherokees] to write home to their friends, . . ." Harris informed his superiors after completing the journey, "telling them of their health, their welfare & their hopes, & pointing out faithfully the advantages of their present over their abandoned homes." He furthermore "impressed upon their minds that our misfortunes had been our destiny & that charity forbade our attaching censure to any human agent whatever."[7]

Cherokees who remained in the East were not persuaded.[8] Tom Foreman cited the recent experience as a warning to his countrymen not to take the money that administration officials offered for enrolling them in deportations. "These men might as well carry a poisoned cup to your mouths and say drink this & I will give you so much money," Foreman exclaimed. "Or let me give you money to allow me to kill you!"[9] Around sixteen thousand Cherokees would remain in the East until forced to leave in 1838.

Another party of westward travelers suffered severely. During the pandemic, the Mormons attempted to build their Kingdom of Zion near the town of Independence in Jackson County, Missouri. While mainstream Protestants preached that the disease called for individual reform that would gradually prepare the way for the millenium, Mormonism's founder and prophet, Joseph Smith, saw it as God's direct intervention to immediately destroy nonbelievers and bring the return of Jesus Christ.[10] The *Evening and Morning Star*, which the Mormons published in Independence, echoed Smith's teachings about the pandemic. "The time is short for the Gentiles; not a moment should be lost," the editors declared about non-Mormons at the height of the second wave. "It is the time to save men's souls, and . . . pray for deliverance while the destroying angel spreads the pestilence over the whole earth."[11]

The Mormons' views infuriated their neighbors in Missouri. On July 20, 1833, a mob attacked the *Evening and Morning Star*'s offices, destroyed the printing press, tarred and feathered two of the sect's leaders, and ordered members of the church to leave the county. Over the next three months, irate neighbors fired bullets into Mormon homes, set their hay bales on fire, and committed other violent acts against them. On November 3, a gunshot felled a Gentile. Members of the nonmainstream sect were blamed, and a mob destroyed more than two hundred Mormon houses and drove more than one thousand Mormons into Clay County.[12]

All of this happened against the backdrop of cholera's ravages. The *Yellowstone* had passed Independence with infected passengers back in early July and exacerbated tensions. The Baptist missionary Isaac McCoy characterized the Mormons as gleeful. "One of them, an intimate acquaintance of mine," the Baptist declared in a public statement, "appeared to be elated with hopes, that the accomplishment, of their predictions was now at hand; that this plague was for the destruction of the wicked, whilst they, the righteous, would escape." To be sure, the mob acted on many motives, which McCoy admitted, especially on the mistaken belief that the religious sect welcomed free people of color and aimed to destroy slavery. Mormon views that cholera was doing the Lord's work, the missionary described, "were too obvious to pass unnoticed."[13]

Mormons did not give up. During the first half of 1834, Joseph Smith gathered among his Michigan and Ohio followers an armed force of 205 men along with 25 women and children. They were ready to take back their Zion, by force if necessary.

Vibrio had other plans for them. In June, Smith's army crossed paths with cholera before entering Jackson County. On the morning of the twenty-fifth, dozens awoke in their encampment with the dreaded symptoms, and by nightfall several had died.[14] The victims, one survivor recalled, were "no strangers" but fellow believers who "were endeared to us by the tenderest ties that bind heart to heart and soul to soul."[15] Within a week's time, fifteen had perished at the camp and had been hastily buried in a nearby creek bank.[16] The prophet disbanded his army, and his followers gave up on their attempt to regain Jackson County.

Joseph Smith saw that God was teaching him and his followers a lesson. The Almighty had punished them, he charged, for their "fractious and unruly spirits."[17] Brigham Young, a member of the Mormon army, later used the experience as an example of God's power and the necessity of following the directives of church leaders.[18] In 1997, long after their final expulsion from the state of Missouri in 1839, Mormons erected a monument in Independence to memorialize the founding members of their church.[19] Like so many other Americans, they fell to a global killer that did not care if its victims were sober and righteous.

One month after striking the Mormons, *Vibrio* found another vulnerable group in the western prairies—the Osages. The Osage Nation, at one time, had dominated a vast area between the Missouri and Arkansas valleys. They planted crops in the valleys, hunted on the plains, and grew wealthy and powerful through voluminous trade with the French and Spanish. By 1834, however, their power had waned as the United States forcibly removed Indigenous peoples into western Missouri and western Arkansas and as Euro-American settlers followed. The federal government coerced the Osages to sign treaties that ceded land and kept their villages concentrated in southeastern Kansas and northeastern Oklahoma along the Neosho and Verdigris rivers. There, they struggled to produce sufficient harvests, frequently failed in their western hunts amid increasing competition, and had less to offer Euro-American traders for the goods that they needed. "You have brought poverty to us," the hungry Osages told a Presbyterian missionary.[20]

Vibrio thus found the Osages in a particularly vulnerable condition. On July 25, some returned to their villages on the upper Neosho River from settlements in Missouri. The Reverend Nathaniel Dodge, who worked in the nearby Boudinot Mission station, claimed they had gone "for whisky, which kept them in a general commotion & as soon as they returned cholera set in & carried them off by scores." Families scattered in all directions, but some never got the chance to leave. "Many of their Chiefs and head men are dead," Dodge reported. "Almost or quite whole families in some instances have been swept away in a sudden manner."[21]

The disease spread south, and on August 15 it broke out at the Hopefield mission in the Lower Neosho Valley. It quickly killed sixteen Osages and the superintendent of the station, Reverend William Montgomery.[22] His wife, Harriet, died a few days later, although the Reverend Abraham Redfield, who relayed the sad news, claimed her cause of death to be "bilious remittent fever."[23] Neither the missionaries nor federal agents in the area indicated any significant spread beyond the Osages, but the damage within that Indigenous nation had been severe, taking as many as four hundred lives before the outbreak burned itself out in September (table 14.1).[24] Not surprisingly, the

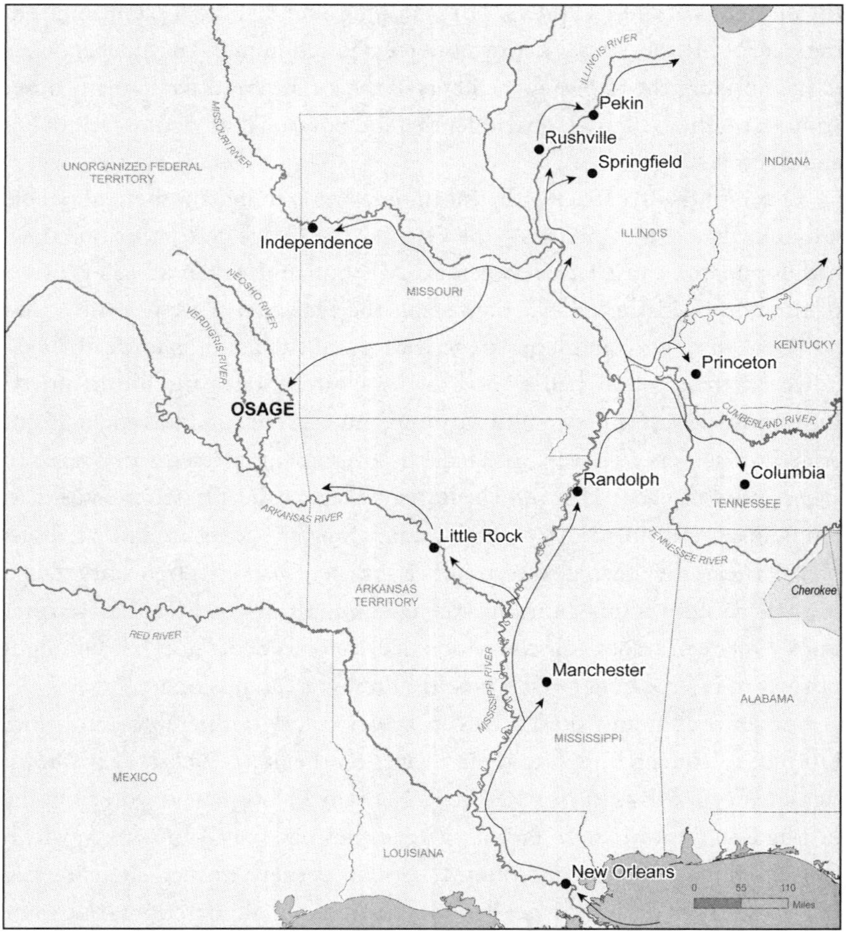

Third-Wave Outbreaks in the West, 1834. Map by Franchesca Rodriguez, Geospatial Center, Stony Brook University.

Table 14.1 Reported Cholera Mortality in the West, 1834

Location	Reported Deaths
Manchester (Yazoo City), MS	40
Randolph, TN	40
Columbia, TN	18
Princeton, KY	33
Cherokees on Arkansas River	50
Mormons in Jackson County, MO	15
Osages, Indian Territory	400
Springfield, IL	17
Rushville, IL	27
Pekin, IL	17
Total	657

Osages did not come back to the missions, and by 1837 Protestant missionaries had abandoned their efforts.[25]

While penetrating the western prairies, *Vibrio* advanced into the midsection of the country like two pincers. One was a continuation of the surge up the Mississippi, which veered eastward up the Ohio River and again reached Pittsburgh. Along the way, it swept through Fallston, Pennsylvania, where newspapers reported that a "virulent and destructive" disease came on quickly and led to the evacuation of "nearly the entire population."[26] The other pincer came from the east as trans-Atlantic shipping again brought the deadly bacteria from Europe.[27] The steadily increasing volume of steamboat traffic carried the pathogen through several places along the Great Lakes and took it all the way to the Menominees in what is today Wisconsin.[28] "The cholera was raging so badly that in many houses three or four were down with it at the same time," Father Theodorus van den Broek witnessed while working in the Indigenous nation. He and two nuns buried an untold number of the deceased, leading him to describe the disease as "so vehement that human assistance was no longer sufficient to help all." One stricken Menominee Catholic woman was out of reach and could not have the last sacrament administered to her. Witnesses saw her opening her mouth and giving the "sign of receiving Holy Communion" and striking her breast right before she died.[29]

Sandwiched between the two pincers was the state of Ohio, where cholera revisited some places and exacted devastating losses in new ones.[30] For example, a canal boat dropped off an incapacitated passenger at Zoar, where residents tried to nurse him back to health, to no avail. Local spread soon followed, leading to a total of fifty-six burials within a few weeks. Zoar had just three hundred residents, mostly German separatists who had founded the town seventeen years earlier.[31]

Detroit also got caught between the pincers and suffered even worse casualties than it had two years before. The population had boomed since 1832, and when cholera returned, it indiscriminately took victims from a large pool of nonimmune people.[32] Nearly one hundred people had perished within a few days in early August, including an associate editor of the *Courier*, a physician, a military officer, and a city alderman.[33] As the outbreak peaked, people desperate to protect themselves broke into a hearse house to take chloride of lime that had been warehoused there.[34] Aaron Hulin arrived in Detroit on September 17 and found a universal state of mourning. He visited the graveyard and learned that the deceased were not the poor, drunken wretches who were supposed to die but those who just "a few days before were

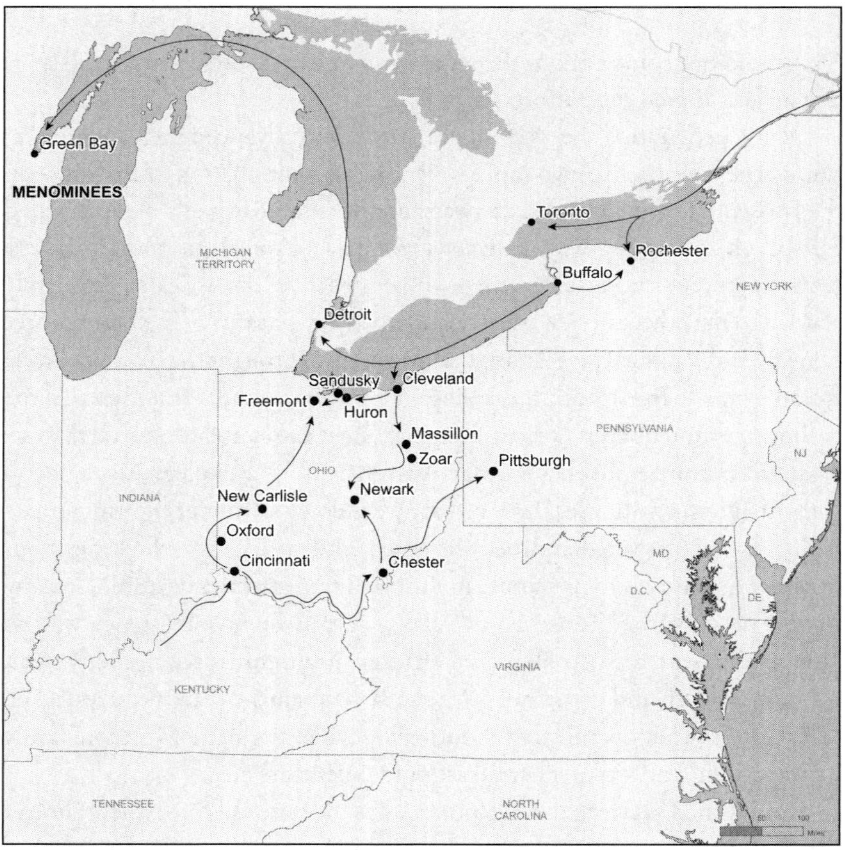

Third-Wave Outbreaks in the Midwest, 1834. Map by Franchesca Rodriguez, Geospatial Center, Stony Brook University.

Table 14.2 Reported Cholera Mortality in the Midwest, 1834

Location	Reported Deaths
Fulton, OH	35
Cincinnati, OH	55
Butler County, OH (Includes Oxford)	72
New Carlisle, OH	25
Chester, OH	10
Fallston, PA	19
Pittsburgh, PA	44
Rochester, NY	58
Buffalo, NY	182
Cleveland, OH	100
Massillon, OH	12
Zoar, OH	56
Huron, OH	43
Sandusky, OH	27
Lower Sandusky (Now Freemont), OH	15
Newark, OH	19
Detroit, Michigan Territory	350
Total	1,122

engaged in active & busy life!" They were "once possessed of tender feelings warm sensibilities & a good heart."[35] By the end of August, 350 among 5,000 people in the city had fallen to the disease (table 14.2).[36]

As the pathogen swirled in the West, outbreaks erupted in several places on the nation's Eastern Seaboard from Massachusetts to Georgia.[37] Since their subscribers were "beginning to talk about the Cholera again," the editors of the New York *Commercial Advertiser* suggested in late July, they should read Dr. David M. Reese's *Treatise on the Epidemic Cholera*. No one, they declared, had produced a better volume than him on "this appalling disease."[38] The scourge took sober victims during this return visit as well as its previous one, though, leaving the *Commercial Advertiser* to search for explanations. The editors described Justice William W. Cowan, who had died of cholera on August 17, as "temperate and regular in his habits, and perhaps as unlikely . . . to fall a victim to the malady, as any person that could be named in the city." An unnamed source assured them that Cowan had the misfortunate of "eating potatoes that had wilted."[39]

Vibrio found ideal conditions to proliferate in the Savannah Valley. On August 29, heavy rain poured on the area's rice plantations, and within two days, five enslaved people were taken on William Wightman's estate, some ten miles away from the city of Savannah.[40] Thereafter, outbreaks erupted on one planation after another in the area as well as the adjacent Ogeechee Valley.[41]

As if to give a warning to their readers of what might be coming their way, Charleston's editors published numerous letters from the cholera-stricken area. Readers of the *Courier* learned that cholera had burned through all enslaved workers and killed an untold number within ten days on P. T. Merchant's estate.[42] "The disease is extending in all directions," one observer claimed, including along the Carolina side of the river. "You can form no idea of the dreadful ravages of this scourge."[43] "It pains me to inform you that out of twenty-five cases on one plantation, four have died," an overseer wrote to his employer. "They were invaded so violently, and the collapse succeeded so immediately, that they were beyond hope in an hour from the time they were seized."[44]

Desperate for anything that would work, enslavers subjected their captives to a barrage of medical treatments. One letter from Georgia recorded, "the lancet [was] resorted to with good effect."[45] Physician Richard Arnold admitted he "felt stunned by [cholera's] rapid course" and found the use of camphor and opium to be "*positively dangerous*."[46] Yet he later claimed not to lose a patient when using other heroic methods.[47] One physician used a salt and mustard concoction, while another had his patients drink a saltwater emetic. "What has been used on one plantation with success," one observer noted, "failed on another."[48]

Along with the dire accounts of mass mortality came the predictable victim blaming. Heavy casualties, white overseers and physicians claimed, stemmed from the resistance of enslaved people to treatment. "This morning, at Dr. Daniel's, one of the women had absolutely to be run down, before she could be made to take medicine," one manager complained to his absentee employer, lamenting that "medicine half an hour before wou'd have probably saved her." The manager asserted he would remain vigilant in his efforts to prevent any more deaths, stating, "I dose if they complain of a finger's ache."[49] A doctor reported that on one plantation he saved all that he could administer treatment to, but some inevitably died because of lack of surveillance and their own supposed obstinance. "From the fatigue of the Nurses, the absence of the Overseer from the negro houses, and the singular aversion on the part of all to make known their illness," the doctor said of afflicted people, "they were by morning found beyond the possible action of medicine."[50]

In a letter to the editor of Savannah's *Georgian*, "Medicus" proclaimed that "boldly" administering calomel and bleeding would be effective, but administering such treatment on a plantation's captive labor force was challenging at best. "Their own prejudices, superstitions and reckless imprudences present so many obstacles in the way of the Physician," Medicus explained, "that he can have no plan properly effected." He further lambasted enslaved nurses as "incompetent." The anonymous doctor revealed that people of color did not share his faith in heroic medicine and that they would try to free their friends and loved ones from care that they (correctly) saw as ineffective and torturous. Planters, Medicus implored, should remove their ill to the woods, keep them under an armed guard, and thereby eliminate intercourse with healthy people who would "attempt to violate every indispensable prescription."[51]

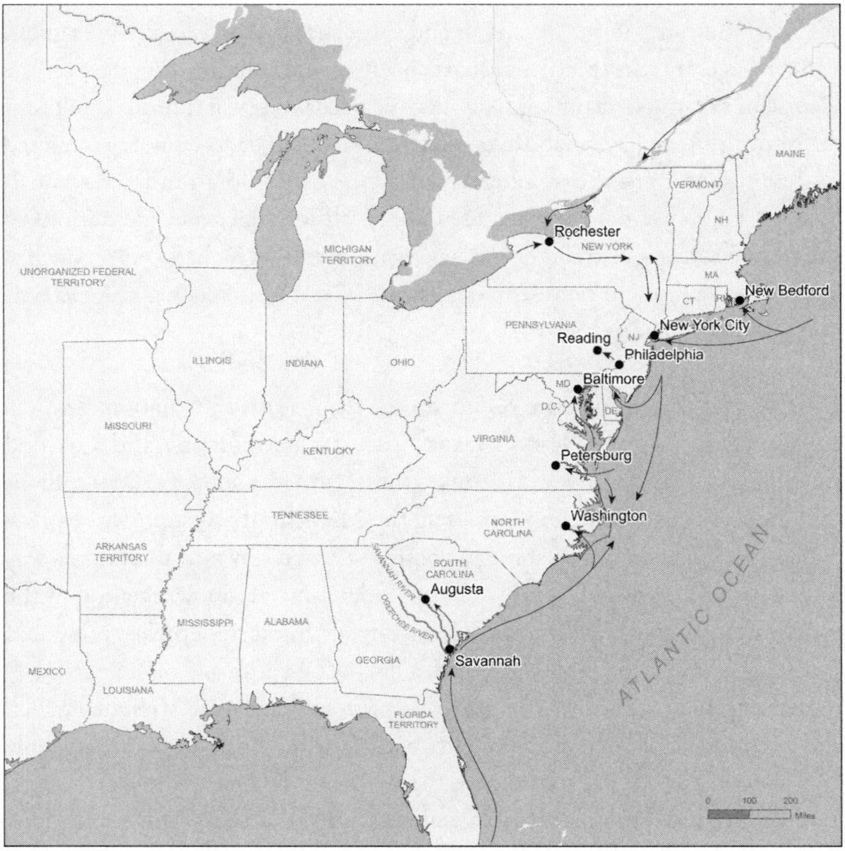

Third-Wave Phase on the Eastern Seaboard, 1834. Map by Franchesca Rodriguez, Geospatial Center, Stony Brook University.

Table 14.3 Reported Cholera Mortality in the East, 1834

Location	Reported Deaths
New Bedford, MA	9
New York City	1,021
Albany, NY	59
Poughkeepsie, NY	16
Savannah and Ogeechee Valleys	1,000
Philadelphia	151
Petersburg, VA	10
Baltimore	71
Total	2,337

Total mortality in the Savannah and Ogeechee valleys was anyone's guess. "The ravages of the pestilence have been terrific among the slaves," one Georgian remarked, claiming that "between six and seven hundred" fell to it on "about" fifteen Savannah River plantations.[52] A later assessment circulated in the press and put the number at an even seven hundred in the Savannah Valley.[53] Planter James Petigru added the deaths on Ogeechee plantations to the public totals and thought the aggregate number reached "near 1,000," a figure that he thought represented between 16 and 20 percent of the enslaved population (table 14.3).[54]

The spring of 1835 brought no respite for the pandemic-weary nation. Cholera continued to lurk in New Orleans, infected newcomers, and boarded steamboats headed upriver.[55] It took an unrecorded number of Memphians to their graves and branched out along the Mississippi's western and eastern tributaries.[56] It returned to some previously stricken towns and found its way to new prey. This fourth wave, to be sure, demonstrated a weakening in the pandemic's geographic reach and deadly impact, but it nonetheless presented shocking examples of cholera's power to defy expectations.[57]

Among the many towns to receive a visit was Palmyra, Missouri, which had been in the pandemic's crosshairs back in 1833. On June 14, four people died suddenly in the town, and with the horror of the first outbreak still fresh in their minds, residents fled. "An almost universal scattering took place, the inhabitants fleeing in every direction—in carriages, on horseback, on foot regardless of property or friends, or connections," one account described.

Seven out of every eight inhabitants reportedly took flight, leaving very few people for *Vibrio* to infect. Still, twenty people, some described as the town's "best citizens," perished.[58]

Vibrio produced its most significant mortality of 1835 in Russellville, Kentucky, a town of little more than one thousand people. The postmaster reported that sixty people died in just a four-day period in late July.[59] Another resident sent an urgent message to nearby Bowling Green that they had only one doctor in their town and "not an oz. of Calomel in the place."[60] The ensuing mass exodus included William Morton, who only made it as far as a bridge on the outskirts when debilitating symptoms set in. He died within a few hours after returning to his house.[61] James Burgess "became almost deranged" when the pathogen took away two of his children, leading him to flee with surviving members of his immediate family. He left three "apprentices" lying incapacitated in their beds.[62] All three were people of color, and they all perished.[63] They were not the only deceased left unattended in their homes and unburied for days.[64] Soon a list of the deceased circulated in the newspapers, and it included the names of some of the most "respectable" people in the town, including Charles Rhea, editor of the *Messenger*.[65]

The pathogen invaded the Russellville home of Louisa and Austin Caldwell. They lost two of their children and desperately tried to find a place of refuge for themselves, their surviving children, and their enslaved servants. Louisa called upon a relative who lived on a farm outside of the town. Her relative did not even open the door but instead shouted at them through the window that they should go back to town. She then went to the rural home of an acquaintance, but the owner would only allow the white people and one servant to enter. The family gave up and returned to their house, finding it looted and the disease lingering in their neighborhood. Austin contracted it and came close to death before recovering. Several of the Caldwells' enslaved people were not so fortunate. Mima and Jacob fell to the disease at some unknown point of the frantic experience, while Kenzia accompanied her enslavers throughout the entire ordeal, only to become one of the last casualties of the Russellville outbreak.[66]

When the Russellville *Messenger* resumed publication, it gave an estimate of the number of fatalities at "about 103." Mima, Jacob, and Kenzia's names did not appear in print.[67] The historian Nancy Baird later examined the records and counted 147 people, or about 15 percent of the entire town's population, as falling to cholera.[68]

Vibrio did quick and deadly work in Versailles a couple of weeks after it struck Russellville. Just twelve miles west of Lexington, the town of eight hundred to one thousand people had escaped the devasting 1833 wave.[69] On August 16, 1835, it suddenly became clear that its residents would not be so lucky again. That morning, dozens of people became sick, and by Monday evening, thirty-six had died. Amid the calamitous escalation, an express rider arrived in Lexington declaring that some of "the most respectable citizens" were stricken and imploring physicians to come help. Ten more people died on Tuesday.[70] Nine physicians from Lexington as well as three from Frankfort rushed to the neighboring town, but very few residents were left to attend to.[71] Like other terror-stricken communities, all who could flee the pestilence did so. The pathogen's failure to give early notice with premonitory symptoms, its rapidity in taking people to their graves, and its indiscriminate selection of victims, according to one resident, "added much to the horrors of the scene." Within a ten-day period, fifty-nine fatalities occurred (table 14.4).[72]

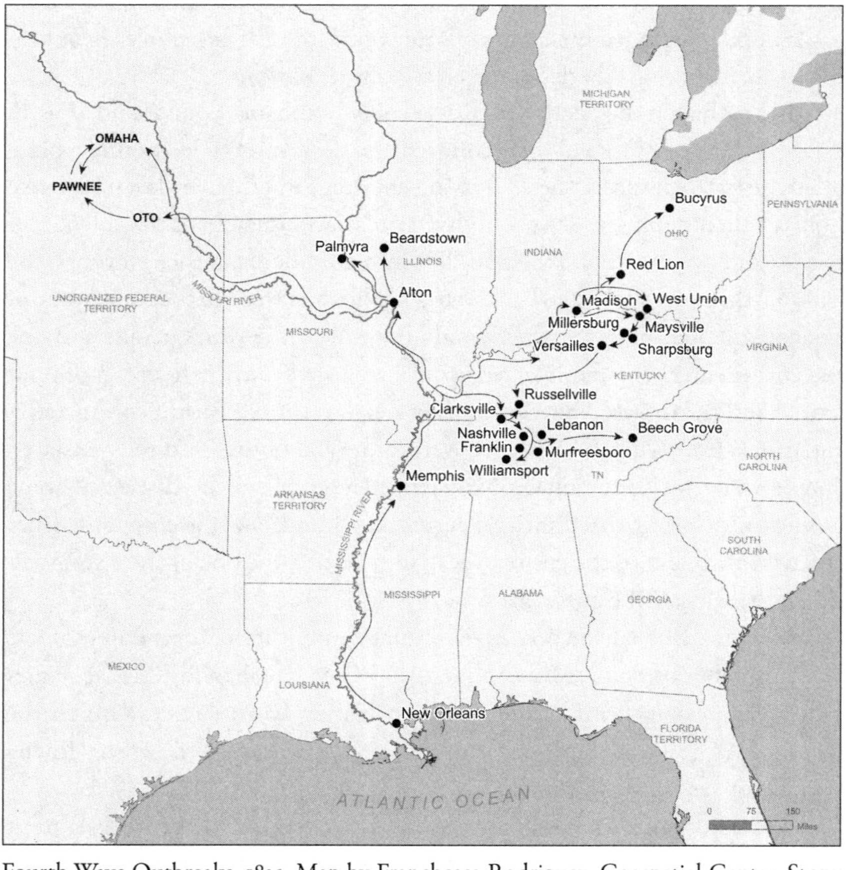

Fourth-Wave Outbreaks, 1835. Map by Franchesca Rodriguez, Geospatial Center, Stony Brook University.

Table 14.4 Reported Cholera Mortality, 1835

Location	Reported Deaths
New Orleans, LA	145
Alton, IL	21
Beardstown, IL	14
Palmyra, MO	20
Madison, IN	40
Red Lion, OH	18
Bucyrus, OH	9
Nashville, TN	60
Lebanon, TN	16
Murfreesboro, TN	30
Clarksville, TN	23
Franklin, TN	16
Beech Grove, TN	7
Williamsport, TN	19
Maysville, KY	30
Sharpsburg, KY	15
Millersburg, KY	11
Russellville, KY	147
Versailles, KY	59
Total	700

Soon after its sweep through Versailles, the 1835 wave evaporated. The pathogen's ascent up the Ohio stopped well short of the river's forks, it stayed away from the East Coast, and no major outbreak occurred in any state in the union in September or beyond. Vague news of an outbreak far to the west proved to be the last flicker of the year. A "gentleman" arrived in St. Louis on September 14 after descending the Missouri and told of cholera's "ravages among the Pawnee and Otto Indian tribes." He was not sure, but he thought that the pestilence had struck the neighboring Omaha people as well.[73] *Vibrio* had, in fact, plagued passengers on steamboats ascending the river in July, making the man's story plausible.[74] A letter from a military officer provided further confirmation. He had traveled from Fort Leavenworth to deliver the Otos and Omahas payments that the federal government owed them. "Both tribes were in very low spirits, having lost a great many last summer by the cholera," he reported. At an Omaha village in which he stayed, the officer heard mourners "crying constantly; sometimes twenty or thirty would be crying around our lodge at the same time."[75]

For months to come cholera news was eerily quiet. *Vibrio* went into its usual winter slumber and then failed to reemerge when warm weather came in 1836. Americans read no reports of the disease creeping up from New Orleans or breaking out in new places as they had during previous springs. Some newspapers even predicted an end to the pandemic.[76] "Having done its dread offices the minister of wrath seems to have been recalled," the *Gazette* of Alexandria, Virginia, asserted, "and leaves behind only the remembrance of the desolation that marked its progress and followed its path."[77]

Amid the calm, residents of Charleston, South Carolina, went about their usual summer routine. Many wealthy people left their urban homes for higher, drier, and cooler locations, while enslaved people and free people of color who were ordinarily a slight majority in the city composed an even larger portion of the resident population. Few of the city's thirty-one thousand residents probably expected any danger from a malady seemingly gone from the nation.

Cholera snuck in, however. It likely came aboard one or more ships that departed from Caribbean or Central American ports where *Vibrio* continued to proliferate. It found its way into the city and then, aided by late-August rains, washed into shallow wells that satiated the thirsts of the city's black majority and working-class white residents.[78] Elites, of course, customarily turned up their noses at these sources, as they supplied a smelly, foul-tasting brew, and instead relied upon cisterns, thus confining the earliest infections to the enslaved and impoverished.[79] The first cases may have, in fact, been invisible to civic leaders, who only slowly came to the realization that their city's turn with the global killer had begun.

By August 29, the outbreak had become obvious enough that T. Y. Simons, the chairman of the board of health, had to break the bad news. He did so with the same dismissiveness and victim blaming as municipal authorities in other large cities regularly displayed. He declared that "some" cholera cases had proved fatal, but "most of those who have suffered, have been irregular in their habits and intemperate, and many of them did not obtain medical aid until at a late period." He then listed shrimp and watermelon among the forbidden foods that the afflicted had supposedly consumed. The chairman stressed to residents the importance of temperance, prudence, and keeping calm and admonished enslavers to police the habits and bodies of their black workers.[80]

As the outbreak escalated, it increasingly took people it was not supposed to, but one would hardly know it by reading the city's newspapers. Charleston's press stuck to the narrative that the illness exclusively fell on people of color and poor white people and refrained from giving a cause of death to supposedly respectable people who died during the outbreak. A notice in both the *Courier* and *Mercury*, for example, invited friends and relatives to the funeral of William Debow at his mother's house on September 10.[81] His mother, Mary, passed one day after saying goodbye to her son, yet not until over two weeks later was there a rare public acknowledgment that cholera had taken their lives. The writer of a joint obituary, probably a family member, listed them as victims of "the prevailing epidemic," while remembering Mary as "a kind and affectionate mother [and] a good christian" and William as "a strictly upright man, and honorable in all his dealings beloved by all who knew him."[82]

Benjamin Elliot, a property broker whose transactions involved both land and enslaved people, passed the same day as Mary Debow did.[83] "Our community held no individual more amiable, upright and honorable," the editors of the *Mercury* said of him two days after his death, while omitting any reference to the cause.[84] An obituary published two weeks later vaguely referred to his surprising and unexpected passing, which had to make any reader suspect cholera. "The unerring hand of death striking at a shining mark, has laid him low," his eulogizers proclaimed, adding that he "ranked high amongst the highest in public esteem."[85]

The outbreak appeared to plateau during its third week. From the eleventh to the eighteenth, the board of health recorded thirty-seven deaths, only three more than the previous week.[86] Beliefs circulated, however, that city officials did not fully capture the novel malady's full impact. William Mazyck Porcher informed his acquaintance that doctors did not reveal all cases, despite the threat of a heavy fine, and that the number of deaths was probably three times larger than had been reported so far. He based his estimation on his observation of three "negro burial grounds" he lived in sight of. Porcher, a plantation owner and enslaver, could not fully comprehend what he observed, but he did touch on the profound grief that people of color must have felt. They experienced many "melancholy deaths," he described, as one-third to one-half of the cases quickly terminated in death. For his part, Porcher had grown "sick of the cursed thing" and hated "to meet any body for fear they may begin to talk about it."[87]

The city responded to aspersions to their failure to keep accurate records. On September 20, the city council passed a resolution that the board of health use sexton reports "of the several burial yards" to present a more accurate account of the outbreak's toll.[88] The outbreak, at least on paper, seemed to escalate. Total fatalities rose to fifty-one for the week that ended on the twenty-fifth.[89] Among the deceased was Frederick S. Elsworth, president of the Charleston Fire Engine Company, who passed on the twenty-first.

Company members publicly expressed their lament for "the sudden and early departure of their much respected associate" and remembered him for "his many amiable traits of character and conduct." Members would wear a mourning band on their left arm for a month. Neither the company's eulogy nor a funeral notice mentioned a cause of death, while a later obituary merely stated that he died of an illness "which was short but very painful."[90] The businessman Jacob Schirmer, in his diary, however, listed Elsworth as one of cholera's many victims.[91]

It is doubtful that the Charleston Board of Health ever had a clear view of the full scope of the unfolding tragedy. In many households, owners medicated themselves and the people they enslaved. Arthur Middleton, for example, informed his New York City relative that he had converted their kitchen into a hospital and replaced the drinking ware on their sideboard with "phials of every kind of mixture." He himself came down with "spasmodic symptoms" and at one point lost hope of seeing his relative again but had recovered enough to compose a letter. His brother, meanwhile, treated three of his enslaved people, with one dying and two surviving. This was proof enough to Arthur of the efficacy of medicine, when applied "within an hour of the attack."[92]

Other Charlestonians, however, had proved not to be proactive. Some enslavers lost between five and ten of their "servants," according to Middleton, and "still a good many whites also have been carried off." He specifically referred to the passing of Robert Gibbes. Middleton claimed cholera seized him after eating the "worst food for supper" on the night of September 24. He awoke the following morning with the terrible illness and was a corpse by nightfall.[93] Notices of the forty-nine-year-old Gibbes's death in local papers gave no cause for his demise.[94]

On September 26, the board of health recorded a one-day high of fourteen fatalities.[95] "*Cholera* today has been distressing," Jacob Schirmer recorded on September 27. "Persons hunting for Doctors in every direction."[96] Ninety-four deaths were recorded for the week that ended October 2, the highest weekly total of the calamity.[97] Almost certainly not counted in this sad record was Claudia Bull, the two-year-old daughter and only child of Mr. and Mrs. William Bull. She, along with five people the Bulls enslaved, perished during a forty-eight-hour period that ended on October 1. Again, her cause of death did not see the light of day, although people privately knew it to be cholera.[98]

October's cooling weather encouraged beliefs that the outbreak would rapidly wind to a close. The board of health decided to cease daily reporting on the fourth, after a noticeable abatement of cases.[99] The city council also tried to bring the outbreak to a visible end by stepping up efforts to police people of color. On October 8, the council outlawed certain mourning customs that free and enslaved black people practiced. They could only gather and "set up with any dead body" with permission of their owners or employers and then with the official approval of the city. In such cases, only a limited number of people could assemble, and the mourners had to conduct their "proceedings . . . in a quiet and orderly manner, so as not to disturb the neighbors."[100]

As was the case in other cities, the desire to declare an end to the outbreak preceded the actual finale. Cholera took its time, exacted mortality for several more weeks, and preyed upon surprising victims. Colonel George Warren Cross died on October 27 "after a short illness of scarcely twenty hours," according to his obituary. The fifty-three-year-old Cross had served as chairman of the Trustees of the Female Academy of South Carolina Society at the time of his death, and with his passing, his city "lost one of her best sons." The obituary further added that he had suffered from an "excessively" violent disease that "greatly aggravated" his loved ones.[101] Robert Dewar Bacot, then a student in New York, knew Cross well enough that his friend back in Charleston thought he ought to know of the man's passing. "I think he died of Cholera," Bacot's friend wrote, "but am not sure."[102] Bacot's cousin described the colonel's death as due to "a spasm in the stomach."[103]

Charleston had officially recognized 380 cholera deaths, with 59 being white people and 321 people of color.[104] The number was certainly an undercount, but by how much no one knows.

Several hundred more people perished on plantations in the South Carolina Lowcountry. Cholera took the lives of thirty-one people whom Thomas Capers enslaved on Daniel Island, on the opposite side of the Cooper River from Charleston.[105] Twenty-two enslaved people died on the Farr estate on the same island, and their names are known to us because white people had been fighting over possession of them after their owner had died years earlier. Dean, Mary, Bristol, Bella, Peter, Maria, Prince, Hannah, Lucy, Celia, Simon, Harry, and Bess were to go to Thomas Capers, but cholera cut their lives short. Another claimant was to get Quash, Lukey, Paul, Marcus, Pompey, Judy, Harriet, Tom, and Betty, but they, too, would not survive the pandemic.[106]

Vibrio found its way into plantations along the South and North Santee rivers. Colonel Thomas Pinckney and other absentee planters of the South Santee called on the services of the Charleston physician Dr. Thomas M. Logan to attend their enslaved workers. The doctor claimed great success. "The disease has become more manageable & I flatter myself that in a few days I shall have the pleasure of informing you of its disappearance," he wrote to an enslaver who employed him.[107] He arrived after cases had peaked and after overseers had moved most of their captive laborers to higher and drier pinelands, however, suggesting that few of the enslaved people he treated had active *Vibrio* infections. Like so many other Americans during the pandemic, they survived despite heroic medicine rather than because of it.

On October 28, Logan returned to Charleston and told the editors of the *Courier* that the scourge had "entirely disappeared" from the South Santee and that 178 enslaved people and two white people had died there from the disease.[108] About a week later, the *Courier* received reports that 245 enslaved people and two white people had perished on the North Santee.[109] With the known deaths on the Lowcountry plantations added to those that occurred in Charleston, the pandemic's final assault added another 862 fatalities to its morbid tally.

Thomas Grimké, his wife, Sarah, and their children were not among the fatalities reported to have happened in Grimké's home state in 1836. They nonetheless experienced cholera in a way that thousands of other American families did.

After leaving his home back in the summer of 1834, Grimké went through Philadelphia to visit his sisters and to deliver a couple of public talks, including an address on September 4 to the Young Men's Temperance Society.[110] On the eleventh, Grimké checked into a Pittsburgh hotel and wrote Daniel Drake for the second time, asking the doctor about the health of the Buckeye State.[111] The doctor responded that cholera outbreaks had ceased and it was safe to continue his journey, but Grimké did not wait around to receive the doctor's letter. The distinguished Charlestonian arrived in Cincinnati on September 20, when he met Drake in person for the first time.

Grimké was the toast of southern Ohio. On September 23, he delivered his address at Miami University championing the virtues of American discourse over that of classical Greek. On the twenty-fifth, he arrived back in Cincinnati and spent more than two weeks dining with local elites and delivering speeches, including a temperance address at Lyman Beecher's church. On October 10, Grimké's visit to Cincinnati came to a close. His brother was expecting him in Columbus, and he had to get on his way. That day, he and Drake had a meal together, "drank a glass of wine made on the neighboring hills," toasted "the perpetual union of Carolina and Ohio," and then said goodbye.

On October 11, Grimké awoke in Springfield, Ohio, after his long journey the day before. He boarded the stage and soon experienced a sudden urge to evacuate his bowels. After one unplanned stop, the driver could not take the rapidly deteriorating man any farther and dropped him off at a tavern twenty-five miles short of Columbus. The tavern owners provided a room and implored him to take some calomel. He refused, claiming he would not take the drug without advice from a doctor.[112] After more purging and cramping, he took a dose of laudanum that a fellow traveler offered him, and he fell into a stupor.[113] Meanwhile, his brother Frederick, who was awaiting his arrival in Columbus, greeted the incoming stage, learned why Thomas was not aboard, and frantically rode to see him. "He recognized me when I went up to his bedside," Frederick wrote, "and a lovely smile beamed upon his face when he saw me. But Oh it was only for a moment, he could hardly articulate only a few broken sentences expressive of acute pain he endured." He did not make it to daylight, perishing in the early morning hours of October 12.[114]

The Charleston *Courier*'s lengthy obituary appeared in newspapers throughout the nation. "Our community was yesterday filled with deep gloom and sorrow, by the melancholy and unlooked for tidings of the decease of this excellent and truly distinguished man," the *Courier* eulogized Grimké, who "fell a victim to a sudden and speedily fatal attack of the Asiatic Cholera." The newspaper lauded the reformer for his "literary and political performances, and his zeal and activity in the cause of religion, benevolence and human improvement," claiming him to be "a patriot, after the order of Washington."[115] While cholera remained firmly associated with intemperance in public discourse, no outlet tried to hide the fact that cholera had taken Grimké's life. None cast aspersions on his morality or invented an explanation for why such an esteemed man had succumbed to the disease.

Dr. Drake had the unenviable task of detailing Grimké's last weeks to his widow, Sarah, and explaining why he, of all people, had perished from such a loathsome disease. The physician thought nothing of the wine the two men had shared on the day of their separation and instead reassured Sarah that her husband had enthralled all who met him and had exercised the prudence expected from one with his status. "From the time of his arrival to that of his departure he enjoyed perfect health," the doctor explained. "At dinner he [ate] with a good appetite but temperately. I had no fears for him." Instead, Drake pointed to what he increasingly thought of as the most logical explanation for why cholera seemed to have come on suddenly. Rain, followed by a plunge in temperature on the day he left, threw his body into disequilibrium. "He rode all night, not I presume sufficiently protected from the change of weather," Drake explained, "and in the morning the fatal malady was awakened in his system."[116]

In wave after wave, the pandemic had continued to baffle Americans. Drake was no closer to an explanation for cholera than he had been back in October of 1832, and he could only chalk up the death of his friend to the weather. Grimké's wife and sisters may have taken some comfort in knowing that he had endeared himself to his Ohio hosts. That knowledge could not erase the sorrow they felt, however. "The awful scene of my Beloved's last moments are ever before me," Sarah wrote to her sister-in-law Angelina, "Oh my dear sister it is a harrowing thought that causes every pore to bleed." Her husband, she mourned, died "in a strange land, and (save a Brother at the close) friendless."[117] Angelina poured her grief into poetry, writing three pages of verse to her surviving brothers and sisters and three pages to her mother, revealing her anguish for later historians to read in the archive. To her mother, she wrote:

> Whilst journeying thro' this vale of tears.
> Well may thou query, who the void shall fill?
> Ah Mother, there are voids in human hearts,
> Which earthly objects <u>cannot</u> fill—there are losses
> Which the soul sustains, that <u>never</u> are supplied.[118]

The Grimké family's sorrow, of course, was not singular. Thomas's wife and children escaped the Charleston outbreak of 1836, and his sisters went on to become ardent abolitionists and pioneers in the women's rights movement, but Thomas's death certainly remained painful for the years to come. The Grimkés' mournful words could have been those of anyone who had lost a loved one to the scourge. A mysterious killer had been on the loose for five years. A diverse array of people fell to cholera, from those suffering the worst injustices of Jacksonian America to the affluent and confident who thought they could perfect the republic through individual reform. Survivors from all walks of life, including those whose voices were not left in the archives, were left to mourn loved ones whose lives cholera had cut tragically short.

Conclusion

AFTER CHOLERA DISAPPEARED from Charleston in the fall of 1836, it would remain away from the nation until 1848. In that year, *Vibrio* swept across Europe in another global pandemic, and by December, ships carrying infected passengers began to arrive in New Orleans. The pathogen surged up the Mississippi Valley in the first of several repetitive waves of the nation's second pandemic of the disease, an event that lasted into the 1850s. Cholera outbreaks again ravaged multiple communities and diverse peoples in all the nation's states and territories, from the far North to the Deep South and from the East Coast to California.

As the second pandemic began, old medical treatises published as early as 1832 were repackaged and reprinted. These promoted the familiar and flawed beliefs: atmospheric influences and miasma were still pointed to as the most likely cause; quarantines and travel restrictions were ridiculed as superstitious and ineffective; the filthy, debauched, and inebriated were warned that they would be singled out, while the temperate, prudent, and clean were comforted that their behavior protected them; and those who thought they were becoming ill were advised to seek out heroic medical intervention at the slightest indications of digestive unease. Ideas were again expressed and circulated that the enlightened and prosperous population of the United States would be in for a light blow. It was not to be, of course. *Vibrio* took thousands more American lives.[1]

Even Thomas Grimké's death back in 1834 had not discernibly altered the contest over the first pandemic's meaning. Anti-alcohol advocates lamented the loss of their fallen comrade, but cholera remained too useful to them in their war against liquor. J. Wilson's "Temperance Hymn," for example, continued to be sung into 1835. Originally composed in anticipation of 1834's jubilee day and published in the New York *Evangelist*, the new anthem

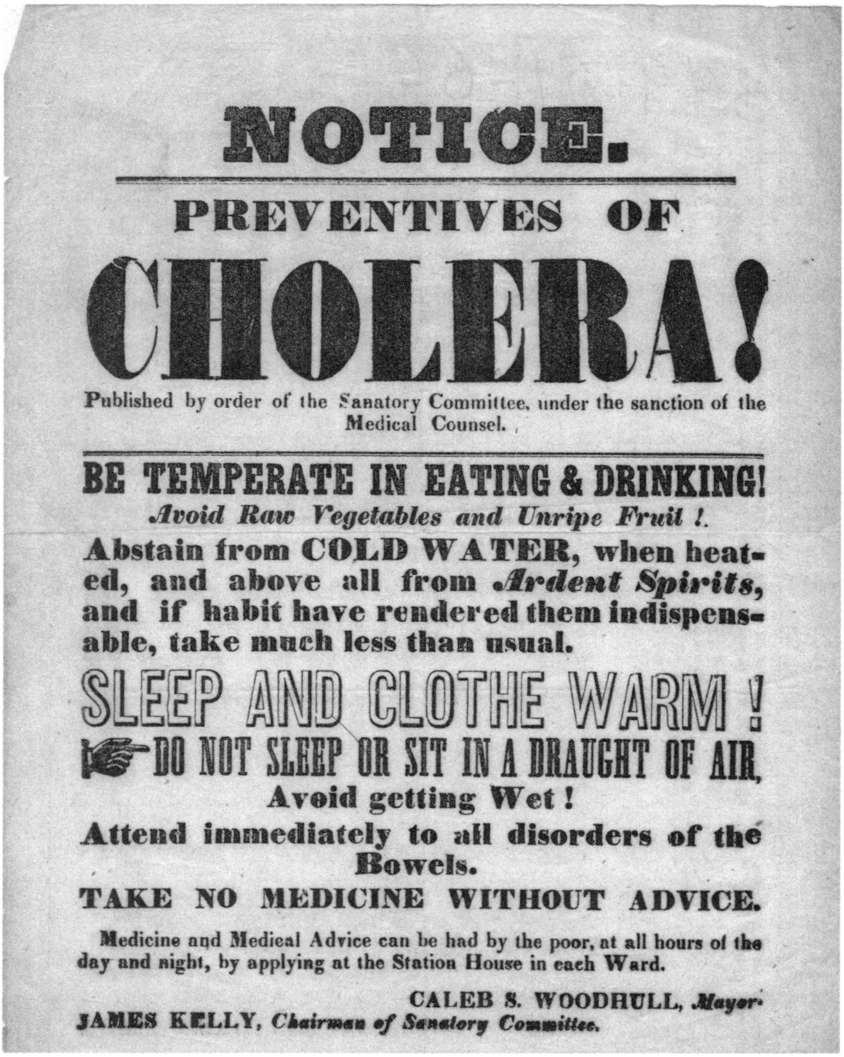
NOTICE.

PREVENTIVES OF

CHOLERA!

Published by order of the Sanatory Committee, under the sanction of the Medical Counsel.

BE TEMPERATE IN EATING & DRINKING!

Avoid Raw Vegetables and Unripe Fruit !.

Abstain from COLD WATER, when heated, and above all from *Ardent Spirits*, and if habit have rendered them indispensable, take much less than usual.

SLEEP AND CLOTHE WARM !

DO NOT SLEEP OR SIT IN A DRAUGHT OF AIR,

Avoid getting Wet !

Attend immediately to all disorders of the Bowels.

TAKE NO MEDICINE WITHOUT ADVICE.

Medicine and Medical Advice can be had by the poor, at all hours of the day and night, by applying at the Station House in each Ward.

CALEB S. WOODHULL, *Mayor.*

JAMES KELLY, *Chairman of Sanatory Committee.*

New York City Notice. Preventives of Cholera! Placard, 1849. When another pandemic reached the United States in the late 1840s, local health officials resorted to the same warnings about the disease that cast it in the same role it was presumed to have played during the previous decade. U.S. National Library of Medicine, 64730880R.

circulated widely.[2] It urged women to awake and speak out against liquor consumption and included in its fifth stanza a stark warning:

> Daughter of nations! the world is in mourning
> For hundreds of thousands by drunkenness slain!
> And millions of mortals to dust are returning,
> For *cholera* follows in alcohols train!!

Daughter of nations, the world is in mourning;
O let not the judgments of heaven be vain!

The reality that cholera was a mysterious disease that proved more indiscriminate than advertised could not displace the fantasy that the temperance movement had perpetuated.

The medical establishment joined the chorus. Dr. Reuben Dimond Mussey, for example, composed his "Essay on Ardent Spirits, and Its Substitutes as a Means of Invigorating Health" over the course of 1833. The Pennsylvania State Temperance Society offered a cash prize to the writer of the best dissertation on the origins and efficacy of the medical use of alcohol. Mussey, a University of Pennsylvania–trained MD and professor at Dartmouth College, submitted his work by the deadline of January 1, 1834, and then he waited. Over the next seven months, entries were read by nine judges, a virtual who's who of medicine and social reform in America at the time: Dr. Parker Cleaveland, professor of chemistry and materia medica at Bowdoin College; William Goodhill, senior editor of the *Genius of Temperance*; Van Brugh Livingston, scion of one of America's most famous families; Reverend W. W. Niles, an agent for the American Temperance Society; Dr. Thomas Sewall, professor of anatomy and physiology at Columbian College in Washington, DC; Dr. Benjamin Silliman, professor of chemistry at Yale College; Roberts Vaux, president of the Pennsylvania State Temperance Society; Dr. John C. Warren, professor of anatomy and surgery at Harvard University; and Reverend Francis Wayland, president of Brown University.

Mussey's efforts paid off. On July 17, 1834, the society announced that his submission was one of two winners. Each author would receive a $300 cash prize, and the two essays would be published.[3] Duff Green, editor and owner of the Washington newspaper the *United States Telegraph*, printed the winning pieces a year later in a single volume titled *Temperance Prize Essays*. The American Temperance Society also publicized the results of the competition and included excerpts from Mussey's work in its annual report for 1835, which were appended in the newly published compilation, *Permanent Temperance Documents*. His achievement was an early step in a long and successful career path that culminated in his presidency of the American Medical Association in 1850.

Mussey unsurprisingly argued that alcohol was never good, not even in small amounts used for medicinal purposes. Its habitual use, moreover, made one susceptible to all known diseases, including the most recent to afflict great harm on humanity. Cholera, he argued, provided the most "appalling evidence...of the pernicious influence of intoxicating liquors in preparing the human constitution for its attack."[4]

The Dartmouth professor employed frequently cited examples to make his case. In Russia, "persons given to drinking have been swept away like flies." "A physician of Warsaw" discovered that, out of every hundred cholera victims, ninety "had been addicted to the free use of ardent spirits." A "great proportion" of the thousands of fatalities in Paris "were intemperate or profligate." [5] In Montreal, "not a drunkard who has been attacked has recovered, and almost all the victims have been at least moderate drinkers."[6] In New York City's Park Street Hospital, only six individuals among the 204 cholera patients were found to be temperate. Albany provided Mussey's coup de grâce, as it did for so many other anti-alcohol crusaders. There, only two members of temperance societies could be supposedly counted among the city's cholera victims. Water, he concluded, was "the natural and proper drink of man," and adding even a little alcohol to it converted it into poison.[7]

From start to finish, the production of Mussey's essay unfolded amidst cholera's dark backdrop. The Dartmouth doctor never observed the deadly disease firsthand; his home state was among the few places to escape the pandemic's multiple waves. He nonetheless did his research and composed his essay with the traumas of 1832 fresh in people's minds and with a second round of *Vibrio* clobbering the Trans-Appalachian West. The contest's judges, moreover, evaluated his contribution as the third wave was finding new communities to victimize. Mussey's essay went to press and was incorporated into the permanent record of the American Temperance Society amid a fourth wave of the global killer.

With each round, the number of fatalities within the families of judges, doctors, ministers, editors, legislators, military officers, businessmen, and other elites added up. Numerous deaths among respectable women and men provided compelling evidence that cholera could inflict harm on anyone. Outbreaks in Cincinnati, New Orleans, and Lexington as well as in small towns, such as Palmyra and Russellville and numerous others, occurred in ways that confounded beliefs that prudence, temperance, and cleanliness would keep people safe. Mass mortality occurred among enslaved people who had neither the means nor the opportunity to drink liquor in significant quantities. The disease struck Indigenous peoples being deported west and those living on the prairies, demonstrating that the scourge would hardly be confined to the urban poor.

Contrary evidence and alternative explanations never seemed to cross Mussey's mind. As he wrote his essay, suggestions that cholera actually spread through the water had been made and could faintly be heard amid the anti-alcohol noise. His views, like those of many of his peers, had been firmly established before June 1832 and would not change as cholera defied expectations.

Praise for Mussey's essay bore out the endurance of the preconceived narrative of how the pandemic would unfold. "It is more likely to be long used as a text book . . . ," the New York *Observer* remarked about *Temperance Prize Essays*, "and to be of more *permanent* benefit than any work which has yet issued from our press on this subject."[8] *The Moral Reformer and Teacher on the Human Constitution*, a new health journal published in 1835, also heralded Mussey's work. A letter to the editor signed W. G. described cholera's victims succumbing to the desperate hope that alcohol would ward off illness, making their supposed cure worse than the disease. "*God of nature*," W. G. claimed, "first punished the *intemperate* of mankind by the *cholera*." The writer was impressed by Mussey's "array of facts that cannot be questioned, and arguments that cannot be resisted."[9] In an 1836 manual for the "young men of the United States," the American Temperance Society highlighted Mussey as an authority who proved cholera's predilection for the inebriated.[10]

Lucius M. Sargent, one of the most prolific temperance writers at the time, invoked Mussey's essay in his 1836 critique of Episcopal Bishop John H. Hopkins's defense of wine. Hopkins claimed that wine consumption in Spain, Italy, and France did not lead to ill social effects. "It is stated by Professor Mussey, in his prize essay," Sargent countered, that "a great proportion" of cholera victims "were intemperate or profligate."[11]

As the pandemic waned and then ceased, anti-alcohol crusaders continued to pinpoint alcohol consumption as the cause of cholera deaths, but they did some reframing. The disease may have been bad but not nearly as damaging as intoxicating beverages continued to be. In the introduction to its annual report for 1835, the American Temperance Society cast liquor as "more malignant than any other epidemic pestilence," being "far more loathsome, infectious and destructive" than typhus, smallpox, yellow fever, and cholera combined.[12] The Reverend William Ellery Channing, the leading figure in Unitarianism and outspoken opponent of habitual drinking, echoed this view. In his temperance jubilee address of 1837, he told a Boston audience that stamping out inebriation was more important than preparing for another "visitation" of disease.[13] Was alcohol, he rhetorically asked, "not an evil more terrible than pestilence, the actual, frequent result of the use of spirituous liquors?"[14]

With their need to promote the benefits of sobriety, temperance advocates belittled the significance of the pandemic. For example, in 1837 the

Pennsylvania State Temperance Society criticized Philadelphia's authorities for taking drunkenness's toll lightly in comparison to their response to cholera five years earlier. The organization wanted the state's constitution to be amended to allow for prohibition, and it used examples of unequal responses to different threats to public health. "The whole city trembled, and the note of preparation to meet the dreaded stranger was heard every where," the society claimed about the first wave of the pandemic. "But here we walk amid the dying and the dead by a more fearful plague, and no man is alarmed. Our fellow-citizens go down to a death from day to day infinitely more loathsome than by the cholera, and no man is concerned."[15]

One year later, delegates to the Western Reserve Temperance Convention in Ohio listed bubonic plague along with "Asiatic cholera" as dangers less deadly than the "retailing of alcoholic drinks," which they condemned as "vending delirium and poisoning human beings for wages."[16] Around the same time, the executive committee of the New York State Temperance Society complained that cholera's previous "sweep" along with gambling and other banes "combined, have not, in our beloved country, produced a tithe of the desolation and woe, the loss of property, health, reputation, happiness, and life" that the liquor trade had.[17]

No one, of course, knew for sure just how many Americans the pandemic had swept away, but it was certainly more than the 28,404 fatalities that can be tabulated from available sources (table 15.1). Many towns and cities quit reporting deaths before outbreaks ceased, did not monitor the pathogen when it returned, and spared a significant number of people from being forever remembered as dying from a disease that supposedly selected degraded victims. Much of the mortality among laborers in work zones, enslaved people on rural plantations, travelers between stops, and Indigenous peoples living in the prairies did not make it into known counts. Cholera also visited several small towns and villages throughout the nation and its territories

Table 15.1 Reported Cholera Mortality in the United States, 1832–1836

First Wave, 1832 (from table 10.1)	18,014
Second Wave, 1833 (from tables 13.1 and 13.2)	4,712
Third Wave, 1834 (from tables 14.1, 14.2, and 14.3)	4,116
Fourth Wave, 1835 (from table 14.4)	700
Fifth Wave, 1836 (Charleston, SC total)	862
Total	28,404

whose tragedies did not get the press's attention at the time or escaped historians' retrospective notice. The scourge certainly took at least thirty thousand lives and likely a few thousand more.

Incomplete knowledge of cholera's demographic toll should not obscure how terrifying cholera proved to be. It exacted mass mortality in short spans of time in several locations, especially in the small towns of Kentucky, Tennessee, and Missouri. In many cases, the proportion of populations lost in American cities and towns far exceeded that lost in European metropolises (table 15.2). Cholera demonstrated its power to cause terror and inflict trauma on numerous US communities in successive waves that Americans were happy to be done with.

Table 15.2 Population Losses in Select European, Canadian, and US Outbreaks

City/Town	Date	Population	Deaths	Percentage Loss
Lancaster, KY	1833	570	116	20.3
Zoar, OH	1834	300	56	18.7
Shelbyville, TN	1833	600	109	18.2
Palmyra, MO	1833	700	104	14.8
MONTREAL	1832	28,000	3,515	14.8
Russellville, KY	1835	1,000	147	14.7
QUEBEC CITY	1832	28,000	3,451	12.3
New Orleans	1832	57,000	6,000	10.5
Lexington, KY	1833	6,000	489	8.2
Detroit, Michigan Territory	1834	5,000	350	7.0
Norfolk, VA	1832	10,000	405	4.1
Richmond, VA	1832	17,000	478	4.1
PARIS, FRANCE [a]	1832	785,000	18,000	2.3
Cincinnati, OH	1832	30,000	571	1.9
New York City, NY	1832	225,000	3,515	1.6
MOSCOW, RUSSIA[b]	1830	305,000	4,588	1.5
SAINT PETERSBURG, RUSSIA[c]	1831	443,000	6,449	1.5
LONDON, UK[d]	1832	1,570,000	5,275	0.3

[a] Delaporte, *Disease and Civilization*, 5.

[b] McGrew, *Russian and the Cholera,* 88–89, 161 (outbreak ended in January 1831).

[c] Barabanova, "The First Cholera Epidemic in St. Petersburg"; McGrew, *Russia and the Cholera,* 123.

[d] D. Barry, "On the Statistics of Epidemic Cholera," in *Transactions of the Statistical Society of London,* vol. 1, pt. 1 (1837): 88; Durey, *The Return of the Plague*, 52.

Powerful public voices, however, continued to diminish the pandemic after it had ended just as they saw it before it began. It was nothing for Americans to fret much about in the first place but instead a selective predator that reinforced beliefs that morality and self-discipline were the key to America's democratic experiment. These voices tragically darkened the light shone on the nation's injustices and inequities, ignored the pain that tens of thousands of Americans suffered, and hid the horror that many people lived through.

Cholera still persuaded some people that it was something other than what it was scripted to be. Dr. Charles Wilkins Short of Lexington, Kentucky, added his voice to that of Dr. Daniel Drake in bucking the medical consensus but waited until five years after the scourge had ravaged his home city. His 1838 essay, "A Brief Historical Sketch of the Origin and Progress of Cholera Asphyxia," characterized the entire pandemic as a severe, unforgettable, and indelible event. "Its extensive prevalence; the rapidity of its movements; its great mortality; its disregard to all extraneous circumstances of time, place and situation," he argued about cholera, "are points in which it differs from, and exceeds all other pestilences which have ever devastated mankind."[18]

Short summarized the deadly malady's tour through his nation with remarkable candor. Some of his medical colleagues, he reminded readers, believed "that a loathsome disease, which had its origin in the poverty, filth and squalid wretchedness of the old world, would be disarmed of its terrors, so soon as it alighted on the land of Freemen."[19] Cholera's ravages in New York City, Cincinnati, and New Orleans in 1832 dispelled such "unfounded confidence," as did its impact on Lexington the following year. The doctor explained that he did not have space "to dwell on the horrors of the pestilence as they were manifested" in his home city, but he did feel "a sacred regard to truth" that forbid him from concealing "painful and humiliating confessions."[20]

Lexington's healthy reputation, Short maintained, gave his medical peers false confidence that the disease would not come. Yet the disease did come, and the city's hundreds of victims constituted "more than a decimation of its inhabitants." The scourge also laid bare "the slanderous reports" of "its selecting its victims alone from the poor, the profligate, and the intemperate." These beliefs "lulled" Lexingtonians "into fatal security" and resulted in "a larger number of sober, useful, and wealthy citizens" dying in higher proportion "than in any other town or city of the Union."[21] The same pattern happened in numerous small towns in Kentucky, Tennessee, Ohio, Indiana, and Missouri. The 1835 outbreak in Versailles, Kentucky, provided an especially vivid example of the falsity of expectations that the United States would only experience a light blow. "The onset there was perhaps as violent and sudden as any recorded in the annals of Cholera," Short concluded.[22]

The Kentucky medical professor did not even capture the full extent of the pandemic's ravages. He made a vague reference to mass mortality in Philadelphia's Arch Street Prison but did not mention the numerous other incarcerated people who had fallen to the disease. He did not include the terrible destruction that the disease had done to canal and railroad construction workers in Maryland, New Jersey, and Pennsylvania. He overlooked how devastating it had been to people of color in Virginia, Maryland, and the Deep South; he failed to acknowledge how catastrophic it had been for Choctaws and Cherokees being deported; and he omitted Charleston's experience, which had punctuated the pandemic. Dr. Short still knew cholera to be an "awful scourge" and never associated its wrath with a punishment inflicted on the habitual drinker. "It has gradually passed from our borders, never we trust to return," he hopefully concluded. [23]

Short's essay remained an anomaly, however. He had provided what appeared to be the last and ignored interpretation of the first pandemic. Between 1838 and 1848, American medical journals were largely devoid of anything other than descriptions of heroic therapies that supposedly had worked during the pandemic. It seemed most doctors wanted to put cholera behind them and hope, as Short did, that it would not return.

Many Americans did not have the luxury of forgetting. The Reverend John Scripps of Rushville, Illinois, was one of these individuals. Cholera broke out in his town on Friday, July 4, 1834, killing eleven people within four days and causing an estimated seven hundred of the town's nine hundred people to flee.[24] Scripps stayed put, nursed the ill, and survived to recount the scary event.[25]

He and his Methodist congregants, he remembered in recollections he wrote in 1858, planned an Independence Day of "of joy and festivity." They invited the entire town to partake in "piles of cakes, confectionaries and other luxuries." "The youths were particularly animated and active," he related. "But O! What a gloomy reverse of all we had meant," he exclaimed about his feelings as he woke up on the fourth. "The first salutations of that morning announced to our ears the soul-harrowing fact that... the Angel of Death was among us." William McCreery (a state senator) and C. V. Putnam, two of town's "halest, robust citizen," had suddenly fell to the disease and would not make it to the end of the day. Others became sick and perished over the weekend. On Sunday, Scripps recounted hearing "heart rending wailings of survivors of their departed loved ones" and "the agonizing groans and moaning of yet other victims writhing in excruciating pangs." These sounds "combined to incite intense terror."

Scripps did not want to write too many details about the people who perished. Those "who yet survive the horrors of that period" need not have "painful reminiscences" about their departed friends and family members reawakened. He did, however, name three youths—Daniel Sherwood, John R. York, and William Willis. They bravely stayed behind when panicked residents sought refuge "among their more distant country friends" or "in encampments in the far off woods." Sherwood, York, and Willis helped establish a hospital, assisted a town physician in caring for the sick and dying, and then paid the ultimate price. "Deaths more or less were of daily occurrence," Scripps recalled about the passing of the three youths and other townspeople. "Some passed off comparatively calm; but most part in convulsive struggles and extreme agonies. I was with them and among them daily to render what aid I could, and hope never again to witness such scenes of horror."

Toward the end of the outbreak, Scripps came down with the disease himself. He had tried to adhere to "dietetic restrictions," but found it difficult given that farmers in the countryside would not come into town with fresh food. "I had probably the most severe attack and became reduced lower than anyone else who recovered, but certainly had far better attention," he claimed. A young physician attended him, two friends sat by his bedside, and he luckily survived. The same was not the case for the Reverend Jewel, "the only minister left in town besides myself," and Mr. Madison Worthington; both died during the last week of July. Their deaths "closed up ... the astounding horrors of our cholera scenes," Scripps concluded.

As in other stricken towns, the total number of fatalities cannot be known as many occurred among those who fled. Rushville's town records recorded twenty-seven burials, which for Scripps was an astonishing number in such a brief period of time for a small town. His town's graveyard stood "almost tenantless" before that fateful July, he claimed. "But the awful devastations of a few short days made it populous, a perfect Golgotha."[26]

Scripps's recollections, of course, do not stand alone. Combined with other memoirs as well as diaries, letters, and news articles, these sources reveal a more complete understanding of cholera than many in Jackson's America wanted to be known. Together, they paint a picture of haunting times as Americans dealt with a mysterious and indiscriminate killer. They bear witness to a pathogen capable of producing terror and mortality in the United States just as it did in other parts of the world. Ignoring this evidence was a choice, and tragically it was a choice that too many powerful people made.

Notes

ABBREVIATIONS

COCCR	Chesapeake and Ohio Canal Company Records
CPM	College Park, Maryland
Duke	David M. Rubenstein Rare Book and Manuscript Library, Duke University, Durham
FHS	Filson Historical Society, Louisville
GTS	General Theological Seminary, New York
HNOC	Historical New Orleans Collection, New Orleans
HSP	Historical Society of Pennsylvania, Philadelphia
KHS	Kansas State Historical Society, Topeka
LRCTU	Louisiana Research Collection, Howard-Tilton Memorial Library, Tulane University, New Orleans
LSU	Special Collections, Hill Memorial Library, Louisiana State University, Baton Rouge
MHS	Maryland Historical Society, Baltimore
NARA	National Archives and Records Administration
NYHS	Patricia D. Klingenstein Library, New York Historical Society
Oberlin	Oberlin College Archives, Oberlin, Ohio
RG	Record Group
SCHS	South Carolina Historical Society Archives, Addlestone Library, College of Charleston
UNC-SHC	Southern Historical Collection, Wilson Library, University of North Carolina at Chapel Hill
UVA	Albert and Shirley Small Special Collections Library, University of Virginia, Charlottesville
VHS	Virginia Historical Society, Richmond

WLCL	William L. Clements Library, University of Michigan, Ann Arbor
WMU	Special Collections Research Center, William and Mary University, Williamsburg

INTRODUCTION

1. Tuscaloosa (AL) *Spirit of the Age*, July 4, 1832; Sarah Haynesworth Gayle, *The Journal of Sarah Haynsworth Gayle, 1827–1835*, ed. Sarah Woolfolk Wiggins and Ruth Smith Truss (University of Alabama Press, 2013), 212.
2. Entry between June 17 and June 28, 1832, in Thomas Knight's Writing Book, 1829–1832, Misc. Mss. Box 22, fo. 22, Kislak Center for Special Collections, University of Pennsylvania, Philadelphia.
3. Elam Tilden to Samuel Tilden, June 18, 1832, Samuel Tilden Papers, Box 1, fo. 11, Manuscripts and Archives Division, New York Public Library, New York.
4. Alfred Robinson to Conway Robinson, June 27, 1832, Moncure Robinson Papers, Mss. 65 R56, 77–14, Box 3, fo. 20. 01, WMU (emphasis in the original).
5. Mrs. Delila [Hurd] to Louisa Cocke, June 26, 1832, John Cocke Papers, Mss. 640, Box 71, UVA.
6. Alexander Smith Johnson to [Mother Mrs. Alexander B. Johnson], June 20, 1832, Alexander Bryan Johnson Papers, Box 1, Sterling Library Manuscripts and Archives, Yale University, New Haven, CT.
7. James Savage to Benjamin Lincoln, June 24, 1832, Lincoln Family Papers, WLCL.
8. Jabez Colt to Roswell Colt, June 20, 1832, Colt Papers, Special Collections, Alexander Library, Rutgers University, New Brunswick, New Jersey.
9. Martha Jefferson Randolph to Ellen Wayles Coolidge, June 21, 1832, Ellen Wayles Randolph Coolidge Correspondence, Mss. 9090, Box 3, UVA.
10. Joseph Coolidge, Jr., to Martha Randolph, June 29, 1832, Ellen Wayles Randolph Coolidge Correspondence, Mss. 9090, Box 3, UVA.
11. Reformed Church in America, General Synod, *The Acts and Proceedings of the General Synod of the Reformed Dutch Church in North America at New York, in June, and Albany, October, 1832* (General Synod, 1832), 91.
12. Andrew Jackson to John F. Schermerhorn, June 12, 1832, in *The Papers of Andrew Jackson, Volume 10, 1832*, ed. Daniel Feller, Thomas Coens, and Laura-Eve Moss (University of Tennessee Press, 2016), 302.
13. United States, Congress, *Register of Debates in Congress . . . of the First Session of the Twenty-Second Congress* (Gales and Seaton, 1833), 1130–32 (quote on 1130).
14. Congress, *Register of Debates in Congress . . . of the First Session of the Twenty-Second Congress*, 1132.
15. Adam Jortner, "Cholera, Christ, and Jackson: The Epidemic of 1832 and the Origins of Christian Politics in Antebellum America," *Journal of the Early Republic* 27 (Summer 2007): 233–64.

16. The 1830 US Census recorded a total of 12,858,670 people, while the 1840 US Census came in at 17,069,453. On average for the decade, the United States added an additional 420,343 people per year, making the total in 1832 approximately 13,706,707. For 1830 total population, see US Census Office, *Abstract of the Returns of the Fifth Census* (Duff Green, 1832), 51, and for 1840, US Census Office, *Compendium of the Enumeration of the Inhabitants and Statistics of the United States, As Obtained at the Department of State, from the Returns of the Sixth Census* (Thomas Allen, 1841), 368. I will occasionally refer to populations of major US cities, and these are based on calculations using an annual rate of growth derived from comparing 1830 and 1840 census data. These can be found in Campbell Gibson, "Population of the 100 Largest Cities and Other Urban Places in the United States: 1790–1990," Working Paper POP-WOP0327, United States Census Bureau, June 1998, https://www.census.gov/library/working-papers/1998/demo/POP-twps0027.html.
17. Charles Rosenberg's *The Cholera Years: The United States in 1832, 1849, and 1866* (University of Chicago Press, 1962) has stood as the oft-cited, seminal book on the pandemic as it struck during the 1830s. While Rosenberg successfully argued that the disease reinforced convictions that Americans had about their social order, he generalized the national experience from what happened in New York City during 1832. Since *The Cholera Years*, works on the topic have tended to be local or state-level studies or have focused on particular medical or political aspects of the pandemic. See Joseph Warring, "Asiatic Cholera in South Carolina," *Bulletin of the History of Medicine* 40 (September 1966): 459–66; Stuart Galishoff, "Cholera in Newark, New Jersey," *Journal of the History of Medicine and Allied Sciences* 25 (October 1970): 438–48; Nancy D. Baird, "Asiatic Cholera's First Visit to Kentucky: A Study in Panic and Fear," *Filson Club Historical Quarterly* 48, no. 3 (1974): 228–40; Ruth C. Carter, "Cincinnatians and Cholera: Attitudes Toward the Epidemics of 1832 and 1849," *Queen City Heritage* 50, no. 3 (1992): 32–48; Marshall S. Berdan, "The Pestilence That Walketh in Darkness: The Cholera Epidemic of 1832," *Virginia Cavalcade* 43, no. 1 (1993): 14–23; Donald Hutslar, "'God's Scourge': The Cholera Years in Ohio," *Ohio History* 105 (Summer/Autumn 1996): 174–91; Greg Olson, "Plague on the Prairie: The Cholera Epidemic of 1833 and Its Impact on One Illinois Town," *Illinois Heritage* 5, no. 1 (January–February 2002): 6–9; James Z. Schwartz, "'A Melancholy and Trying Season': Cholera and the Conflict over Cultural Boundaries in Early Michigan," *Journal of the Early Republic* 26 (Spring 2006): 95–116; John B. Osborne, "Preparing for the Pandemic: City Boards of Health and the Arrival of Cholera in Montreal, New York, and Philadelphia in 1832," *Urban History Review* 36 (Spring 2008): 29–42; Ashleigh R. Tuite, Christina H. Chan, and David N. Fisman, "Cholera, Canals, and Contagion: Rediscovering Dr. Beck's Report," *Journal of Public Health Policy* 32 (August 2011): 320–33; Louise B. McCabe, "Cholera, Germantown, 1832: Suspicion and Science," *Germantown Crier* 64 (Spring 2014): 21–25; Sarah Schuetze,

"Mapping a Demon Malady: Cholera Maps and Affect in 1832," *Common-Place: The Interactive Journal of Early American Life* 17, no. 1 (Fall 2016), https://commonplace.online/article/mapping-a-demon-malady/; David Petriello, "'A People So Well Fed and So Clean': The 1832 Cholera Pandemic in New Jersey," *NJS: An Interdisciplinary Journal* (Winter 2020): 91–115.

18. The general literature on Jacksonian America is quite vast, but two massive syntheses dominate the field: Sean Wilentz's 1,044-page *The Rise of American Democracy: Jefferson to Lincoln* (Norton, 2005) and David Walker Howe's 904-page *What God Hath Wrought! The Transformation of America, 1815–1848* (Oxford University Press, 2007). Both give cholera only cursory treatment. Wilentz mentions the 1830s pandemic on a single page (p. 372) and suggests that it merely presented a minor impediment to "a spirited mass campaign" supporting Andrew Jackson's re-election. David Walker Howe's *What God Hath Wrought!* slides cholera into two pages (pp. 469–70), wherein he summarizes the prayer debate and says of the pandemic, "of course the poor suffered the most" (p. 470).
19. The lack of literature on cholera at the time that Wilentz and Howe wrote their respective works was unfortunate because the pandemic supports one of their respective interpretations more than the other. Wilentz tries to convince readers that positive developments toward the ultimate democratization of American political culture characterizes Jackson's America. He cautions readers from underappreciating this progress due to the pervasiveness of slavery, racism, Indian Removal, and patriarchy. Howe, by contrast, characterizes the unprogressive aspects of Jacksonian America as a consequence of an exclusive white male democracy. Cholera vividly exposed those glaring contradictions to democracy that Howe emphasized and that Wilentz downplayed.
20. David A. Sack, MD, professor at Johns Hopkins Bloomberg School of Public Health, personal communications with the author, April 4, 2019, and December 8, 2020. For a clinical overview of cholera, see Suman Kanungo et al., "Cholera," *The Lancet* 399 (April 2022): 1429–40.
21. Sonia Shah, *Pandemic: Tracking Contagions, from Cholera to Ebola and Beyond* (Sarah Crichton Books/Farrar, Straus and Giroux, 2016), 45.
22. Shah, *Pandemic*, 45.
23. While cholera in Jackson's America has not received singular treatment, several works have treated cholera more globally, reconstructed the several pandemics that have occurred up to the present day, and detailed medical and public health responses. Shah's *Pandemic* is an accessible introduction to the ecological and medical history of the topic, while at the same time a gripping account of how cholera should alert us to the dangers of emerging infectious diseases today. My starting point, though, goes back to Charles Rosenberg's "Cholera in Nineteenth-Century Europe: A Tool for Social and Economic analysis," *Comparative Studies in Society and History* 8 (July 1966): 452–63. I take up Rosenberg's challenge to use the lens of cholera to understand the United States in the 1830s in more depth. Christopher Hamlin's *Cholera: The Biography* (Oxford University Press, 2009) has

been particularly informative to my analysis. Focusing on cholera writers of the nineteenth century, Hamlin illuminates the fact that educated western Europeans and Americans saw cholera as a threat to a liberal political order, as a challenge to progress itself, something my study fundamentally agrees with. A deeper dive into the American experience in the 1830s reveals the extent to which the affluent and powerful purposefully tried to obscure cholera's illuminating light on the dark side of liberalism. My work also provides an added dimension to what Samuel K. Cohn, Jr., has demonstrated in his *Epidemics: Hate and Compassion from the Plague of Athens to AIDS* (Oxford University Press, 2018). Cohn recounts several episodes of riots and collective violence during cholera outbreaks, which have largely involved peasant and working-class protests against the medical policing by public authorities. These protests occurred in both tyrannical and liberal regimes and even after the causative agent and mechanism in which it spread became widely known. Cohn did not find causal connections between epidemics and revolutionary movements but rather the opposite: political mobilization and repression accelerated the progress of cholera. A similar phenomenon happened in the United States in the 1830s: cholera did not cause or substantially change the historical processes of Jacksonian America as much as xenophobia, exploitation, ethnic cleansing, and human trafficking enhanced the lethal trajectory of cholera. On cholera outside of the United States, see Roderick McGrew, *Russia and the Cholera, 1823–1832* (University of Wisconsin Press, 1965); R. J. Morris, *Cholera, 1832: The Social Response to an Epidemic* (Holmes & Meier, 1976); Margaret Pelling, *Cholera, Fever, and English Medicine, 1825–1865* (University of Oxford Press, 1978); Michael Durey, *The Return of the Plague: British Society and the Cholera, 1831–1832* (Gill and Macmillan, 1979); François Delaporte, *Disease and Civilisation, the Cholera in Paris, 1832*, trans. A. Goldhammer (Harvard University Press, 1986); Geoffrey Bilson, *A Darkened House: Cholera in Nineteenth-Century Canada* (University of Toronto Press, 1989); Richard J. Evans, "Epidemics and Revolutions: Cholera in Nineteenth-Century Europe," *Past & Present* 120 (August 1988): 123–46; Evans, *Death in Hamburg: Society and Politics in the Cholera Years, 1830–1910* (Oxford University Press, 1987); Frank Snowden, *Naples in the Time of Cholera, 1884–1911* (Cambridge University Press, 1995); Kseniya Barabanova, "The First Cholera Epidemic in St. Petersburg," *Arcadia* (2014), no. 6. Environment & Society Portal, Rachel Carson Center for Environment and Society, https://doi.org/10.5282/rcc/5385. Other scholars have explored cholera in the context of imperialism. See David Arnold, "Cholera and Colonialism in British India," *Past & Present* 113 (1986): 118–51; Viyah Prashad, "Native Dirt/Imperial Ordure: The Cholera of 1832 and the Morbid Resolutions of Modernity," *Journal of Historical Sociology* (1994): 243–60; Warwick Anderson, "Excremental Colonialism: Public Health and the Poetics of Pollution," *Critical Inquiry* 21 (1995): 640–69; and Mark Harrison, "A Dreadful Scourge: Cholera in Early Nineteenth-Century India," *Modern Asian Studies* 54, no. 2 (2020): 502–33.

24. On alcohol consumption and the movement to curtail it during the first half of the nineteenth century, see W. J. Rohrbaugh, *The Alcoholic Republic: An American Tradition* (Oxford University Press, 1981); Ian R. Tyrell, *Sobering Up: From Temperance to Prohibition in Antebellum America, 1800–1860* (Greenwood Press, 1979); and Matthew Warner Osborn, *Rum Maniacs: Alcoholic Insanity in the Early American Republic* (University of Chicago Press, 2014).
25. M. V. Singer and C. Leffmann, "Alcohol and Gastric Acid Secretion in Humans: A Short Review," *Scandinavian Journal of Gastroenterology*, suppl. 146 (1988): 11–21, https://doi.org/10.3109/00365528809099126; S. Chari et al., "Alcohol and Gastric Acid Secretion in Humans," *Gut* 34, no. 6 (1993): 843–47, https://doi.org/10.1136/gut.34.6.843; S. Chari Jiaqi Pan et al., "Alcohol Consumption and the Risk of Gastroesophageal Reflux Disease: A Systematic Review and Meta-analysis," *Alcohol and Alcoholism* 54, no.1 (January 2019): 62–69, https://doi.org/10.1093/alcalc/agy063; "Is Alcohol Harming Your Stomach?," https://www.drinkaware.co.uk/facts/health-effects-of-alcohol/general-health-effects/is-alcohol-harming-your-stomach.
26. "WHO Regional Director's Statement on Cholera Outbreaks," November 2, 2022, https://www.emro.who.int/media/news/who-regional-director-for-the-eastern-mediterraneans-statement-on-cholera-outbreaks.html.
27. Pioneering works in recovering the experiences of diverse people during a pandemic are Elizabeth Fenn's *Pox Americana: The Great Smallpox Epidemic of 1775–82* (Farrar, Straus and Giroux, 2001) and Nancy Bristow's *American Pandemic: The Lost Worlds of the 1918 Influenza Pandemic* (Oxford University Press, 2012).

CHAPTER 1

1. Boston *Traveler,* December 28, 1830; New York *Commercial Advertiser*, December 28, 1830; New York *Spectator*, December 29, 1830; Philadelphia *Daily Chronicle*, December 29, 1830; Baltimore *Gazette and Daily Advertiser*, December 30, 1830; Charleston (SC) *Courier*, January 5, 1831; Cincinnati *National Republican and Daily Mercantile Advertiser*, January 8, 1831.
2. New York *Spectator*, December 31, 1830.
3. Boston *New England Palladium* in Philadelphia *United States Gazette for the Country*, January 11, 1831; Concord *New-Hampshire Statesmen*, January 8, 1831.
4. On the growth and development of the newspapers, see Gerald Baldasty, *The Commercialization of News in the Nineteenth Century* (University of Wisconsin Press, 1992), 11–35; Stephen W. Campbell, *The Bank War and the Partisan Press: Newspapers, Financial Institutions, and the Post Office in Jacksonian America* (University of Kansas Press, 2019).
5. New York *Journal of Commerce*, August 10, 1831.
6. Diebitsch's death received abundant coverage in the US press. See New York *Journal of Commerce*, August 10, 1831; New York *Evening Post*, August 11, 1831; New York *Spectator*, August 16, 1832; Baltimore *American and Commercial Daily*

Advertiser, August 15, 1831; Washington (DC) *Globe*, August 15, 1832; Keene (NH) *Farmer's Museum*, August 19, 1831; Haverhill (NH) *Essex Gazette*, August 20, 1831; Montpelier *Vermont Watchman and State Gazette*, August 23, 1831; Tuscaloosa *Alabama State Intelligencer*, September 3, 1831.

7. New York *Spectator*, July 1, 1831; New York *Spectator*, September 6, 1832; New York *Spectator*, September 20, 1832.
8. New York *Spectator*, August 16, 1831.
9. New York *Commercial Advertiser*, October 14, 1831.
10. New York *Spectator*, August 12, 1831.
11. Boston *Commercial Gazette*, July 18, 1831; New York *Commercial Advertiser*, July 19, 1831; Norwich (CT) *Courier*, July 20, 1831; Philadelphia *United States Gazette for the Country*, July 22, 1831; New York *Spectator*, July 22, 1831; Washington (DC) *Globe*, July 22, 1831; Brattleboro (VT) *Messenger*, July 23, 1831; Lowell (MA) *Mercury*, July 23, 1831; Newport (RI) *Mercury*, July 23, 1831; Amherst (NH) *Farmer's Cabinet*, July 23, 1831; Columbus *Ohio Monitor*, August 3, 1831.
12. Chelsea *Vermont Advocate*, September 15, 1831; Philadelphia *National Gazette*, October 15, 1831; Philadelphia *National Gazette*, November 22, 1831.
13. Reports of the Hungarian peasants' revolt appeared in the Augsburg newspaper *Allgemeine Zeitung* in August and early September, began to circulate in British newspapers in September, and reached US newspapers in mid-October. The version quoted is from London *Courier*, September 17, 1831, in Philadelphia *National Gazette*, November 5, 1831. This version also appeared in Philadelphia *Inquirer*, November 2, 1831; New York *Spectator*, November 8, 1831; Providence (RI) *Manufacturers' & Farmers' Journal*, November 14, 1831; Worcester *Massachusetts Spy*, November 16, 1831; and Sandusky (OH) *Clarion*, December 7, 1831. An earlier account circulated, referring to the peasants having the "insane notion that the physicians sought to poison the poor people by order of the Government...woe to the physician or nobleman who falls into the hands of the infuriated peasantry." See Newport (RI) *Mercury*, October 15, 1831; Dover (NH) *Enquirer*, October 18, 1831; Woodstock (VT) *Mercury*, October 21, 1831; Washington (PA) *Review and Examiner*, October 22, 1831; Lawrenceburg (IN) *Western Statesman*, October 28, 1831; and Detroit *Free Press*, October 20, 1831.
14. New York *Spectator*, August 30, 1831.
15. Philadelphia *National Gazette*, September 2, 1831; Newport (RI) *Mercury*, September 3, 1831; Washington (DC) *National Intelligencer*, September 5, 1831; Hagerstown (MD) *Mail*, September 9, 1831; Leesburg (VA) *Genius of Liberty*, September 10, 1831; Boston *Liberator*, September 10, 1831.
16. New York *Spectator*, January 13, 1832.
17. New York *Spectator*, August 12, 1831.
18. New York *Spectator*, September 6, 1832.
19. New York *Spectator*, October 28, 1831.
20. Philadelphia *National Gazette*, November 8, 1831; Baltimore *Gazette*, November 10, 1831; New York *Evening Post*, November 10, 1831; Philadelphia *United States Gazette*, November 11, 1831; Washington (DC) *United States Telegraph*, November 14, 1831.

21. New York *American*, December 5, 1831; Jamestown (NY) *Journal*, December 14, 1831.
22. On quarantine practices in the United States pre–germ theory, see David S. Barnes, "Cargo, 'Infection,' and the Logic of Quarantine in the Nineteenth Century," *Bulletin of the History of Medicine* 88 (Spring 2014): 75–101.
23. New York *Evening Post*, August 6, 1831.
24. New York *Spectator*, August 16, 1831.
25. New York *Spectator*, September 20, 1832.
26. New York *Spectator*, September 23, 1831; New York *Spectator*, October 4, 1831.
27. Providence *Rhode-Island American*, September 16, 1831; Nantucket (MA) *Inquirer*, September 17, 1831; Gloucester (MA) *Telegraph*, August 13, 1831; New Bedford (MA) *Gazette*, September 19, 1831; Portland (ME) *Advertiser*, September 20, 1831; Providence *Rhode-Island Republican*, November 8, 1831; Savannah *Georgian*, September 27, 1831; Salem (MA) *Gazette*, October 18, 1831; Washington (DC) *Daily National Journal*, August 16, 1831; Baltimore *Gazette*, September 14, 1831.
28. Providence (RI) *Patriot*, August 10, 1831.
29. Smith gave his lecture on November 9, 1831. It was thereafter published and marketed in pamphlet form. Mather J. Smith, *A Discourse on the Epidemic Cholera Morbus of Europe and Asia* (J. Seymour, 1831). New York newspapers gave it positive notice. See New York *Commercial Advertiser*, November 26, 1831; New York *Advertiser*, November 29, 1831; New York *Spectator*, November 29, 1831; New York *Evening Post*, November 29, 1831.
30. "Causes of the Epidemic Cholera," *Journal of Health* 3, no. 2 (September 21, 1831): 27–30 (quote on 30). Excerpts published in Worcester *Massachusetts Spy*, February 15, 1832.
31. "Sanitary Cordon," *Journal of Health* 3, no. 5 (November 9, 1831): 75–76.
32. New York *Advertiser*, February 3, 1832.
33. Hartford (CT) *American Mercury*, February 6, 1832; Baltimore *Gazette*, February 6, 1832; New York *Spectator*, February 7, 1832; Hartford *Connecticut Courier*, February 7, 1832; New Haven *Connecticut Journal*, February 7, 1832; Salem (MA) *Gazette*, February 7, 1832; Auburn (NY) *Free Press*, February 8, 1832; Northampton (MA) *Hampshire Gazette*, February 8, 1832; Lynchburg *Virginian*, February 13, 1832.
34. New York *Spectator*, January 6, 1832.
35. US Congress, *Cholera Morbus*, 22d Cong., 1st sess., January 20, 1832, House Report 226, quotes on 34–35.
36. US Congress, *Cholera Morbus*, 22d Cong., 1st sess., January 20, 1832, House Report 226; Washington (DC) *Daily Globe*, April 9, 1832.
37. The Baltimore *Gazette*, January 2, 1832, published the exact same article as the New York *Daily Advertiser* but did not attribute its piece to another source and did not title it "Horrors of Cholera Morbus." Papers that reprinted the *Advertiser*'s article with attribution and with the word "Horrors" in the title include Boston

Columbian Centinel, January 4, 1832; Worcester (MA) *National Aegis*, January 11, 1832; Gardiner (ME) *Christian Intelligencer and Eastern Chronicle*, January 13, 1832; Newport (RI) *Mercury*, January 14, 1832; Portsmouth *New-Hampshire Gazette*, January 17, 1832; Boston *Liberator*, January 28, 1832; Springfield (IL) *Sangamo Journal*, February 16, 1832.

38. Boston *Courier*, January 21, 1832; Providence (RI) *Patriot*, January 28, 1832; Worcester *Massachusetts Spy*, February 1, 1832; Newport *Rhode-Island Republican*, February 7, 1832; Hallowell (ME) *American Advocate*, February 8, 1832; Brattleboro (VT) *Messenger*, February 11, 1832; Frederick (MD) *Herald*, February 18, 1832.
39. New York *Evening Post*, January 21, 1832.
40. Hartford (CT) *Times*, February 6, 1832; Portsmouth (ME) *Journal*, February 18, 1832; Hartford (CT) *Episcopal Watchman*, February 21, 1832; "Further Quarantine Regulations," *Boston Medical and Surgical Journal* 6, no. 6 (March 28, 1832): 111.
41. Eve's life and career are discussed in R. A. Halley, "Paul Fitzsimons Eve, A.M., M.D., LL.D.," *American Historical Magazine and Tennessee Historical Quarterly* 9, no. 4 (October 1904): 281–342.
42. Charleston (SC) *Courier*, February 28, 1832, also in Savannah *Georgian*, March 3, 1832; Augusta (GA) *Constitutionalist*, March 13, 1832.
43. "The Cholera Not Contagious," *Journal of Health* 3, no. 10 (January 25, 1832): 147–62.
44. Philadelphia *National Gazette*, February 11, 1832. Other newspapers circulated the *Gazette*'s editorial. See Boston *Post*, February 18, 1832; Providence (RI) *Microcosm*, February 18, 1832; Newport (RI) *Mercury*, February 18, 1832; Pittsburgh (PA) *Weekly Gazette*, February 21, 1832; Hartford *Connecticut Mirror*, February 25, 1832; Nantucket (MA) *Inquirer*, February 25, 1832; Dover (NH) *Enquirer*, March 6, 1832.
45. Benjamin C. Mifflin, *Charles Mifflin, M.D., with an Account of his Ancestors and Ancestral Connections* (Riverside Press, 1876).
46. US newspapers carried advertisements for a variety of medical treatises on cholera, many of them that espoused the noncontagion theory. See advertisement in Boston *Courier*, March 12, 1832, for Henri Scoutetten, *A Medical and Topographical History of the Cholera Morbus: Including the Mode of Prevention and Treatment*, trans. A. S. Doane (Carter and Hendee, 1832). Also in Philadelphia *National Gazette*, March 22, 1832; Charleston (SC) *Courier*, March 30, 1832; Pittsburgh (PA) *Weekly Gazette*, May 18, 1832; and Savannah *Georgian*, May 29, 1832. The Scoutetten work was accompanied by a map showing in red the spread of cholera from South Asia through Europe and across the English Channel to the British Isles. The text frequently refers to the terror of the pandemic, and the red ink lines, according to Sarah Schuetze, enhanced fear of the creeping pandemic. See Schuetze, "Mapping a Demon Malady: Cholera Maps and Affect in 1832."
47. Originally published in New York *Daily Advertiser*, and then carried by a variety of US newspapers: New York *American*, March 6, 1832; Philadelphia *Daily Chronicle*,

March 7, 1832; Baltimore *American*, March 10, 1832; Philadelphia *National Gazette*, March 10, 1832 (and again on March 13, 1832); New York *Observer*, March 10, 1832; Hartford (CT) *Episcopal Watchman*, March 13, 1832; Alexandria (VA), *Gazette*, March 14, 1832; Jamestown (NY) *Journal*, March 21, 1832. A truncated version that emphasized cholera's preference for poor people can be found in the Northampton (NH) *Gazette*, March 14, 1832.

48. New York *Spectator*, May 11, 1832.
49. Baltimore *Gazette*, May 24, 1832; New York *Spectator*, May 25, 1832; New York *Commercial Advertiser*, May 29, 1832; Hartford *Connecticut Courant*, May 29, 1832; New Haven *Connecticut Journal*, May 29, 1832; condensed versions in Hartford (CT) *American Mercury*, May 28, 1832; Charleston (SC) *Courier*, May 30, 1832.
50. New York *American*, May 7, 1832; Philadelphia *Daily Chronicle*, May 8, 1832; Philadelphia *The United States Gazette*, May 8, 1832; Baltimore *Gazette*, May 9, 1832; Boston *Daily Advertiser*, May 9, 1832; New *York Spectator*, May 11, 1832; Portsmouth (NH) *Journal of Literature and Politics*, May 12, 1832; Windsor *Vermont Republican and American Journal*, May 12, 1832; Charleston (SC) *Courier*, May 14, 1832; Portland (ME) *Eastern Argus*, May 15, 1832.
51. New York *Spectator*, May 29, 1832 (emphasis in original). See also New York *American*, May 28, 1832; Philadelphia *National Gazette*, May 31, 1832; Albany (NY) *Argus*, June 1, 1832: New Haven (CT) *Columbian Register*, June 2, 1832. Total deaths are according to Delaporte, *Disease and Civilization*, 5.
52. Boston *Courier*, June 4, 1832; Alexandria (VA) *Gazette*, June 5, 1832; Charleston (SC) *Mercury*, June 9, 1832; Savannah *Georgian*, June 11, 1832; Woodstock (VT) *Mercury*, June 15, 1832.
53. New York *American*, June 5, 1832; Philadelphia *National Gazette*, June 6, 1832; Baltimore *American*, June 7, 1832; Boston *Courier*, June 7, 1832; New York *Spectator*, June 8, 1832; Albany (NY) *Argus*, June 8, 1832; Alexandria (VA) *Gazette*, June 8, 1832; Boston *Traveller*, June 8, 1832; Washington (DC) *Globe*, June 8, 1832; Charleston (SC) *Southern Patriot*, June 12, 1832; Lansingburgh (NY) *Gazette*, June 12, 1832; Bennington (VT) *Gazette*, June 12, 1832; Pittsburgh (PA) *Weekly Gazette*, June 12, 1832; Geneva (NY) *Courier*, June 13, 1832; Savannah *Georgian*, June 13, 1832.
54. Rosenberg, *The Cholera Years*, 15.
55. The pamphlet was published in full in Philadelphia newspapers: *Daily Chronicle*, May 17, 1832; *National Gazette*, May 18, 1832; and *United States Gazette*, May 22, 1832. Editors outside of Philadelphia published it in whole or provided readers extensive extracts and summaries. See Baltimore *American*, May 22, 1832; Alexandria (VA) *Gazette*, May 23, 1832; Richmond (VA) *Constitutional Whig*, May 25, 1832; Boston *Columbian Centinel* in Springfield (MA), *Weekly Republican*, June 30, 1832; Bangor (ME) *Penobscot Journal*, July 3, 1832.
56. First appearing in New York *Observer*, April 28, 1832, and then reprinted in Boston *Christian Watchman*, May 4, 1832; Worcester (MA) *Family Visitor*, May 8, 1832; Bridgeton (NJ) *West Jersey Observer*, May 12, 1832; Boston *Recorder*, May 16, 1832;

Poughkeepsie (NY) *Independence*, May 16, 1832; Hudson *Ohio Observer*, May 17, 1832; New Echota (Cherokee Nation) *Cherokee Phoenix*, May 19, 1832; Gettysburg (PA) *Republican Banner*, May 22, 1832; Boston *Youth's Companion, & Weekly Family Visitor*, May 26, 1832; Albany (NY) *Temperance Recorder*, June 5, 1832.

57. American Temperance Society, *Fifth Report of the American Temperance, Presented at the Meeting in Boston, May, 1832* (Aaron Russell, 1832), 80. Excerpted and published in Alexandria (VA) *Gazette*, May 2, 1832.

58. Original publication in the New York *Journal of Commerce* and then picked up and republished in various religious and not explicitly religious periodicals: Providence (RI) *American and Gazette*, April 3, 1832; Norwich (CT) *Courier*, April 4, 1832; Providence (RI) *Microcosm*, April 7, 1832; Charles Town *Virginia Free Press*, April 12, 1832; Haverhill (MA) *Gazette*, April 14, 1832; Macon (GA) *Telegraph*, April 14, 1832; Eastport (ME) *Sentinel*, April 18, 1832; Philadelphia *Daily Chronicle*, April 19, 1832; Belfast *Maine Working Men's Advocate*, April 19, 1832; Bridgeton (NJ) *West Jersey Observer*, April 21, 1832; Woodstock (VT) *Observer*, April 24, 1832; Piqua (OH) *Courier and Enquirer*, April 25, 1832; Morristown (NJ) *Jerseyman*, April 25, 1832; Pittsburgh (PA) *Weekly Gazette*, May 8, 1832; Somersworth (NH) *Great Falls Journal*, May 12, 1832; Little Rock *Arkansas Times and Advocate*, May 30, 1832; "No Great Loss Without Some Small Gain," *Christian Magazine: Conducted Under the Supervision of the Associate Reformed Synod of New-York* 1, no. 5 (May 1832): 159.

CHAPTER 2

1. Boston *Post*, June 21, 1832; New York *Evening Post*, June 22, 1832; Boston *Investigator*, June 22, 1832; Boston *Statesman*, June 23, 1832; Philadelphia *Daily Chronicle*, June 23, 1832; Baltimore *American*, June 25, 1832; Gettysburg (PA) *Republican Banner*, June 26, 1832; Binghamton (NY) *Broome Republican*, June 28, 1832; Belfast *Maine Working Men's Advocate*, June 28, 1832; Lynchburg *Virginian*, July 2, 1832; Nashville *National Banner*, July 3, 1832; Halifax (NC) *Roanoke Advocate*, July 5, 1832.

2. Some papers did not reprint the letter verbatim but did relay news that "an Irish emigrant died at Montpelier." See New York *Commercial Advertiser*, June 23, 1832; then reprinted in Baltimore *American*, June 26, 1832; Alexandria (VA) *Gazette*, June 26, 1832; Hartford *Connecticut Courant*, June 26, 1832; New York *Spectator*, June 26, 1832; Boston *Columbian Centinel*, June 27, 1832; Worcester *Massachusetts Spy*, June 27, 1832; Portland (ME) *Christian Mirror*, June 28, 1832; Pawtucket (RI) *Chronicle and Manufacturers' and Artizans' Advocate*, June 29, 1832; Amherst (NH) *Farmer's Cabinet*, June 30, 1832; Boston *Trumpet and Universalist Magazine*, June 30, 1832; Charleston (SC) *Courier*, July 2, 1832.

3. Salem (MA) *Gazette*, June 26, 1832. Summary of this article in Lowell (MA) *Observer*, June 30, 1832; Boston *Christian Watchman*, June 29, 1832; New Haven (CT) *Columbian Register*, June 30, 1832; Worcester *Massachusetts Spy*, July 4, 1832.

4. New York *Commercial Advertiser*, June 28, 1832. Also published in Philadelphia *Daily Chronicle*, June 29, 1832; Baltimore *American*, June 30, 1832; Alexandria (VA) *Gazette*, July 2, 1832; New York *Spectator*, July 3, 1832; Lynchburg *Virginian*, July 5, 1832.
5. Hidetaka Hirota, *Expelling the Poor: Atlantic Seaboard States and the Nineteenth-Century Origins of American Immigration Policy* (Oxford University Press, 2017), 19; see also Kerby A. Miller, *Emigrants and Exiles: Ireland and the Irish Exodus to North America* (Oxford University Press, 1985), 204.
6. Kevin Kenny, *The American Irish: A History* (Longman, 2000), 54; Miller, *Emigrants and Exiles*, 215.
7. Miller, *Emigrants and Exiles*, 207.
8. Kenny, *The American Irish*, 52–54.
9. Jacobson, *Whiteness of a Different Color: European Immigrants and the Alchemy of Race* (Harvard University Press, 1998), 27–49.
10. Kenny, *The American Irish*, 58; Miller, *Emigrants and Exiles*, 254.
11. Kenny, *The American Irish*, 58–59; Miller, *Emigrants and Exiles*, 255–56; Hirota, *Expelling the Poor*, 21.
12. Hirota, *Expelling the Poor*, 21.
13. Kenny, *The American Irish*, 58–59. On the grueling conditions, see also Miller, *Emigrants and Exiles*, 255–56; Hirota, *Expelling the Poor*, 21.
14. Liverpool (UK) *Courier*, June 20, 1832, in Oxford (UK) *Jackson's Oxford Journal*, June 23, 1832.
15. Liverpool (UK) *Mercury*, June 15, 1832.
16. Sheffield (UK) *Sheffield and Rotherham Independent*, June 23, 1832.
17. Liverpool (UK) *Mercury*, June 15, 1832.
18. Liverpool (UK) *Courier*, June 20, 1832, in Oxford (UK) *Jackson's Oxford Journal*, June 23, 1832.
19. "Cholera in the Ship Brutus," *Medico-Chirurgical Review, and Journal of Practical Medicine* 17, no. 33 (July 1, 1832): 285.
20. Shah, *Pandemic*, 45.
21. Philadelphia *National Gazette*, June 5, 1832.
22. John M. Woodworth, *The Cholera Epidemic of 1873 in the United States* (Government Printing Office, 1875), 563.
23. Bilson, *A Darkened House*, 9–12.
24. Woodworth, *The Cholera Epidemic of 1873*, 563.
25. Schenectady (NY) *Cabinet*, June 20, 1832.
26. Philadelphia *National Gazette*, June 19, 1832.
27. Bilson, *A Darkened House*, 24.
28. Albany (NY) *Argus*, June 22, 1832.
29. Bilson, *A Darkened House*, 24.
30. "Rising Population and Immigration," Le Canada: A People's History/Une Histoire Populaire, accessed February 20, 2025, https://www.cbc.ca/history/EPCONTENTSE1EP7CH1PA2LE.html; Bilson, *A Darkened House*, 24.

31. Bilson, *A Darkened House*, 28–29 (quote on 28).
32. Mary McLean Walsh, Memoirs, in "Inspiring Emigrant Letters Home to Ireland from America in the Famine Era," IrishCentral, accessed February 20, 2025, https://www.irishcentral.com/roots/history/letters-ireland-america-famine. See also Miller, *Exiles and Emigrants*, 262.
33. Mary McLean Walsh, Memoirs.
34. Bilson, *A Darkened House*, 48.
35. Mr. Buchanan's Report, December 12, 1832, Report, in Emigration to North America and Australia; British Parliamentary Papers, 1833, XXVI, (141), pp. 299–319; CMSIED 1200341, available online in Documenting Ireland: Parliament, People and Migration database, https://www.dippam.ac.uk/ied/records/37852.
36. "Beck's Report on Cholera, Made to His Excellency Gov. Throop, August, 1832," *Transactions of the Medical Society of the State of New York, Vol. 1, 1832–1833* (Webster and Skinners, 1833), 352.
37. Albany (NY) *Argus*, June 22, 1832; New York *Evening Post*, June 22, 1832.
38. Plattsburgh (NY) *Republican*, June 23, 1832.
39. Plattsburgh (NY) *Republican*, June 23, 1832.
40. Bellows Falls *Vermont Chronicle*, June 22, 1832.
41. New York *Evening Post*, June 18, 1832; Albany (NY) *Argus*, June 19, 1832; Burlington (VT) *Weekly Free Press*, June 22, 1832.
42. Bellows Falls *Vermont Chronicle*, June 22, 1832.
43. New York Board of Health, *Report of the Commissioners Employed to Investigate the Origin and Nature of Epidemic Cholera in Canada* (Peter Van Pelt, 1832), 19.
44. Benjamin Lincoln to Theodore Lincoln, June 17, 1832, Benjamin Lincoln Papers, Harvey Cushing/John Hay Whitney Medical Library, Yale University, New Haven.
45. New York *Evening Post*, June 16, 1832.
46. Lansingburgh (NY) *Gazette*, June 19, 1832.
47. Albany (NY) *Argus*, June 22, 1832.
48. The Albany *Argus* published this information in an extra issue on the evening of June 15. The extra issue has not been found, but it was received by New York City newspapers and reprinted. See New York *Evening Post*, June 16, 1832.
49. Albany (NY) *Argus*, June 22, 1832.
50. Middlebury (VT) *People's Press*, June 26, 1832.
51. Albany (NY) *Argus*, June 19, 1832.
52. Entry for June 17, 1832, in Almon Underwood Journal, WLCL.
53. Entry for June 18, 1832, in Almon Underwood Journal, WLCL.
54. "Beck's Report on Cholera," 352; Albany (NY) *Argus*, June 22, 1832.
55. Albany (NY) *Argus*, June 19, 1832.
56. Albany (NY) *Argus*, June 19, 1832.
57. Albany (NY) *Argus*, June 22, 1832.
58. Albany (NY) *Argus*, June 22, 1832.
59. Philadelphia *Cholera Gazette*, September 19, 1832, 166–69.

60. New York *Evening Post*, June 22, 1832.
61. New York Board of Health, *Origin and Nature of Epidemic Cholera in Canada*, 14–24.

CHAPTER 3

1. Samuel R. Johnson and E. Johnson to Mr. and Mrs. Peter Roosevelt, June 21, 1832, Samuel Roosevelt Johnson Papers, Box 2, GTS (emphasis in original). Samuel's half-uncle, Peter Roosevelt, adopted him after both of his parents passed away when he was one year old. Little is known about Peter Roosevelt. Neither Theodore nor Franklin Delano were direct descendants.
2. Anicartha Miller to Margaret Youle, June 20, 1832, Anicartha Miller Letters, NYHS.
3. Mary Suckley to George Suckley, June 19, 1832, Suckley Family Papers, Box 2, WLCL.
4. Philip Hone, *Diary of Philip Hone, 1828–1851*, ed. Bayard Tuckerman (Dodd, Mead, and Company, 1889), I, 56.
5. The US Census records 202,589 people in New York City in 1830 and 312,710 in 1840. (See Gibson, "Population of the 100 Largest Cities.") Assuming New York grew, on average, by about 11,000 people per year during the 1830s, the city had about 225,000 at the start of the pandemic. Scholarly and journalistic accounts of New York and cholera in 1832 claim as many as 250,000. See "Disasters, New York City, Cholera Epidemic of 1832," NYCdata, Weissman Center for International Business, Baruch College City University of New York, 2021, https://www.baruch.cuny.edu/nycdata/disasters/cholera-1832.html; John Noble Wilford, "How Epidemics Helped Shape the Modern Metropolis," *New York Times*, April 15, 2008.
6. New York *Evening Post*, June 16, 1832.
7. New York *Morning Courier and Enquirer*, June 18, 1832.
8. Rosenberg, *The Cholera Years*, 20–25.
9. Dudley Atkins, ed., *Reports of Hospital Physicians and Other Documents in Relation to the Epidemic Cholera of 1832* (G.&C.&H. Carvill, 1832), 9–10; Rosenberg, *The Cholera Years*, 25–26.
10. Rosenberg, *The Cholera Years*, 26.
11. Atkins, *Reports of Hospital Physicians*, 10.
12. Rosenberg, *The Cholera Years*, 26 n. 21.
13. New York *Standard*, July 2, 1832, reprinted in Geneva (NY) *Gazette and Mercantile Advertiser*, July 11, 1832.
14. New York *Journal of Commerce*, July 2, 1832.
15. New York *Morning Courier and Enquirer*, July 2, 1832.
16. New York *Evening Post*, July 2, 1832.
17. New York *American*, July 2, 1832.
18. New York *Commercial Advertiser*, July 3, 1832.

19. New York *Evening Post*, July 3, 1832.
20. James R. Manley, *Letters Addressed to the Board of Health, and to Richard Riker, Recorder of the City of New-York* (Peter Van Pelt, 1832), 17.
21. John Pintard, *Letters from John Pintard to His Daughter, Eliza Noel Pintard Davidson, 1816–1833* (New York Historical Society, 1911), 66.
22. E. E. Briggs to Jeremiah Briggs, July 4, 1832, Jeremiah Briggs Letters, Manuscripts and Archives Division, New York Public Library, New York.
23. New York *Mercury*, July 4, 1832; New York *Journal of Commerce*, July 4 and July 7, 1832.
24. New York *Commercial Advertiser*, July 5, 1832.
25. New York *Commercial Advertiser*, July 7, 1832.
26. New York *Commercial Advertiser*, July 7, 1832.
27. William Price to James Clapp, July 8, 1832, Kernan Family Papers, Box 1, Rare and Manuscripts Collections, Carl A. Kroch Library, Cornell University, Ithaca.
28. Abby Wood to Sarah Morse Haynsworth, July 10 [1832], Haynsworth Family Paper Papers, 1229: 25/28/5, SCHS.
29. New York *Evening Post*, July 13, 1832; N. Willis to Captain Briggs, July 22, 1832, Jeremiah Briggs Letters, Manuscripts and Archives Division, New York Public Library, New York; Samuel R. Johnson to William Shelton, July 31, 1832, Samuel Roosevelt Johnson Papers, Box 3, GTS.
30. Samuel R. Johnson to Mr. and Mrs. Peter Roosevelt, July 5, 1832, Samuel Roosevelt Johnson Papers, Box 2, GTS.
31. Mrs. Peter Roosevelt to S. R. Johnson, July 7, 1832, Samuel Roosevelt Johnson Papers, Box 2, GTS.
32. Pintard, *Letters*, 67.
33. Pintard, *Letters*, 71.
34. New York *Commercial Advertiser*, July 9, 1832.
35. Shah, *Pandemic*, 64–67.
36. Shah, *Pandemic*, 66.
37. New York *American*, July 9, 1832; New York *Evening Post*, July 10, 1832.
38. New York *Evening Post*, July 11, 1832.
39. James Lee to William H. Wilson, July 9, 1832, Wilson Family Papers, Box 34, WLCL (emphasis in original).
40. Christopher C. Yates, *Observations on the Epidemic Now Prevailing in the City of New-York; Called the Asiatic or Spasmodic Cholera; with Advice to the Planters of the South, for the Medical Treatment of Their Slaves* (George P. Scott and Co., 1832), 26.
41. Pintard, *Letters*, 72.
42. Lyman Beecher, *Six Sermons on the Nature, Occasions, Signs, Evils, and Remedy of Intemperance* (American Tract Society, 1827), 7–8, 44.
43. Beecher wrote his letter sometime between cholera's appearance in Canada and its arrival in New York City. It was first published in the Cincinnati *Standard* and then later published as a stand-alone piece by the American Tract Society, which

advertised it for sale two weeks into the outbreak in New York City. See New York *Evangelist*, July 14, 1832. It was also published in whole or in part in periodicals, including the one quoted from: Lyman Beecher, "An Appeal on the Subject of Cholera," *Christian Advocate* 10 (August 1832): 356–61, quotes on 356, 358, 357, 359, 360–61.

44. Samuel R. Johnson to Mr. and Mrs. P. Roosevelt, July 10 (morning), 1832, Samuel Roosevelt Johnson Papers, Box 2, GTS.
45. New York *Morning Courier and Enquirer*, July 14, 1832.
46. New York *Evening Post*, July 14, 1832.
47. New York *Evening Post*, July 14, 1832.
48. James Riker, Jr., Diary and Reminiscences, 1836–1868, Unpublished Mss., NYHS. Riker began making regular entries into his diary in 1836 but started with a retrospective account of his life up to that year.
49. Pintard, *Letters*, 73–74.
50. New York *American*, July 21, 1832.
51. New York *Evening Post*, July 16, 1832.
52. New York *Spectator*, July 19, 1832.
53. Poughkeepsie (NY) *Independence*, July 18, 1832; Boston *Traveler*, July 27, 1832 ("vagrants"); Philadelphia *Inquirer*, July 23, 1832 ("abandoned women"); Silas D. Canfield to Mahlon Canfield, July 24, 1832, Canfield-Dickerson Family Papers, Box 12, fo. 5, New Jersey Historical Society, Newark ("poorer classes"); Philadelphia *Inquirer*, July 23, 1832; John Lamb to Mary Lamb, July 22, 1832, James M. Willcox Papers, Box 1, Duke; Hiram Corson, *Reminiscences of the Cholera Epidemic of 1832: And Notes on the Treatment of the Disease at That Time [Reprinted from the Philadelphia Medical Times for Aug. 9 and Sept. 6, 1884]* (n.p., n.d.), 2; John Colt to Roswell Colt, July 29, 1832, Roswell L. Colt Family Papers, Special Collections, Alexander Library, Rutgers University, New Brunswick, New Jersey ("abandoned, drunken female from 5 points"); Silas Canfield to Mahlon Canfield, July 31, 1832, Canfield-Dickerson Papers, Box 12, fo. 5, New Jersey Historical Society, Newark.
54. Rosenberg, *The Cholera Years*, 32.
55. New York *American*, July 17, 1832.
56. New York *Morning Courier and Enquirer*, July 18, 1832.
57. New York *Evening Post*, July 23, 1832.
58. Pintard, *Letters*, 75.
59. Thomas Masters to Martha C. Master, July 19, 1832, Masters-Taylor-Wilbur Papers, Box 2, WLCL.
60. Atkins, *Reports of Hospital Physicians*, 153.
61. Atkins, *Reports of Hospital Physicians*, 151.
62. Samuel W. Francis, "Biographical Sketches of Distinguished Living New York Physicians, X. Isaac Wood, M.D.," *Medical and Surgical Reporter* 15 (July–December 1866): 454–58, quotes on 456.

63. David Oshinsky, *Bellevue: Three Centuries of Medicine and Mayhem at America's Most Storied Hospital* (Doubleday, 2016), 42–43.
64. New York *Commercial Advertiser*, July 21, 1832.
65. New York *American*, July 10, 1832.
66. Judith Roosevelt to Samuel R. Johnson, July 18, 1832, Samuel Roosevelt Johnson Papers, Box 3, GTS.
67. New York *Evening Post*, July 20, 1832. The board of health report of July 21, 1832, lists a death on the corner of Desbrosses and Greenwich streets. Presumably this was of Judith Roosevelt. New York *Evening Post*, July 23, 1832.
68. Samuel R. Johnson to William Shelton, July 31, 1832, Samuel Roosevelt Johnson Papers, Box 3, GTS.

CHAPTER 4

1. Kristin O'Brassill-Kulfan, *Vagrants and Vagabonds: Poverty and Mobility in the Early American Republic* (New York University Press, 2019), 134, 149.
2. Samuel Jackson, "Report Embracing a View of Principal Facts Connected with the Prevalence of Malignant Cholera in Philadelphia in 1832, Made to the Consulting Medical Board," in Philadelphia *Cholera Gazette* 1, nos. 15 and 16 (November 21, 1832), 249.
3. Pennsylvania General Assembly, *Report of the Committee Appointed to Investigate the Local Causes of Cholera in the Arch Street Prison* (Henry Welsh, 1833), 5–6.
4. Philadelphia *Inquirer*, July 6, 1832; Philadelphia *Daily Chronicle*, July 6, 1832; Philadelphia *Poulson's American*, July 6, 1832; Philadelphia *National Gazette*, July 7, 1832; Philadelphia *United States Gazette*, July 7, 1832.
5. Jackson, "Report Embracing a View of the Principal Facts," in Philadelphia *Cholera Gazette* (November 21, 1832), 245–46.
6. On the rain in Philadelphia on the twenty-ninth, see entry for July 29, 1832, in Deborah Norris Logan Diary, Vol. 14, 1832–1834, Logan Family Papers (Collection 379), Box 41, HSP (hereafter cited as Logan Diary); Philadelphia *Daily Chronicle*, July 30, 1832; Philadelphia *Inquirer*, July 31, 1832.
7. Philadelphia *National Gazette*, July 31, 1832.
8. John Lamb to Mary Lamb, July 31, 1832, James M. Willcox Papers, Box 1, Duke.
9. Philadelphia *Gazette*, August 6, 1832.
10. On rainfall, see entries for August 4 and 5, 1832, in Logan Diary. A table of cases and deaths from July 29 through August 13 is given in Corson, *Reminiscences of the Cholera Epidemic of 1832*, 2.
11. Entry of August 6, 1832, in Logan Diary; Philadelphia *Inquirer*, August 8, 1832, August 10, 1832.
12. Corson, *Reminiscences of the Cholera Epidemic of 1832*, 4.
13. John B. Osborne, "Preparing for the Pandemic: City Boards of Health and the Arrival of Cholera in Montreal, New York, and Philadelphia in 1832," *Urban History*

Review 36 (January 2008): 39; see also John B. Osborne, "Cholera," in *Encyclopedia of Greater Philadelphia*, accessed June 22, 2020, https://philadelphiaencyclopedia.org/archive/cholera/.

14. Philadelphia *Inquirer*, August 3, 1832; Osburn, "Preparing for the Pandemic," 37.
15. John Watson and Willis Hazard, eds., *Annals of Philadelphia, and Pennsylvania, in the Olden Time: Being a Collection of Memoirs, Anecdotes, and Incidents of the City and Its Inhabitants and of the Earliest Settlements of the Inland Part of Pennsylvania*, vol. 3 (E. S. Stuart, 1891), 393.
16. Philadelphia *Inquirer*, August 3, 1832; Osburn, "Preparing for the Pandemic," 37.
17. Philadelphia *Inquirer*, August 8, 1832. Doctors who signed the letter were as follows: Joseph Parrish, N. Chapman, Samuel Jackson, Thomas Harris, Richard Harlan, Ch. D. Meigs, Ch. Lukens, W. E. Horner, O. H. Taylor.
18. Philadelphia *Inquirer*, August 8, 1832.
19. New York *American*, August 10, 1832 (its own words and the reprinted doctors' letter). Baltimore *Gazette*, August 9, 1832, reprinted from preamble from Philadelphia *Inquirer* and then the doctors' letter. See also New York *Evening Post*, August 9, 1832; Gettysburg (PA) *Adams Sentinel*, August 14, 1832; Litchfield (CT) *Enquirer*, August 16, 1832.
20. New York *Evening Post*, August 8, 1832; Philadelphia *Daily Chronicle*, August 9, 1832; Philadelphia *Poulson's American*, August 10, 1832; Baltimore *Gazette*, August 14, 1832; Newburyport (MA) *Herald*, August 14, 1832; Lancaster (PA) *Examiner*, August 16, 1832; Poughkeepsie (NY) *Journal*, August 15, 1832; Portsmouth (NH) *Gazette*, August 28, 1832; St. Johnsbury (VT) *Weekly Messenger and Connecticut and Passumpsic River Valley Advertiser*, September 4, 1832.
21. New York *Commercial Advertiser*, August 14, 1832.
22. Utica (NY) *Sentinel and Gazette*, August 21, 1832.
23. Maria Miller to Isabella Bloomfield, September 11, 1832, Oneida County History Center, photocopy provided by Janice Reilly.
24. Utica (NY) *Sentinel and Gazette*, August 21, 1832.
25. Entry of August 23, 1832, in Board of Health, Minute Books, 1832, Utica, NY, Uticana Collection, BHE 1, Oneida County History Center; Utica (NY) *Sentinel and Gazette*, August 14, 1832, August 21, 1832.
26. Amos H. Hosmer to Asa and Mary Davis, March 12, 1833, Amos H. Hosmer letter, MS 2958.4780, NYHS.
27. The *Observer*'s brief account was taken up and reprinted in several papers with little variation: New York *Commercial Advertiser*, September 7, 1832; New York *Evening Post*, September 7, 1832; Boston *Courier*, September 10, 1832; Salem (MA) *Gazette*, September 11, 1832; New York *American*, September 11, 1832; Washington (DC) *National Intelligencer*, September 11, 1832; Alexanderia (VA) *Gazette*, September 11, 1832; Northampton (MA) *Hampshire Gazette*, September 12, 1832; New Haven (CT) *Columbian Register*, September 15, 1832; Windsor *Vermont Republican*, September 15, 1832; Lynchburg *Virginian*, September 17, 1832; Nashville *National Banner*, September 19, 1832.

28. Utica (NY) *Sentinel and Gazette*, September 4, 1832.
29. Utica (NY) *Sentinel and Gazette*, September 11, 1832.
30. Entry for September 3, 1832, in Board of Health, Minute Books, 1832, Utica, NY.
31. Poughkeepsie (NY) *Independence*, July 4, 1832.
32. Hunting Sherrill, *An Essay on Epidemics: As They Appeared in Dutchess County, from 1809 to 1824: . . . with an Appendix, Containing an Account of the Epidemic Cholera, as It Appeared in Poughkeepsie in 1832* (Booth & Smith, 1832), 11.
33. Hunting Sherrill, *On the Pathology of Epidemic Cholera* (S. Wood and Sons, 1835), 10.
34. Poughkeepsie (NY) *Independence*, July 18, 1832; Poughkeepsie (NY) *Journal*, July 18, 1832.
35. Poughkeepsie (NY) *Independence*, July 25, 1832; Poughkeepsie (NY) *Journal*, July 25, 1832.
36. New York *Evening Post*, July 25, 1832.
37. Sherrill, *On the Pathology of Epidemic Cholera*, 11.
38. Sherrill, *On the Pathology of Epidemic Cholera*, 10.
39. Sherrill, *An Essay on Epidemics*, 12.
40. Poughkeepsie (NY) *Independence*, August 1, 1832.
41. Sherrill, *On the Pathology of Epidemic Cholera*, 16.
42. Poughkeepsie (NY) *Journal*, August 1, 1832.
43. New York *Evening Post*, August 4, 1832.
44. Sherrill, *On the Pathology of Epidemic Cholera*, 15–16. Newspapers at the time of the outbreak perpetuated an estimate of "about 220" inmates. The source of the estimate was never made clear. See New York *Evening Post*, August 4, 1832. Sherrill had visited the poorhouse during the outbreak and examined its records afterward, and thus his estimate seems more reliable.
45. Poughkeepsie (NY) *Independence*, August 8, 1832. Perhaps due to a later publication schedule, the *Journal* of August 8, 1832, put the number of dead in the poor house at fifty.
46. Poughkeepsie (NY) *Dutchess Republican*, August 8, 1832, in New York *Commercial Advertiser*, August 8, 1832; Philadelphia *Daily Chronicle*, August 9, 1832; Baltimore *American*, August 10, 1832; Philadelphia *Inquirer*, August 10, 1832; Alexandria (VA) *Gazette*, August 11, 1832; Newburyport (MA) *Herald*, August 14, 1832; Providence (RI) *American*, August 14, 1832; Salem (MA) *Gazette*, August 14, 1832; Saratoga Springs (NY) *Sentinel*, August 14, 1832; Richmond (VA) *Constitutional Whig*, August 14, 1832; Charleston (SC) *Courier*, August 16, 1832; Jackson (TN) *Southern Statesman*, August 25, 1832.
47. Henry Noble McCracken, *Blithe Dutchess: The Flowering of an American County from 1812* (Hastings House, 1958), 313.
48. New York *Spectator*, August 13, 1832.
49. Sherrill, *On the Pathology of Epidemic Cholera*, 26. Sherrill claimed to find this number in the poorhouse's records.
50. Albany (NY) *Argus*, August 24, 1832.

51. Newark (NJ) *Daily Advertiser*, July 12, 1832.
52. Newark (NJ) *Daily Advertiser*, July 17, 1832.
53. Newark (NJ) *Daily Advertiser*, July 16, 1832.
54. Newark (NJ) *Daily Advertiser*, July 19, 1832.
55. Newark (NJ) *Daily Advertiser*, July 16, 1832.
56. [Unsigned] to Mrs. Patrick, August 1, 1832, American Science and Medicine Collection, WLCL.
57. Newark (NJ) *Daily Advertiser*, July 20, 1832.
58. Newark (NJ) *Daily Advertiser*, July 21, 1832, July 23, 1832.
59. Newark (NJ) *Daily Advertiser*, August 1, 1832. The *Daily Advertiser* listed James as a nine-year-old, but his age at the time was eight according to ancestry.com, which noted his death in October. https://www.ancestry.com/discoveryui-content/view/190145611:60541?tid=&pid=&queryId=8ee1304a2eac8c7de909083f4b4a4412&_phsrc=MNh102&_phstart=successSource.
60. Newark (NJ) *Daily Advertiser*, August 3, 1832, August 6, 1832, August 10, 1832, August 18, 1832, August 20, 1832, August 22, 1832, August 23, 1832, and September 15, 1832.
61. Samuel H. Pennington, "Report for the Eastern District," in *The Rise, Minutes, and Proceedings, of the New Jersey Medical Society, Established July 23d, 1766* (Jennings & Hardham, 1875), 301–8 (quote on 308).
62. Pennington, "Report for the Eastern District," 303.
63. Charles Lawrence, *History of the Philadelphia Almshouses and Hospitals from the Beginning of the Eighteenth to the Ending of the Nineteenth Centuries . . .: Showing the Mode of Distributing Public Relief Through the Management of the Boards of Overseers of the Poor, Guardians of the Poor and the Directors of the Department of Charities and Correction* (1905), 116, 118–19.
64. Philadelphia *Cholera Gazette*, August 15, 1832.
65. Philadelphia *Daily Chronicle*, August 13, 1832.
66. Lawrence, *History of the Philadelphia Almshouses*, 120–21.
67. Lawrence, *History of the Philadelphia Almshouses*, 119.
68. Philadelphia *Cholera Gazette*, November 25, 1832.
69. Rosenberg, *Cholera Years*, 29.
70. Boston *Christian Herald*, August 8, 1832.
71. Boston *US Catholic Intelligencer*, August 17, 1832.
72. Boston *US Catholic Intelligencer*, September 14, 1832.
73. Boston *Traveler*, October 30, 1832.
74. Lemuel Shattuck, *Report of the Sanitary Commission of Massachusetts, 1850* (Harvard University Press, 1948), 80.
75. A. K. Hoffman, "Communication from A.K. Hoffman, M.D. Physician of the Sing Sing State Prison, December 25, 1832," *Transactions of the Medical Society of the State of New York*, vol. 2 (E. W. and C. Skinner, 1835), 91.
76. New York *American*, July 20, 1832.

77. New York *Evening Post*, July 21, 1832.
78. Albany (NY) *Argus*, July 27, 1832.
79. Hoffman, "Communication from A.K. Hoffman," 91.
80. New York *American*, August 10, 1832.
81. Hoffman, "Communication from A.K. Hoffman," 91.
82. New York *Commercial Advertiser*, August 30, 1832.
83. "On the Apartment for Criminals and Untried Prisoners, in the Arch Street Jail," *Hazard's Register of Pennsylvania* 11, no. 12 (March 23, 1833): 177–84. This was a reprint of an official publication: *Report of the Committee Appointed to Investigate the Local Causes of Cholera in the Arch Street Prison, in the City of Philadelphia* (Henry Welsh, 1833).
84. "On the Apartment for Criminals and Untried Prisoners," 177. That the bacteria spread by way of crowding and poor hygiene rather than a contaminated water source seems more likely as Arch Street Prison stood along the main water lines of the Fairmount Water Works and would not have received water from a nearby and contaminated source. Kristin O'Brassill-Kulfan, personal communication, September 29, 2023.
85. "On the Apartment for Criminals and Untried Prisoners," 177.
86. Jessie Reading Burden, "Report on Arch Street Prison," in *Report of the Committee Appointed to Visit the Eastern Penitentiary* (Henry Welsh, 1833), 18; "On the Apartment for Criminals and Untried Prisoners," 177 ("bewildered").
87. Kristin O'Brassill-Kulfan, "'People First': Interpreting and Commemorating Houselessness and Poverty," *The Public Historian* 45 (February 2023): 29.
88. "On the Apartment for Criminals and Untried Prisoners," 178.
89. "On the Apartment for Criminals and Untried Prisoners," 177.
90. Richard Harlan to John James Audubon, quoted in Richard Rhodes, *John James Audubon: The Making of an American* (Knopf, 2004), 368.
91. "On the Apartment for Criminals and Untried Prisoners," 178.
92. Philadelphia *Inquirer*, August 6, 1832.
93. "What Shall We Do?" *Journal of Health* 3, no. 23 (August 8, 1832), 357.
94. This article is attributed to the Philadelphia *Sunday Morning Courier* of August 11 and reprinted in Philadelphia *Daily Chronicle*, August 13, 1832.
95. Philadelphia *The United States Gazette*, August 8, 1832.
96. Philadelphia *The United States Gazette*, August 11, 1832.

CHAPTER 5

1. Entries for August 11, August 18, August 24, and August 25, 1832, in Ann M. Van Wart Journals, 1832–1837, vol. 1, WLCL
2. Entries for August 13, August 26, and August 28, 1832, in Ann M. Van Wart Journals, 1832–1837, vol. 1, WLCL
3. Lydia and Charles G. Finney to Parents, July 15, 1832, Finney Papers, Box 3, Oberlin.
4. Lydia and Charles G. Finney to Parents, July 15, 1832, Finney Papers, Box 3, Oberlin.

5. Ad ran continuously in New York *Commercial Advertiser* from July 24 to August 14, 1832.
6. New York *Morning Courier and Enquirer*, July 25, 1832.
7. New York *Truth Teller* in Boston *US Catholic Intelligencer*, August 3, 1832.
8. New York *Commercial Advertiser*, July 26, 1832; New York *Mercury*, August 8, 1832.
9. New York *Evangelist*, August 4, 1832.
10. Tho[mas] H. Skinner to C. G. Finney, July 29, 1832, Finney Papers, Box 3, Oberlin.
11. Charles G. Finney, *Memoirs of Rev. Charles G. Finney. Written by Himself* (A. S. Barnes & Company, 1876), 320.
12. Silas Mathews to C. G. Finney, August 11, 1832, Finney Papers, Box 3, Oberlin; Luther Myrick to C. G. Finney, September 3, 1832, Finney Papers, Box 3, Oberlin.
13. Lewis Tappan to C. G. Finney, August 17, 1832, Finney Papers, Box 3, Oberlin.
14. William Green, Jr., to Charles Finney, August 25, 1832, Finney Papers, Box 3, Oberlin.
15. Pintard, *Letters*, 74.
16. John Pintard to Samuel Bayard, July 19, 1832, Pintard Papers, Box 3, fo. 6, NYHS; Pintard, *Letters*, 74 (quote).
17. Pintard, *Letters*, 75.
18. John Pintard to Samuel Bayard, July 26, 1832, Pintard Papers, Box 3, fo. 6, NYHS.
19. Pintard, *Letters*, 82 and 86.
20. John Pintard to Samuel Bayard, July 19, 1832, Pintard Papers, Box 3, fo. 6, NYHS.
21. John Pintard to Samuel Bayard, July 26, 1832, Pintard Papers, Box 3, fo. 6, NYHS.
22. Pintard, *Letters*, 76.
23. Pintard, *Letters*, 77.
24. Pintard, *Letters*, 78.
25. Pintard, *Letters*, 78.
26. Pintard, *Letters*, 80. The cause of Bristed's death was identified as cholera in the New York *Journal of Commerce*, August 2, 1832, but was not identified in other newspapers. See New York *American*, August 2, 1832; New York *Commercial Advertiser*, August 2, 1832; New York *Mercury*, August 8, 1832.
27. Pintard, *Letters*, 82.
28. Pintard, *Letters*, 86–87.
29. Pintard, *Letters*, 91–92.
30. Ewing seemed to be well known at the time, but he appears largely absent from historical work. He was educated at the College of New Jersey (later Princeton), studied law, and created a prosperous practice in Trenton. He served as a Federalist in New Jersey's State Legislature. For more information, see "Biography of Charles Ewing," Ewing Township, accessed December 10, 2023, https://www.ewingnj.org/charlesewing.
31. New York *Commercial Advertiser*, August 7, 1832.

32. Silas D. Canfield to Mahlon Canfield, August 7, 1832, Canfield-Dickerson Family Papers, Box 12, fo. 5, New Jersey Historical Society, Newark.
33. Salem (NJ) *Messenger*, c. August 8 (original not found) but reprinted in Philadelphia *Daily Chronicle*, August 11, 1832; New York *Commercial Advertiser*, August 13, 1832; Richmond (VA) *Enquirer*, August 14, 1832; Bridgeport (CT) *Spirit of the Times*, August 15, 1832; Providence (RI) *Microcosm*, August 18, 1832; Wilkes-Barre (PA) *Wyoming Republican and Herald*, August 22, 1832; Staunton (VA) *Spectator*, August 24, 1832.
34. New York *Commercial Advertiser*, August 13, 1832.
35. New York *Commercial Advertiser*, August 15, 1832.
36. Trenton *New Jersey State Gazette*, August 18, 1832.
37. P. R. Livingston to Samuel Southard, August 8, 1832, Southard Papers, Box 41, fo. 5, Firestone Library Special Collections, Princeton University; Trenton *Emporium and True American*, August 11, 1832.
38. Garret D. Wall to Samuel Southard, August 23, 1832, Southard Papers, Box 42, fo. 7, Firestone Library Special Collections.
39. Marleen Barr, "Deborah Norris Logan, Feminist Criticism, and Identity Theory: Interpreting a Woman's Diary Without the Danger of Separatism," *Biography* 8, no. 1 (1985): 12–24.
40. Entries of May 3, May 13, May 25, June 29, and July 2, 1832, in Logan Diary.
41. Entry for July 7, 1832, in Logan Diary.
42. Entry for August 4, 1832, in Logan Diary.
43. Entry for August 6, 1832, in Logan Diary.
44. For more on the estate, see Stenton: A House of Learning, Past and Present, accessed December 10, 2023, https://www.stenton.org/cultural-landscape-1.
45. Entry for August 7, 1832, in Logan Diary; Deborah Norris Logan to Sarah Miller Walker, August 19, 1832, Maria Dickinson Logan Collection (Collection 382), HSP.
46. Entry for August 8, 1832, in Logan Diary.
47. Entry for August 9, 1832, in Logan Diary.
48. Philadelphia *Poulson's American*, August 8, 1832.
49. Deborah Norris Logan to Sarah Miller Walker, August 19, 1832, Maria Dickinson Logan Collection (Collection 0382), HSP.
50. Philadelphia *Poulson's American*, August 21, 1832.
51. Entry for August 22, 1832, in Logan Diary.
52. Entry for August 28, 1832, in Logan Diary.
53. Entry for August 30, 1832, in Logan Diary.
54. Entry for August 31, 1832, in Logan Diary.
55. New York *Evening Post*, August 22, 1832.
56. New York *Morning Courier and Enquirer*, August 28, 1832.
57. New York *American*, August 30, 1832.

58. New York *Evening Post*, September 11, 1832.
59. Finney, *Memoirs*, 320.
60. Oberlin (OH) *Oberlin Evangelist*, May 9, 1849.
61. Pintard, *Letters*, 92.
62. Pintard, *Letters*, 92.
63. Pintard, *Letters*, 95–96.
64. Pintard, *Letters*, 167.
65. Samuel Lewis Southard, *An Eulogium upon the Hon. Charles Ewing: Late Chief Justice of New Jersey* (D. Fenton, 1832), 11, 12.
66. John W. Barber and Henry Howe, *Historical Collections of the State of New Jersey* (S. Tuttle, 1846), 303. Ewing also had a township named after him in 1834: https://www.livingplaces.com/NJ/Mercer_County/Ewing_Township.html.
67. Entry for September 21, 1832, in Logan Diary.
68. Entry for September 22, 1832, in Logan Diary.
69. Entry for September 23, 1832, in Logan Diary.
70. Entry for September 23, 1832, in Logan Diary.
71. Diary of Deborah Bowman, Chester County Historical Society, West Chester, Pennsylvania.
72. Entry for September 24, 1832, in Logan Diary.
73. Entry for September 26, 1832, in Logan Diary.
74. Deborah Norris Logan to Sarah [Miller Walker], October 1, 1832, Maria Dickinson Logan Collection (Collection 382), HSP.
75. The cartographer and publisher Henry Schenk Tanner of Philadelphia compiled statistics from official reports, medical treatises, newspapers, and other sources to tabulate the number of deaths occurring globally up to the middle of September 1832 in his *Geographical and Statistical Account of the Epidemic Cholera*. His work is a good starting place to understand mortality patterns, but he rushed his work to publication before the outbreaks in the United States ceased, and his figures undercount mortality in the nation. This book relies on other sources for many of the areas that are focused on as follows: Shattuck, *Report of the Sanitary Commission*, 80 (Boston); "Annual Bill of Mortality," in New York, *Commercial Advertiser*, January 21, 1833 (New York City); William E. Rowley, "The Albany Microscope: Gadfly for Jacksonian Democracy," *New York History* 71, no. 2 (April 1990): 182–83 (Albany); Albany (NY) *Argus*, August 22, 1832 (Poughkeepsie); Hoffman, "Communication from A. K. Hoffman," 91 (Sing Sing); Pennington, "Report for the Eastern District," 301–8 (Newark); and Samuel Jackson, "Personal Observations and Experience of Epidemic or Malignant Cholera in the City of Philadelphia," *American Journal of Medical Sciences* 11 (February 1833): 292 (Philadelphia).
76. Atkins, *Reports of Hospital Physicians*, 11. This was advertised for sale on November 13. See New York *Evening Post*, November 13, 1832; New York *Spectator*, November 15, 1832; New York *Commercial Advertiser*, November 15, 1832.
77. Samuel Jackson, "Report Embracing a View of the Principal Facts," in Philadelphia *Cholera Gazette*, November 21, 1832, 244–52, quotes on 248.

78. James Riker, Jr., Diary and Reminiscences, 1836–1868, Unpublished Mss., NYHS.

CHAPTER 6

1. Alison Goodyear Freehling, *Drift Toward Dissolution: The Virginia Slavery Debate of 1831–1832* (Louisiana State University Press, 1982), 82–121, 144.
2. Ann Maury to Dr. James M. Morris, March 7, 1832, Richard Morris Papers, Box 2, UVA.
3. Ann Maury to Dr. James M. Morris, July 10, 1832, Richard Morris Papers, Box 2, UVA.
4. Ann Maury to Dr. James M. Morris, August 17, 1832, Richard Morris Papers, Box 2, UVA.
5. New York *Morning Courier and Enquirer*, June 27, 1832.
6. Baltimore *Gazette*, June 29, 1832; Richmond (VA) *Constitutional Whig*, July 3, 1832.
7. Philadelphia *National Gazette*, June 30, 1832; Alexandria (VA) *Gazette*, July 3, 1832; Easton (MD) *Gazette*, July 7, 1832; New Bern (NC) *Spectator*, July 6, 1832; Fayetteville (NC) *Observer*, July 10, 1832; Savannah (GA) *Republican*, July 12, 1832; Charles Town *Virginia Free Press*, July 26, 1832.
8. New York *American*, July 18, 1832, in Richmond (VA) *Enquirer*, July 24, 1832; Vicksburg (MS) *Whig*, August 9, 1832.
9. From New York *Journal of Commerce*, July 18, 1832, in Frederick (MD) *Herald*, July 21, 1832; Alexandria (VA) *Gazette*, July 23, 1832; Richmond (VA) *Constitutional Whig*, July 24, 1832; Charleston (SC) *Courier*, July 26, 1832.
10. Charleston (SC) *Courier*, August 9, 1832; reprinted in Macon (GA) *The Weekly Telegraph*, August 15, 1832.
11. Philadelphia *Cholera Gazette*, August 11, 1832, 63.
12. Yates, *Observations on the Epidemic Now Prevailing in the City of New-York... with Advice to the Planters of the South, for the Medical Treatment of Their Slaves*, 37. Notice of publication or advertised for sale in New York *Evening Post*, August 19, 1832; Baltimore *Gazette*, August 22, 1832; Alexandria (VA) *Gazette*, August 27, 1832; Charleston (SC) *Courier*, September 20, 1832; Savannah *Georgian*, September 18, 1832.
13. Baltimore *Gazette*, August 27, 1832; Hagerstown (MD) *Torch Light*, August 30, 1832; Washington (DC) *United States Telegraph*, August 31, 1832; Washington (DC) *Globe*, September 1, 1832; Richmond (VA) *Enquirer*, September 4, 1832; Philadelphia *National Gazette*, September 4, 1832; Washington (DC) *National Intelligencer*, September 5, 1832; Charles Town *Virginia Free Press*, September 6, 1832; Easton (MD) *Gazette*, September 8, 1832; Fayetteville (NC) *Observer*, September 11, 1832; Lynchburg *Virginian*, September 17, 1832; Frankfort (KY) *Argus*, September 26, 1832; Little Rock *Weekly Arkansas Gazette*, October 31, 1832.
14. John McPherson to William McPherson, August 7, 1832, American Science and Medicine Collection, WLCL; William Gibbons to William Dunham, August 14, 1832, Gibbons Papers, Letterbook 4, Drew University, Madison, New Jersey.

15. Benjamin Wright to John Hartwell Cocke, August 7, 1832, Cocke Family Papers, Box 71, UVA.
16. Entry for July 25, 1832, Common Place Book, 1827–1832, Blow Family Papers, Mss1 B6235a130, sec. 8, VHS.
17. It was not until a retrospective summary of the outbreak that the Norfolk Board of Health confirmed the epidemic had begun as early as July 24. See Norfolk (VA) *American Beacon*, September 18, 1832.
18. Norfolk (VA) *American Beacon*, August 2, 1832.
19. "City of Norfolk Utilities," Official Site of the City of Norfolk, 2025, https://www.norfolk.gov/DocumentCenter/View/74743/Utilities-Pamphlet.
20. Norfolk (VA) *American Beacon*, August 11, 1832.
21. Norfolk (VA) *American Beacon*, August 16, 1832.
22. Norfolk (VA) *American Beacon*, September 18, 1832.
23. Norfolk's population in the 1830 US Census was 9,814, and the city's growth had been stagnant. In 1840, the population reached just 10,920. See Gibson, "Population of the 100 Largest Cities and Other Urban Places in the United States."
24. Conway Whittle II to Francis M. Lewis, August 13, 1832, Conway Whittle Papers, Box 10, fo. 1, WMU; Entries for August 5 and 6, 1832, Louisa Cocke Diary, Cocke Family Papers, Box 193, UVA; Otway B. Barraud to John Hartwell Cocke, [August 5, 1832], Cocke Family Papers, Box 71, UVA; William Kennon to Nancy Randolph, August 13, 1832, William H. Kennon Papers, Box 1, UVA; Thomas [Ready?] to Samuel Downey, September 9, 1832, Samuel Smith Downey Papers, Box 4, Duke.
25. Eliza Vickery to Margaret Prentis, August 10, 1832, Webb-Prentis Papers, Box 9, UVA (emphasis in original).
26. Eliza Vickery to Margaret Prentis, August 20, 1832, Webb-Prentis Papers, Box 9, UVA.
27. Eliza Vickery to Margaret Prentis, August 30, 1832, Webb-Prentis Papers, Box 9, UVA.
28. Eliza Vickery to Margaret Prentis, August 28, 1832, Webb-Prentis Papers, Box 9, UVA; Eliza Vickery to Margaret Prentis, August 30, 1832, Webb-Prentis Papers, Box 9, UVA.
29. John Galt Williamson to Dr. A.D. Galt, September 7, 1832, Galt Papers, Series 2, Box 2, fo. 21, WMU.
30. William Kennon to Nancy Randolph, September 15, 1832, William H. Kennon Papers, Box 1, UVA.
31. Norfolk (VA) *American Beacon*, August 11, 1832, and August 16, 1832.
32. Other Southern papers picked this up: Baltimore *American*, August 15, 1832; Richmond (VA) *Whig and Commercial Journal*, August 17, 1832; Fredericksburg (VA) *Political Arena*, August 21, 1832; Nashville *National Banner*, August 28, 1832.
33. Norfolk (VA) *American Beacon*, September 13, 1832.
34. Norfolk (VA) *American Beacon*, September 18, 1832.
35. Norfolk (VA) *American Beacon*, September 18, 1832.

36. Eliza Vickery to Margaret Prentis, October 11, 1832, Webb-Prentis Papers, Box 9, UVA (emphasis in original).
37. Richmond (VA) *Whig and Commercial Journal*, October 15, 1832. Holt's death notice did not indicate cholera, but residents of Norfolk knew it to be the cause. See Mary Robertson to Louisa Cocke, October 15, 1832, Cocke Family Papers, Box 72, UVA.
38. Norfolk (VA) *American Beacon*, September 11, 1832.
39. Richmond (VA) *Enquirer*, September 14, 1832.
40. Richmond (VA) *Whig and Commercial Journal*, September 8, 1832; Richmond (VA) *Enquirer*, September 11, 1832.
41. Richmond (VA) *Enquirer*, September 11, 1832.
42. Richmond's population in the 1830 US Census was 16,060, and 20,153 in 1840. See Gibson, "Population of the 100 Largest Cities and Other Urban Places in the United States."
43. George Roper to George Crutchfield, September 14, 1832, Crutchfield Family Papers, VHS; Philip M. Tabb to William Patterson Smith, September 13, 1832, William Patterson Smith Papers, Box 3, Duke; Richmond (VA) *Whig and Commercial Journal*, September 13, 1832.
44. Richmond (VA) *Enquirer*, September 21, 1832.
45. Richmond (VA) *Southern Religious Telegraph*, September 21, 1832.
46. Richmond (VA) *Whig and Commercial Journal*, September 20, 1832.
47. Richmond (VA) *Whig and Commercial Journal*, September 22, 1832.
48. Richmond (VA) Department of Public Utilities, *Watering the City of Richmond* (William Byrd Press, 1930).
49. Various real estate advertisements tout connection to the water works. See Richmond (VA) *Enquirer*, July 6, 1832, and October 26, 1832; Richmond (VA) *Constitutional Whig*, November 16, 1832.
50. Richmond (VA) *Whig and Commercial Journal*, September 24, 1832.
51. Richmond (VA) *Constitutional Whig*, October 2, 1832.
52. James V. Wilcox, Jr., to Mary Ann Lamb, September 26, 1832, James M. Willcox Papers, Box 1, Duke.
53. Frank Harris to Frederick Harris, October 21, 1832, Frank A. Harris Papers, Duke.
54. Richmond (VA) *Enquirer*, October 5, 1832.
55. Richmond (VA) *Enquirer*, October 6, 1832.
56. Richmond (VA) *Enquirer*, October 5, 1832.
57. Richmond (VA) *Enquirer*, October 5, 1832.
58. Richmond (VA) *Compiler* in New York *Evening Post*, October 15, 1832. No surviving issues of the *Compiler* published during the fall of 1832 are known to exist, except September 29, 1832, and November 17, 1832, which appear to be available only in the Library of Congress in hardcopy. The author has not viewed these issues. See https://chroniclingamerica.loc.gov/lccn/sn84024698/holdings/.
59. Richmond (VA) *Whig and Commercial Journal*, October 15, 1832.
60. Richmond (VA) *Compiler* in Richmond, *Enquirer*, October 23, 1832.

61. Richard Cary Ambler to John Jaquelin Ambler, November 6, 1832, Ambler Family Papers, Box 16, UVA.
62. Richmond (VA) *Whig*, October 5, 1832.
63. New York *Journal of Commerce*, October 13, 1832.
64. Philadelphia *National Gazette*, October 15, 1832; New York *Mercury*, October 17, 1832; Boston *Columbian Centinel*, October 17, 1832; Portland (ME) *Eastern Argus*, October 17, 1832.
65. Richmond (VA) *Southern Religious Telegraph*, October 19, 1832. This was circulated in full in Northampton (MA) *Hampshire Gazette*, October 31, 1832; Little Rock *Weekly Arkansas Gazette*, December 5, 1832.
66. Richmond (VA) *Southern Religious Telegraph*, November 2, 1832.
67. Richmond (VA) *Constitutional Whig*, October 12, 1832. Some editors chose to reprint the racist piece. See New York *Commercial Advertiser*, October 15, 1832; Philadelphia *Inquirer*, October 15, 1832; New York *Christian Intelligencer*, October 20, 1832.
68. Ann Maury to Dr. James M. Morris, August 17, 1832, Richard Morris Papers, Box 2, UVA.
69. James Maury to James Vass, September 7, 1832, and James Maury to William Maury, September 22, 1832, both in James Maury Letter Book, vol. II, WMU.
70. Ann Maury to Dr. James M. Morris, November 3, 1832, Richard Morris Papers, Box 2, UVA.
71. Ann Maury to Dr. James M. Morris, August 27, 1833, Richard Morris Papers, Box 2, UVA.
72. Ann Maury to Dr. James M. Morris, November 3, 1832, Richard Morris Papers, Box 2, UVA.
73. Randolph Edwin Archer, *The Life of Rev. John Jasper, Pastor of Sixth Mt. Zion Baptist Church, Richmond, Va., from His Birth to the Present Time, with His Theory on the Rotation of the Sun* (R. T. Hill & Co., Publishers, 1884), 12, 7.
74. Henry Box Brown, *Narrative of Henry Box Brown, Who Escaped from Slavery Enclosed in a Box 3 Feet Long and 2 Wide. Written from a Statement of Facts Made by Himself by Charles Stearn* (Brown & Stearns, 1849), 40.
75. James Williams, *Narrative of James Williams, an American Slave, Who Was for Several Years a Driver on a Cotton Plantation in Alabama* (American Anti-Slavery Society; Isaac Knapp, 1838), 26, 27.

CHAPTER 7

1. C. F. Mercer to John Ingle, September 3, 1832, COCCR, Box 6, NARA, CPM.
2. Leesburg (VA) *Genius of Liberty*, September 1, 1832; Frederick (MD) *Herald*, September 1, 1832.
3. Washington (DC) *National Intelligencer*, September 6, 1832. The letter writer could not be anyone other than Mercer. His private letter was also dated September

3 from Leesburg and the travels of the anonymous letter writer matched those that Mercer discussed in his private letter.

4. Henry Boteler to John Ingle, September 4, 1832, COCCR, Box 6, NARA, CPM.
5. Peter Way, *Common Labour: Workers and the Digging of North American Canals, 1780–1860* (Cambridge University Press, 1993), 146–56.
6. R. John Brockman, *Commodore Robert F. Stockton, 1795–1866: Protean Man for a Protean Nation* (Cambria Press, 2009), 77–85.
7. S. Howell to Robert F. Stockton, August 3, 1832, Claude W. Unger Collection, (Collection 1860A), Box 22, fo. 5, HSP.
8. Philadelphia *National Gazette*, August 4, 1832; "Delaware and Raritan Canal and Princeton Basin," Report by Genevieve C. Cobb, October 14, 1973, Delaware and Raritan Canal Files, Historical Society of Princeton.
9. James W. Alexander, *Forty Years, Familiar Letters of James W. Alexander: Constituting, with Notes, a Memoir of His Life* (Scribner, 1870), 193.
10. Benjamin Rice to John H. Cocke, August 23, 1832, John Cocke Papers, Mss. 640, Box 71, UVA.
11. Alexander, *Forty Years, Familiar Letters of James W. Alexander*, 193.
12. Trenton *New Jersey State Gazette*, August 4, 1832.
13. Trenton *New Jersey State Gazette*, August 11, 1832, August 18, 1832.
14. Philadelphia *United States Gazette*, August 8, 1832.
15. Philadelphia *Daily Chronicle*, August 14, 1832; New York *Evening Post,* August 15, 1832; Baltimore *Gazette*, August 16, 1832; Philadelphia *National Gazette*, August 16, 1832; Newark *Daily Advertiser*, August 17, 1832; Washington (DC) *National Intelligencer*, August 18, 1832; Philadelphia *United States Gazette*, August 18, 1832; New York *Spectator*, August 20, 1832; Albany (NY) *Argus*, August 21, 1832; Boston *Columbian Centinel*, August 22, 1832; Northampton (MA) *Hampshire Gazette*, August 22, 1832; Norwich (CT) *Courier*, August 22, 1832; Hagerstown (MD) *Torch Light*, August 23, 1832; Pittsfield (MA) *Sun*, August 23, 1832; Charleston (SC) *Courier*, August 24, 1832; Gardiner (ME) *Christian Intelligencer*, August 24, 1832; Brattleboro (VT) *Messenger*, August 25, 1832; New York *Observer*, August 25, 1832.
16. From the Doylestown *Democrat* in Philadelphia *Inquirer*, August 23, 1832; Philadelphia *Daily Chronicle*, August 23, 1832; Boston *Courier*, August 28, 1832; Providence *Rhode-Island American*, August 28, 1832; Baltimore *Gazette*, August 30, 1832; Dedham (MA) *Patriot*, August 31, 1832; Amherst (NH) *Farmer's Cabinet*, August 31, 1832; Brattleboro (VT) *Messenger*, September 1, 1832; Worcester *Massachusetts Spy*, September 5, 1832.
17. Trenton *New Jersey State Gazette*, September 8, 1832.
18. Summersville (NJ) *Messenger*, July 18, 1832, in New York *American*, July 20, 1832.
19. Trenton *New Jersey State Gazette*, August 11, 1832.
20. Trenton *Emporium and True American*, August 18, 1832.
21. Trenton *New Jersey State Gazette*, August 18, 1832.
22. Trenton *Emporium and True American*, November 3, 1832.

23. Brockman, *Commodore Robert F. Stockton*.
24. Gerald A. Francis, "The Philadelphia & Columbia Railway," The Lower Merion Historical Society, 2025, https://collections.lowermerionhistory.org/home/full-text/contents/columbia-railway/.
25. West Chester (PA) *Village Record and General Advertiser*, September 5, 1832. This account identifies the location as the border between Newlin and West Bradford townships, which is ten miles west of West Chester.
26. The original source of this is merely listed as "*Temp. Adv.*," which was the short-lived *Temperance Advocate and Journal of the Times* published out of West Chester, Pennsylvania. No issues dated to 1832 are known to currently exist. (See Library of Congress, Chronicling America Historic American Newspapers online, https://chroniclingamerica.loc.gov/lccn/sn90069125/.) The West Chester (PA) *Chester County Democrat* reprinted the report in its September 4, 1832, issue. The account identified the company as the "Pennsylvania Railroad," which was also used at the time for the P&C, and the location of the outbreak as "lower down the valley," which would have been in the general direction of Newlin and West Bradford. If the two newspapers were referring to the same location, they probably were referring to the railroad near where it crossed the west branch of Brandywine Creek. This suggests that the first mass burial of railroad workers occurred near Downington rather than East Whiteland, or today's Malvern, as suggested in William E. Watson and J. Francis Watson, *Massacre at Duffy's Cut: Tragedy & Conspiracy on the Pennsylvania Railroad* (The History Press, 2018).
27. West Chester (PA) *Village Record*, August 29, 1832.
28. West Chester (PA) *Temperance Advocate* in *Chester County Democrat*, September 4, 1832 (emphases in the original).
29. West Chester (PA) *Village Record*, August 29, 1832.
30. West Chester (PA) *Village Record*, September 5, 1832.
31. West Chester (PA) *Chester County Democrat*, September 11, 1832.
32. Watson and Watson, *Massacre at Duffy's Cut*, 71.
33. "Humanity Disgraced" in Baltimore's *Gazette*, October 23, 1823; Hagerstown (MD) *Torch Light*, October 25, 1832; Annapolis *Maryland Republican*, October 27, 1832; Easton (MD) *Gazette*, October 27, 1832; Lynchburg *Virginian*, October 29, 1832; York (PA) *Gazette*, October 30, 1832; Gettysburg (PA) *Adams Sentinel*, November 6, 1832; Steubenville (OH) *Jefferson Democrat*, November 7, 1832. See also Wilkes-Barre (PA) *Wyoming Republican*, October 3, 1832; Alexandria (VA) *Gazette*, October 16, 1832.
34. "Unparalleled Barbarity" first appeared in Pottsville (PA) *The Miner's Journal*, November 3, 1832, and this version was then reprinted in New York *Commercial Advertiser*, November 6, 1832; Philadelphia *Inquirer*, November 6, 1832; Philadelphia *Daily Chronicle*, November 6; New York *Evening Post*, November 7; New York *Spectator*, November 8; New Haven *Columbian Register*, November 10; Trenton *Emporium and True American*, November 10, 1832; Portland (ME) *Eastern Argus*,

November 12, 1832; Buffalo (NY) *Patriot and Commercial Advertiser*, November 13, 1832; Richmond (VA) *Enquirer*, November 13, 1832; Delhi (NY) *Delaware Gazette*, November 14, 1832; Worcester *Massachusetts Spy*, November 14, 1832; Litchfield (CT) *Enquirer*, November 13, 1832; Boston *New England Artisan, and Farmer's Mechanic's and Laboring-man's Repository*, November 15, 1832; Boston *Investigator*, November 16, 1832; Brattleboro (VT) *Messenger*, November 17, 1832; Boston *Trumpet and Universalist Magazine*, November 17, 1832; Danville (VT) *North Star*, November 19, 1832; Norwalk (OH) *Huron Reflector*, November 20, 1832; Rutland (VT) *Weekly Herald*, November 20, 1832; Easton (MD) *Eastern-Shore Whig and People's Advocate*, November 20, 1832; Sandusky (OH) *Clarion*, November 21, 1832; Schenectady (NY) *Cabinet*, November 21, 1832.

35. Nashville *National Banner*, November 3, 1832; reprinted in Little Rock (AR) *Times and Advocate*, November 21, 1832.
36. The October 3, 1832, issue does not survive today in any known collection, but it was published and appears to have been mailed out to subscribers outside of Chester County as the poem cannot be found in any prior issues. It is most likely that the editor, Charles Miner, when he retired, pulled the October 3 issue for unclear reasons before he donated the rest of the issues to a local historical society. The issue may have included a version of the "Humanity Disgraced" story or at least alluded to it. William E. Watson and J. Francis Watson suggest that the East Whiteland Horse Company prevented this issue from circulating at least locally because it potentially incriminated individuals in the murders. See Watson and Watson, *Massacre at Duffy's Cut*, 67.
37. The poem, but no other content from the October 3 issue, made it into a remarkable number of newspapers: Washington (DC) *National Intelligencer*, October 5, 1832; New York *American*, October 6, 1832; Fayetteville (NC) *Weekly Observer*, October 9, 1832; Boston *Courier*, October 9, 1832; Philadelphia *Daily Chronicle*, October 9, 1832; Philadelphia *Poulson's American*, October 10, 1832; Boston *Traveller*, October 12, 1832; Newport (RI) *Herald of the Times*, October 18, 1832; Pawtucket (RI) *Chronicle*, October 19, 1832; Charlotte (NC) *Miners' and Farmers' Journal*, October 20, 1832; Litchfield (CT) *Enquirer*, October 25, 1832; Woodstock *Vermont Courier and Farmer's, Manufacturer's, and Mechanic's Advocate*, October 26, 1832; Woodstock (VT) *Mercury*, October 26, 1832; Litchfield (CT) *Enquirer*, October 25, 1832; Boston *Liberator*, October 27, 1832; Savannah *Georgian*, October 29, 1832; Hagerstown (MD) *Torch Light*, November 15, 1832.
38. "Resolution of 9th April, 1833—Pamph. Laws, page 502. RESOLUTION, For the relief of William B. Mitchell," in *Compilation of the Laws of Pennsylvania, Relative to the Internal Improvements: Together with the Canal and Railway Regulations, as Established by the Board of Canal Commissioners* (Barrett and Parke, 1840), 108.
39. Quoted in Watson and Watson, *Massacre at Duffy's Cut*, 45.
40. West Chester (PA) *Village Record*, November 7, 1832.
41. West Chester (PA) *Village Record*, November 14, 1832.

42. New York *Spectator*, November 19, 1832.
43. Pottsville (PA) *Miner's Journal*, November 24, 1832.
44. Rosenberg, *The Cholera Years*, 37; Cohn, *Epidemics*, 187.
45. Margaret Bayard Smith, *The First Forty Years of Washington Society: Portrayed by the Family Letters of Mrs. Samuel Harrison Smith from the Collection of Her Grandson* (Scribner, 1906): 335–40.
46. Washington (DC) *National Intelligencer*, January 8, 1833.
47. Joseph Hollman to John Ingle, September 4, 1832, Thomas McCoy to John Ingle, September 6, 1832, and Benjamin Price to John Ingle, September 5, 1832, all in COCCR, Box 6, NARA, CPM.
48. Purcell to President and Director, September 11, 1832, COCCR, Box 6, CPM.
49. Hagerstown (MD) *Torch Light*, September 6, 1832.
50. Baltimore *Niles Weekly Register*, September 22, 1832, 52.
51. New York *Commercial Advertiser*, October 6, 1832. The letter was dated September 21, 1832, and other papers reprinted it. See Frederick (MD) *Herald*, October 13, 1832, and Annapolis *Maryland Gazette*, October 25, 1832.
52. Mercer to Walter Smith, September 24, 1832, COCCR, Box 6, NARA, CPM.
53. Washington (DC) *National Intelligencer*, October 18, 1832.
54. Washington (DC) *National Intelligencer*, October 24, 1832.
55. Richmond (VA) *Enquirer*, October 9, 1832.
56. Hagerstown (MD) *Torch Light*, October 18, October 25, and November 1, 1832; Charles Town *Virigina Free Press*, October 18, 1832.
57. Alfred Cruger to Mercer, December 10, 1832, Alfred Cruger to President and Directors, December 20, 1832, Gordon to Board of Directors, December 31, 1832, all in COCCR, Box 6, NARA, CPM.
58. [Charles F. Mercer], *Memorial of the Chesapeake and Ohio Canal Company to the General Assembly of Maryland, December 31, 1832* (Washington, 1832), 8.
59. Proceedings of the Stockholders, Volume A, Chesapeake and Ohio Canal Company, 1828 to 1835, 276, COCCR.
60. Delaware and Raritan Canal Commission, "A Brief History of the Delaware and Raritan Canal," accessed February 21, 2025, https://www.nj.gov/dep/drcc/about-canal/history/. There are remnants of headstones in Griggstown Cemetery on Canal Road that are also believed to be markers of nineteen Irish canal workers taken by cholera in 1832. See Janet Muser, *Rocky Hill, Kingston, and Griggstown* (Arcadia Publishing, 1998), 110.
61. State of New Jersey Department of Environmental Protection News Release, March 17, 2003, NJDEP-News Release 03/30 - Honoring the Irish Who Built the D&R Canal. The picture of the stone monument can be found here: https://www.nj.gov/dep/drcc/about-canal/history/.
62. Photo posted on Historical Marker Database online, accessed February 21, 2025, https://www.hmdb.org/Photos1/132/Photo132466o.jpg?11252005.
63. Watson and Watson, *Massacre at Duffy's Cut*, 66.

64. "'Duffy's Cut Part Two' as Team Uncovers Fresh Mass Burial Site," *Derry Journal*, June 5, 2020, https://www.derryjournal.com/news/people/duffys-cut-part-two-as-teamuncovers-fresh-mass-burial-site-2875720. In May 2025, the Watsons exhumed human remains from a steep embankment on the outer edge of the Northwood Cemetery. As of this writing, they continue to investigate the connection of the remains to the 1832 cholera outbreak and possible vigilante violence. See Zoe Greenberg, "Evidence Suggesting a Second Mass Grave of Irish Railroad Workers Is Unearthed in Downington," *Philadelphia Inquirer*, July 15, 2025.
65. Watson and Watson, *Massacre at Duffy's Cut*, 115.
66. Watson and Watson, *Massacre at Duffy's Cut*, 137.
67. Watson and Watson, *Massacre at Duffy's Cut*, 120–22.
68. Watson and Watson, *Massacre at Duffy's Cut*, 132.

CHAPTER 8

1. Frederick Douglass, *Life and Times of Frederick Douglass, Written by Himself*, rev. ed. (DeWolf & Fiske Company, 1892), 108, 109.
2. Baltimore *American*, June 12, 1832.
3. Isaac A. Coles to John Hartwell Cocke, July 22, 1832, Cocke Family Papers, Mss. 640, Box 71, UVA.
4. Douglass, *Life and Times of Frederick Douglass*, 110 (emphasis in original).
5. Horatio Jameson, *A Treatise on Epidemic Cholera* (Lindsay and Blakiston, 1855), 108–9.
6. Peter Hoffman Cruse to John Pendleton Kennedy, August 15, 1832, Peter Hoffman Cruse Papers, VHS.
7. Cruse to Kennedy, August 28, 1832, Cruse Papers, VHS (emphasis in original).
8. Cruse to Kennedy, August 29, 1832, Cruse Papers, VHS.
9. Baltimore *Patriot and Mercantile Advertiser*, August 30, 1832.
10. Horatio G. Jameson, "An Epitome of the More Important Circumstances Connected with the Epidemic Cholera," *Maryland Medical Recorder* 3, no. 1 (1832): 209.
11. Jameson, *Treatise on Epidemic Cholera*, 108.
12. Jameson, *Treatise on Epidemic Cholera*, 109.
13. Jameson, *Treatise on Epidemic Cholera*, 109.
14. James L. Hawkins to Daniel Sprigg, August 13, 1832, Letter to Daniel Sprigg, MHS.
15. H. S. Wells to Dennis Delany, August 13, 1832, Dennis Delany Collection, Small Collections, Box 13, fo. 12, WLCL.
16. Peter Hoffman Cruse to John P. Kennedy, August 15, 1832, Peter Hoffman Cruse Papers, VHS.
17. Philadelphia *The United States Gazette*, August 14, 1832.
18. Entries for August 16–21, 1832, Monroe Journal, Record of Cholera Epidemic, MHS (emphasis in original).

19. Lynchburg *Virginian*, August 27, 1832.
20. Baltimore *Gazette*, August 21, 1832.
21. Baltimore *Gazette*, August 21, 1832.
22. Entry for August 24, 1832, Monroe Journal, Record of Cholera Epidemic, MHS.
23. Cruse to Kennedy, August 24, 1832, Cruse Papers, VHS.
24. Cruse to Kennedy, August 28, 1832, Cruse Papers, VHS.
25. Cruse to Kennedy, September 1, 1832, Cruse Papers, VHS.
26. Baltimore *Gazette*, September 3, 1832.
27. Baltimore *Patriot*, September 6, 1832; Baltimore *American*, September 7, 1832.
28. Katherine A. Harvey, "Practicing Medicine at the Baltimore Almshouse, 1828–1850," *Maryland Historical Magazine* 74, no. 3 (September 1979): 223–37 (number of deaths on p. 226).
29. Entry for August 22, 1832, Monroe Journal, Record of Cholera Epidemic, MHS.
30. Entry for August 26, 1832, Monroe Journal, Record of Cholera Epidemic, MHS.
31. Entry for August 27, 1832, Monroe Journal, Record of Cholera Epidemic, MHS.
32. Baltimore *Gazette*, September 1, 1832. The city government discussed the report on Tuesday, August 28, and Wednesday, August 29. See Baltimore *Gazette and Daily Advertiser*, August 30, 1832.
33. Baltimore *Gazette*, July 28, 1832.
34. On Baltimore water, John H. B. Latrobe, *Picture of Baltimore, Containing a Description of All Objects of Interest in the City; and Embellished with Views of the Principal Public Buildings* (F. Lucas, Jr., 1832), 71–75; Martin Melosi, *The Sanitary City: Environmental Services in Urban America from Colonial Times to the Present* (University of Pittsburgh Press, 2008), 54; and Virginia Hawn, "Baltimore's Reaction to the Cholera Epidemic, Summer, 1832, As Reflected by the City's Newspapers," Report Goucher College, March 2, 1962, MHS.
35. Cruse to Kennedy, [August 24, 1832], Cruse Papers, VHS.
36. Cruse to Kennedy, August 29, 1832, Cruse Papers, VHS (emphasis in original).
37. Cruse to Kennedy, August 28, 1832, Cruse Papers, VHS.
38. Entry for August 31, 1832, Monroe Journal, Record of Cholera Epidemic, MHS; Baltimore, *Gazette*, August 31, 1832.
39. Entries for September 1–3, 1832, Monroe Journal, Record of Cholera Epidemic, MHS (emphasis in original).
40. Martin Robison Delany, *The Condition, Elevation, Emigration, and Destiny of the Colored People of the United States* (Published by the author, 1852), 143–44.
41. "The Colored People. A Day's Account of What They Are Doing and Saying. An Address by Frederick Douglass," *Baltimore Sun*, September 7, 1891.
42. Rt. Rev. James A. Handy, *Scraps of African Methodist Episcopal History* (A. M. E. Book Concern, [1902]), 404; "Lewis G. Wells, M.D." in George F. Bragg, *Men of Maryland* (Church Advocate Press, 1914), 125.
43. Jameson, *Treatise on Epidemic Cholera*, 151.
44. Jameson, *Treatise on Epidemic Cholera*, 151.

45. Baltimore *Republican and Commercial Advertiser*, September 3, 1832.
46. Handy, *Scraps of African Methodist Episcopal History*, 404.
47. Baltimore *Patriot*, September 4, 1832.
48. Cruse to Kennedy, September 1, 1832, VHS.
49. Cruse to Kennedy, September 6, 1832, VHS (emphases in original).
50. G. L. Dulaney to John Pendleton Kennedy, September 17, 1832, Cruse Papers, VHS.
51. Baltimore *Gazette*, September 8, 1832; Baltimore *Niles Weekly Register*, September 8, 1832; Philadelphia *National Gazette*, September 10, 1832; Lynchburg *Virginian*, September 13, 1832; Fayetteville (NC) *Observer*, September 18, 1832.
52. Baltimore *American*, September 8, 1832.
53. Baltimore *Patriot*, September 8, 1832.
54. Baltimore *American*, September 8, 1832.
55. Baltimore *Republican*, September 8, 1832.
56. Entries for September 7–8, 1832, Monroe Journal, Record of Cholera Epidemic, MHS.
57. Entry for September 12, 1832, Monroe Journal, Record of Cholera Epidemic, MHS.
58. Entry for September 13, 1832, Monroe Journal, Record of Cholera Epidemic, MHS.
59. Baltimore *Gazette*, September 13, 1832.
60. Baltimore *Gazette*, September 13, 1832.
61. Baltimore *Gazette*, September 15, 1832.
62. Baltimore *Gazette*, September 26, 1832.
63. T. J. Wilson, Reminiscences: Taken from Memory, and Not from a Diary, 1819–1865, MHS.
64. Horatio G. Jameson, "Consulting Physicians Report, December 31, 1832," in *The Ordinances of the Mayor and City Council of Baltimore, Passed at the Extra Sessions in 1832, and at the January Session, 1833. To Which Is Annexed Sundry Acts of Assembly; Passed at December Session, 1832; A List of the Officers of the Corporation, The Summary of the Register, and the Annual Reports and Returns of the Officers of the Corporation* (Sands & Neilson, 1833), 23.
65. Jameson, *Treatise on Epidemic Cholera*, 110.
66. For table 8.1, figures for Baltimore and the Calverton Almshouse are cited above in this chapter. Norfolk, Smithfield, and Richmond counts are cited where referred to in chapter 6. Totals for Washington, DC, Williamsport, MD, Hagerstown, MD, and Halltown, VA are from chapter 7. The remaining figures draw on Tanner, *Geographical and Statistical Account*, 29–34.

CHAPTER 9

1. Theodore Clapp, *Autobiographical Sketches and Recollections During a Thirty-Five Years' Residence in New Orleans*, 1st ed. (Phillips, Sampson & Company, 1857), 117.

2. Clapp, *Autobiographical Sketches*, 186.
3. Clapp, *Autobiographical Sketches*, 120.
4. Clapp, *Autobiographical Sketches*, 124.
5. Clapp, *Autobiographical Sketches*, 125.
6. Clapp, *Autobiographical Sketches*, 132.
7. Clapp, *Autobiographical Sketches*, 125.
8. Clapp, *Autobiographical Sketches*, 130.
9. Clapp, *Autobiographical Sketches*, 135.
10. Clapp, *Autobiographical Sketches*, 135.
11. Clapp, *Autobiographical Sketches*, 129.
12. "Report from the Major General of the Army, Washington, November 1832," in New York *Commercial Advertiser*, December 22, 1832.
13. Patrick J. Jung, *The Black Hawk War of 1832* (University of Oklahoma Press, 2007), 139–41.
14. Tanner, relying on eastern newspapers, recorded ten deaths in Cleveland before his work went to press. See Tanner, *Geographical and Statistical Account*, 34. For the latter mortality, see Cleveland *Advertiser* in Sandusky *Clarion*, October 10, 1832. An online encyclopedia states that fifty total deaths occurred in Cleveland alone in 1832, but no corroborating evidence for this claim could be found. See "Cholera Epidemic of 1832," *Encyclopedia of Cleveland History*, Case Western Reserve University, accessed November 23, 2025, https://case.edu/ech/articles/c/cholera-epidemic-1832.
15. The estimates were from sixty to one hundred. See Richard Adler, *Cholera in Detroit: A History* (McFarland, 2013), 83.
16. Daniel Drake, *An Account of the Epidemic Cholera, as It Appeared in Cincinnati* (Chronicle Office, 1832), 20. Also published as "Epidemic Cholera in Cincinnati," *Western Journal of Medical and Physical Sciences* 6 (October, November, and December 1832): 321–64. Drake gave the estimate of 30,000, but it matches what would be expected based on a comparison of the 1830 and 1840 censuses, which recorded 24,831 and 46,338 respectively. See Campbell, "Population of the 100 Largest Cities and Other Urban Places in the United States."
17. Cincinnati *Liberty Hall and Cincinnati Gazette*, June 28, 1832 (hereafter cited as Cincinnati *Gazette*). On Drake's life and legacy, see https://med.uc.edu/about/daniel-drake-medal/daniel-drake (accessed October 27, 2025); Emmet Field Horine, *Daniel Drake: Pioneer Physician of the Midwest* (University of Pennsylvania Press, 1961).
18. Daniel Drake, *A Discourse on Intemperance: Delivered at Cincinnati, March 1, 1828, Before the Agricultural Society of Hamilton County and Subsequently Pronounced, by Request to a Popular Audience* (Looker & Reynolds, 1828).
19. Cincinnati *Gazette*, August 30, 1832.
20. Cincinnati *Gazette*, October 11, 1832; Horine, *Daniel Drake*, 262.

21. John Henry, "A Letter on the Cholera as It Occurred in Cincinnati, Ohio, in the Month of October 1832," *Transylvania Journal of Medical and the Associate Sciences* 5, no. 5 (October, November, and December 1832): 512; Benjamin Herr, "Journal, 1830," *German American Annals*, new ser., vol. 1 (January 1903): 22; Cincinnati *Gazette*, January 25, 1832. On Cincinnati's water supply in 1832, see Cincinnati (Ohio) Board of Administration, *The Cincinnati Waterworks: A Paper Submitted by the Board of Administration for the Consideration of the Members of Hamilton County Delegation to the LXXII. General Assembly of Ohio* (Cincinnati Board of Administration, 1896), 10–11; Cincinnati *National Republican* January 5, 1832; Cincinnati *Gazette*, March 1, 1832; Melosi, *Sanitary City*, 37–38.
22. Drake, *Epidemic Cholera, as It Appeared in Cincinnati*, 17.
23. Cincinnati *Daily Journal*, October 19, 1832.
24. Isaac Jewett to Samuel Appleton, October 25, 1832, in Taylor Dunn, ed., "'Cincinnati Is a Delightful Place': Letters of a Law Clerk [Isaac Jewett], 1831–1834," *Bulletin of the Historical and Philosophical Society of Ohio* 10, no. 4 (October 1952): 270.
25. The outbreak appeared to occur, according to Drake, "in all parts of the city, high and low, thickly and thinly peopled, clean and dirty, nearly at the same time." Drake, *Epidemic Cholera, as It Appeared in Cincinnati*, 15.
26. Cincinnati *Daily Journal*, October 19, 1832.
27. Cincinnati *Chronicle and Literary Gazette*, October 26, 1832, in Lynchburg *Virginian*, November 8, 1832.
28. Drake, *Epidemic Cholera, as It Appeared in Cincinnati*, 20.
29. New York *Commercial Advertiser*, November 9, 1832; Maysville (KY) *Eagle*, November 15, 1832, in Alexandria (VA), *Gazette*, November 21, 1832; Portsmouth (NH) *Journal and Rockingham Gazette*, December 1, 1832; Frankfort (KY) *Argus*, November 14, 1832; Theodore Bell, "Remarks on Spasmodic Cholera, as It Appeared in Louisville in October 1832," *Transylvania Journal of Medical and Associate Sciences* 5 (October, November, and December 1832): 542; Harvey Green to Hector Green, November 11, 1832, Green Family Papers, fo. 6, FHS.
30. Henry Clay to Francis T. Brooke, October 18, 1832, in *The Papers of Henry Clay, Vol. 8: Candidate, Compromiser, Whig, March 5, 1829–December 31, 1836*, ed. Robert Seager and Melba Porter Hay (University of Kentucky Press, 1984), 584.
31. Philadelphia *Inquirer*, October 29, 1832; Philadelphia *National Gazette*, October 30, 1832; Lynchburg *Virginian*, November 1, 1832.
32. Henry Clay to James Brown, October 23, 1832, in *Papers of Clay Papers, Vol.* 8, 587.
33. Alexandria (VA) *Gazette*, October 25, 1832.
34. Washington (DC) *National Intelligencer*, October 29, 1832. The US Census recorded a population of St. Louis at 4,977 in 1830 and then 16,469 in 1840, making its population about 7,300 people in 1832 based on an annual numerical increase of approximate 1,150. See Gibson, "Population of the 100 Largest Cities and Other Urban Places in the United States."

35. Boston *Jesuit: Catholic Sentinel*, January 12, 1833.
36. Washington (DC) *National Intelligencer*, November 13, 1832. More than 140 certainly perished, but the number of cholera fatalities in the city during the pandemic remains poorly known. A figure of 300 for 1832 is included in popular histories without any attribution. See Elizabeth Davis, "Historically Yours: St. Louis Cholera Epidemic of 1849," *News Tribune*, July 23, 2019, https://www.newstribune.com/. Another estimate puts the total cholera deaths from 1832 to 1835 at 500 but provides no source for this figure. See Walter J. Daly, "The Black Cholera Comes to the Central Valley of America in the 19th Century—1832, 1849, and Later," *Transactions of the American Clinical and Climatological Association,* 119 (2008): 143–53. The lack of clarity necessitates the lower number of cholera fatalities recorded at the time to be used in table 9.1.
37. Jackson (TN) *Southern Statesman*, October 27, 1832.
38. Chambers, *Conquest of Cholera*, 133; Woodville (MS) *Southern Planter*, November 3, 1832; Natchez (MS) *Courier and Adams, Jefferson, and Franklin Advertiser*, October 26, 1832.
39. Vicksburg (MS) *Whig*, October 25, 1832.
40. Woodville (MS) *Southern Planter*, December 8, 1832.
41. Vicksburg (MS) *Whig*, November 8, 1832.
42. Drake, *Epidemic Cholera, as It Appeared in Cincinnati*, 18 (quote), 19.
43. Drake, *Epidemic Cholera, as It Appeared in Cincinnati*, 18, 19.
44. New Orleans *Bee*, August 11, 1832; Michel Halphen, *Mémoire sur le Cholera-Morbus, compliqué d'une Epidémie de Fièvre Jaune, qui a régné simultanément a la Nouvelle Orléans en 1832* (Paris: 1833), 54. The author wishes to thank Sarah Jourdain for identifying key passages in the work and Nathan Greenhaw for translating the book.
45. New Orleans *Louisiana Courier*, August 1, 1832.
46. New York *Evening Post*, August 27, 1832.
47. S. Frederick Starr and Jack Stewart, "The Rise and Fall of the New Orleans Cistern," Preservation Resource Center of New Orleans, accessed May 2, 2023, https://prcno.org/rise-fall-new-orleans-cistern/; Natchez (MS) *Courier*, July 12, 1833; Halphen, *Mémoire sur le Cholera-Morbus*, 35.
48. New Orleans had a population of 46,082 in the 1830 US Census and was growing rapidly at the time. It reached 102,193 in 1840, indicating that the city added, on average, 5,611 more people each year during the 1830s. A population in 1832 of 57,000, then, is a reasonable estimate. See Gibson, "Population of the 100 Largest Cities and Other Urban Places in the United States."
49. Carolyn Goldsby Kolb, "At the Confluence of Science and Power: Water Struggles of New Orleans in the Nineteenth Century," PhD Dissertation, University of New Orleans, 2006: 62–82. See also Gary A. Donaldson, "Bringing Water to the Crescent City: Benjamin Latrobe and the New Orleans Waterworks System," *Louisiana History: The Journal of the Louisiana Historical Association* 28 (Autumn 1987): 381–96; and "Managing Streets, Utilities, and Municipal Services in Historic New Orleans,"

Preservation Resource Center of New Orleans, accessed April 29, 2023, https://prcno.org/managing-streets-utilities-municipal-services-historic-new-orleans/.

50. Halphen, *Mémoire sur le Cholera-Morbus*, 36.
51. John H. B. Latrobe, *Southern Travels: Journal of John H.B. Latrobe*, ed. Samuel Wilson (Historic New Orleans Collection, 1986): 46–47.
52. Kolb, "At the Confluence of Science and Power," 52.
53. Kathryn Olivarius, *Necropolis: Disease, Power, and Capitalism in the Cotton Kingdom* (Harvard University Press, 2022). On the debate over the supposed innate immunity of Africans and people of African descent, see Mariola Espinosa, "The Question of Racial Immunity to Yellow Fever in History and Historiography," *Social Science History* 38 (Winter 2014): 437–52.
54. New Orleans *Louisiana Courier*, September 29, 1832.
55. New Orleans *Louisiana Courier*, October 6, 1832.
56. New Orleans *Louisiana Courier*, October 20, 1832.
57. The *Experiment* arrived in New Orleans on October 21 after it had dropped off corpses at Memphis, Vicksburg, and Natchez. See New Orleans *Louisiana Courier*, October 22, 1832, and Woodville (MS) *Southern Planter*, November 3, 1832. In a public letter he wrote to Mayor of Mobile, dated November 1, Mayor Prieur claimed cholera arrived aboard three vessels that landed on October 22. See Savannah *Georgian*, November 15, 1832.
58. New Orleans *Louisiana Courier*, October 24, 1832; Halphen, *Mémoire sur le Cholera-Morbus*, 51–52; Woodworth, *The 1873 Cholera Epidemic*, 579. Halphen claimed that the *Constitution* came from St. Louis, but newspapers locate Louisville as the point of the steamboat's departure. See Jackson (TN) *Southern Statesman*, October 27, 1832.
59. New Orleans *Louisiana Courier*, October 24, 1832. Death of seven to cholera: Jackson (TN) *Southern Statesman*, October 27, 1832. Another report claimed twenty-five deaths, including the wife of the captain, who was put ashore at Vicksburg and then died. "A letter to the editor, from a gentleman at Villemont [AR], dated 25th ult." in Little Rock *Arkansas Gazette*, November 8, 1832.
60. C. Dart to Lewis Alderson, November 5, 1832, Lewis Alderson Papers, KHS.
61. Alexandria (VA) *Gazette*, January 4, 1833.
62. Clapp, *Autobiographical Sketches*, 117.
63. New Orleans *Louisiana Courier*, October 27, 1832.
64. The report from the *Argus* was reprinted in the Woodville (MS) *Southern Planter*, November 3, 1832, but was mistakenly dated October 21. From the context of the paper, the report had to be the October 26 issue. It refers to the board of health not giving a report yet, but they would do so on the twenty-sixth, after the paper went to press. Extant issues of the *Argus* during the fall 1832 outbreak are not known to exist. See Library of Congress, Directory of US Newspapers in American Libraries, accessed February 22, 2025, https://www.loc.gov/item/sn83026386/?st=holdings.
65. Woodville (MA) *Southern Planter*, November 3, 1832.

66. New Orleans *Louisiana Courier*, October 27, 1832.
67. New Orleans *Emporium*, October 27, 1832, in Woodville (MS) *Southern Planter*, November 3, 1832.
68. New Orleans *Bee*, October 29, 1832.
69. New Orleans *Bee*, October 30, 1832.
70. Halphen, *Mémoire sur le Cholera-Morbus*, 56.
71. Alexandria (VA) *Gazette*, January 4, 1833.
72. Halphen, *Mémoire sur le Cholera-Morbus*, 54.
73. Madison (IN) *Republican*, November 15, 1832.
74. New Orleans *Bee*, November 8, 1832.
75. New Orleans *Louisiana Courier*, November 2, 1832.
76. New Orleans *Louisiana Courier*, November 5, 1832.
77. Halphen, *Mémoire sur le Cholera-Morbus*, 56.
78. Mayor to President and Members of the City Council, November 1, 1832, New Orleans, Mayor's Messages, New Orleans Conseil de Ville [translations], New Orleans Public Library, AA506.
79. Halphen, *Mémoire sur le Cholera-Morbus*, 57.
80. Halphen, *Mémoire sur le Cholera-Morbus*, 59.
81. New Orleans *Bee*, November 8, 1832.
82. New Orleans *Bee*, November 10, 1832.
83. Cary Robinson to Conway Robinson, February 12, 1833, Moncure Robinson Papers, 01/Mss. 65, 77–14, Box 3, fo. 23, WMU.
84. M. M. Inskeep to Fanny G. Hampton, October 29, 1832, Fanny Leverich Eshleman Craig Collection, Box 1, fo. 13, LRCTU.
85. Thomas Moore to James M. King, December 22, 1832, University of Tennessee Libraries, Volunteer Voices Digital Collections, online https://digital.lib.utk.edu/collections/islandora/object/volvoices%3A14748#page/1/mode/1up.
86. Halphen, *Mémoire sur le Cholera-Morbus*, 61.
87. Halphen, *Mémoire sur le Cholera-Morbus*, 61.
88. Boze composed a bulletin of events that he later sent to his employer, Henri de Ste- Gême, who was an absentee owner living in France. Reference to his bulletin will be by entry date. November 5, 1832, Ste-Gême Family Papers, Mss. 100, fo. 213, p. 5, HNOC.
89. Savannah *Georgian*, November 15, 1832.
90. New Orleans *Commercial Bulletin*, July 2, 1833.
91. New Orleans *Times-Democrat*, September 10, 1893. See also Ambrose Cowperthwaite Fulton, *A Life's Voyage: A Diary of a Sailor and Land, Jotted Down During a Seventy-Years' Voyage* (Published by the author, 1898), 533–34.
92. Published in New Orleans *Times-Picayune*, July 18, 1937, excerpted and published on the Midlo Center for New Orleans Studies at the University of New Orleans website: https://neworleanshistorical.org/items/show/1461 (accessed February 22, 2025).

93. Christine Bordelon, "New Park Celebrates Irish Contributions to New Orleans." *Clarion Herald: Official Newspaper of the Archdiocese of New Orleans*, accessed December 30, 2025, https://clarionherald.org/news/new-park-celebrates-irish-contributions-to-new-orleans.
94. M. M. Inskeep to Fanny G. Hampton, October 29, 1832, Fanny Leverich Eshleman Craig Collection, Box 1, fo. 13, LRCTU.
95. M. M. Inskeep to Fanny G. Hampton, October 29, 1832, New Orleans, Fanny Leverich Eshleman Craig Collection, Box 1, fo. 13, LRCTU.
96. C. Dart to Lewis Alderson, November 5, 1832, Lewis Alderson Papers, KHS.
97. C. Dart to Lewis Alderson, November 24, 1832, Lewis Alderson Papers, KHS.
98. Carl Kohn to Samuel Kohn, December 2, 1832, Carl Kohn Letter Book, HNOC.
99. October 27, 1832, entry in Ste-Gême Family Papers, Mss. 100, fo. 211, p. 13, HNOC.
100. November 11, 1832, entry in Ste-Gême Family Papers, Mss. 100, fo. 214, p. 3, HNOC.
101. New Orleans *Emporium*, November 1, 1832, in Natchez (MS) *Courier*, November 9, 1832.
102. New Orleans *Louisiana Courier*, November 2, 1832 (emphasis in original).
103. New Orleans *Bee*, November 3, 1832.
104. New Orleans *Bee*, November 10, 1832.
105. New Orleans *Advertiser*, November 5, 1832, in Portland (ME) *Eastern Argus*, November 30, 1832.
106. New Orleans *Louisiana Courier*, November 7, 1832.
107. New Orleans *Emporium*, November 13, 1832, in Philadelphia, *Inquirer*, November 27, 1832.
108. New Orleans *Bee*, November 8, 1832.
109. New Orleans *Courier*, November 9, 1832.
110. New Orleans *Bee*, November 17, 1832.
111. November 25, 1832, entry in Ste-Gême Family Papers, Mss. 100, fo. 213, p. 4, HNOC; McDonogh to [?] Shephard, November 21, 1832, Box 8, fo. 25, John McDonogh Papers, LRCTU.
112. William Worthington to John Worthington, November 19, 1832, Van Ness Family Papers, Box 82, fo. 1, NYHS.
113. [Nathan] Morse to Isaac Edward Morse, December 3, 1832, Morse and Wederstrandt Family Papers, Box 1, fo. 4, LRCTU.
114. John Pintard to Samuel Bayard, December 10, 1832, Box 3, fo. 6, Pintard Papers, NYHS.
115. "Eighth 'vial of the wrath of God,'" in New Orleans *Emporium*, November 1, 1832: Natchez (MS) *Courier*, November 9, 1832; Charleston (SC) *Mercury*, November 13, 1832; Richmond (VA) *Constitutional Whig*, November 16, 1832; Baltimore *Gazette*, November 17, 1832; Alexandria (VA) *Gazette*, November 19, 1832; New York *Commercial Advertiser*, November 19, 1832; New York *Morning Courier and*

Enquirer, November 19, 1832; Philadelphia *Poulson's American*, November 19, 1832; Philadelphia *Daily Chronicle*, November 20, 1832; Washington (DC) *United States Telegraph*, November 20, 1832; Annapolis *Maryland Republican*, November 20, 1832; New London *Connecticut Gazette*, November 21, 1832; Norwich (CT) *Courier*, November 21, 1832; Hagerstown (MD) *Torch Light*, November 22, 1832; Lancaster (PA) *Examiner*, November 22, 1832; Hallowell (ME) *American Advocate*, November 23, 1832; Newburyport (MA) *Herald*, November 23, 1832; Portland (ME) *Eastern Argus*, November 23, 1832; Pawtucket (RI) *Chronicle*, November 23, 1832; Hartford *Connecticut Mirror*, November 24, 1832; Boston *Liberator*, November 24, 1832; Brandon *Vermont Telegraph*, November 27, 1832; Gettysburg (PA) *Adams Sentinel*, November 27, 1832; Gettysburg (PA) *Republican Banner*, November 27, 1832; Lawrenceburg (IN) *Western Statesman*, November 30, 1832. This made it into at least one British paper: London *Morning Chronicle*, December 13, 1832. "*Compound of all the evils*" in New Orleans *Louisiana Courier*, November 2, 1832: Nashville *National Banner*, November 15, 1832; Annapolis *Maryland Republican*, November 24, 1832; Washington (DC) *National Intelligencer*, November 26, 1832; Gettysburg (PA) *Adams Sentinel*, December 4, 1832; Baltimore (MD) *Niles Weekly Register*, December 1, 1832.

116. Natchez *Mississippi Free Trader*, November 16, 1832; Charleston (SC) *Courier*, November 21, 1832; Baltimore *American*, November 24, 1832; Baltimore *Gazette*, November 27, 1832; Washington (DC) *National Intelligencer*, November 27, 1832; Vicksburg (MS) *Whig*, November 28, 1832; Lynchburg *Virginian*, November 29, 1832; Annapolis *Maryland Gazette*, November 29, 1832; Cincinnati *Baptist Weekly Journal of the Mississippi Valley*, November 30, 1832; Pittsburgh (PA) *Weekly Gazette*, November 30, 1832; Savannah *Georgian*, November 30, 1832; Boston *Courier*, December 1, 1832; Portland (ME) *Advertiser*, December 3, 1832; Salem (MA) *Gazette*, December 4, 1832; Saratoga Springs (NY) *Sentinel*, December 4, 1832; Charleston (SC) *Courier*, December 5, 1832; Northampton (MA) *Hampshire Gazette*, December 5, 1832; Montpelier *Vermont Patriot and State Gazette*, December 10, 1832.

117. Protest that originally appeared in New Orleans *Emporium*, November 13, 1832, subsequently appeared in Philadelphia *Inquirer*, November 27, 1832; Philadelphia *Daily Chronicle*, November 28, 1832; New York *Morning Courier and Enquirer*, November 29, 1832; Baltimore *Niles Weekly Register*, December 1, 1832; Portland (ME) *Advertiser*, December 3, 1832; Philadelphia *Poulson's American*, December 3, 1832; Portsmouth *New-Hampshire Gazette*, December 4, 1832. Notice of Penrice's death, often entitled "Uncertainty of Life," appeared in Boston *Gazette*, in Portland (ME) *Eastern Argus*, November 30, 1832; New York *American*, December 1, 1832; Newport (RI) *Mercury*, December 1, 1832; Baltimore *Niles Weekly Register*, December 1, 1832; Philadelphia *Daily Chronicle*, December 3, 1832; Philadelphia *Poulson's American*, December 3, 1832; Dover (NH) *Enquirer*, December 4, 1832; New York *American*, December 4, 1832; Worcester (MA) *National Aegis*, December 5, 1832; Pittsfield (MA) *Sun*, December 6, 1832; Burlington (VT) *Weekly Free Press*, December 7, 1832; Morristown (NJ) *Jerseyman*, December

12, 1832; Washington (DC) *National Intelligencer*, December 15, 1832; Columbus *Ohio Monitor*, December 24, 1832.

118. New York *Journal of Commerce*, November 19, 1832; subsequently in Boston *Courier*, November 21, 1832; Albany (NY) *Argus*, November 23, 1832; Gloucester (MA) *Telegraph*, November 24, 1832; Providence (RI) *Microcosm*, November 24, 1832; Rochester (NY) *Union and Advertiser*, November 24, 1832; Saratoga Springs (NY) *Sentinel*, November 27, 1832; Hartford *Connecticut Courant*, November 27, 1832; Middlebury (VT) *Register and Addison County Journal*, November 27, 1832; Northampton (MA) *Hampshire Gazette*, November 28, 1832; Richmond (VA) *Enquirer*, November 30, 1832; Burlington (VT) *Sentinel and Democrat*, November 30, 1832; Hagerstown (MD) *Mail*, December 1, 1832; Montpelier *Vermont Patriot*, December 3, 1832; Norwalk (OH) *Huron Reflector*, December 4, 1832; Preston (UK) *Preston Chronicle and Lancashire Advertiser*, January 5, 1833.
119. Halphen, *Mémoire sur le Cholera-Morbus*, 62.

CHAPTER 10

1. Quoted in Tom Mould, *Choctaw Tales* (University of Mississippi Press, 2004), 154.
2. F. W. Armstrong to George Gibson, December 2, 1832, in *Correspondence on the Subject of the Emigration of Indians, Between the 30th November 1831 and 27th December 1833* (5 vols., Washington, 1834–1835), 1: 401.
3. F. W. Armstrong to Gibson, December 2, 1832, *Correspondence on the Subject of the Emigration of Indians*, 1: 401.
4. Andrew Jackson, Second Annual Message, December 6, 1832, on American Presidency Project, University of California-Santa Barbara, https://www.presidency.ucsb.edu/documents/second-annual-message-3.
5. On Indian Removal, see Claudio Saunt, *Unworthy Republic: The Dispossession of Native Americans and the Road to Indian Territory* (W. W. Norton, 2020). On the Choctaws, see Arthur DeRosier, *The Removal of the Choctaw Indians* (University of Tennessee Press, 1981); Donna L. Akers, *Living in the Land of Death: The Choctaw Nation, 1830–1860* (Michigan State University Press, 2004); Christina Snyder, *Great Crossings: Indians, Settlers, & Slaves in the Age of Jackson* (Oxford University Press, 2017).
6. Quoted in Francis Paul Prucha, ed., *Cherokee Removal: The "William Penn" Essays and Other Writings by Jeremiah Evarts* (University of Tennessee Press, 1981), 192, 209.
7. Talley to Winans, July 5, 1830, William Winans Manuscript Papers, J. B. Cain Archives of Mississippi Methodism, Millsaps-Wilson Library, Millsaps College, Jackson, Mississippi.
8. It has been circulated in popular culture that a Choctaw chief, probably George Harkins, told the editor of the Little Rock *Arkansas Gazette* in 1831 that the removal was "a trail of tears and death." Eventually, "the Trail of Tears" became applied to the general experience of Indian Removal, particularly after the Cherokees called the experience "the trail where they cried." The author has not been

able to find that the *Arkansas Gazette* published the words "a trail of tears and death." On recent use of this, see "First Choctaw Forced Removal Causes Death of Thousands," Investing in Native Communities, accessed April 27, 2024, https://nativephilanthropy.candid.org/events/first-choctaw-forced-removal-causes-death-of-thousands/.

9. Reuben H. Grant to Peter Pitchlynn and Other Choctaw Delegates, December 21, 1854, Peter Pitchlynn Papers, Box 2, fo. 55, Western History Collections, University of Oklahoma.
10. "Treaty with the Choctaw, 1830," in *Indian Affairs: Laws and Treaties*, ed. Charles Kappler, 7 vols. (Government Printing Office, 1904), II, 310–19, quote 313.
11. Kingsbury to Greene, April 26, 1831, American Board of Commissioners for Foreign Missions Archives, Series 18.3.4, vol. 5, no. 11, Houghton Library, Harvard University, Cambridge, MA; Calvin Cushman to Greene, March 16, 1832, American Board of Commissioners for Foreign Missions Archives, Series 18.3.4, vol. 5, no. 198, Houghton Library, Harvard University, Cambridge, MA.
12. Saunt, *Unworthy Republic*, 124–26, 128, 203–5.
13. Colquhoun to Gibson, December 10, 1831, quoted in Grant Foreman, *Indian Removal: The Emigration of the Five Civilized Tribes of Indians* (University of Oklahoma Press, 1972), 60 n18.
14. The deadly consequences of the 1831 deportation are well detailed in Foreman, *Indian Removal*, 65, 68–70; DeRosier, *Choctaw Removal*, 135–37; and Saunt, *Unworthy Republic*, 124–36, 140–42.
15. Andrew Jackson to Anthony Bledsoe Shelby, April 23, 1832 (marked private), *The Papers of Andrew Jackson, Volume 10, 1832*, 250.
16. On the Armstrongs' Jacksonian ties, see Carolyn Thomas Foreman, "The Armstrongs of Indian Territory," *Chronicles of Oklahoma* 30 (Autumn 1952): 292–307.
17. Unsigned letter to Lewis Cass, May 2, 1832, Peter Pitchylnn Collection, Helmerich Center for American Research, Thomas Gilcrease Museum of American Art and Culture, Tulsa, OK.
18. Peter Pitchlynn to Lewis Cass, July 10, 1832, Letters Received by the Office of Indian Affairs, 1824–1881, NARA, RG 75, microfilm 234, reel 185.
19. Robb to Pitchlynn, July 28, 1832, in *Correspondence on the Subject of the Emigration of Indians*, 2: 890.
20. William Armstrong to Gibson, September 10, 1832, in *Correspondence on the Subject of the Emigration of Indians*, 1: 378–79.
21. J. H. Hook to William Armstrong, September 5, 1832, in *Correspondence on the Subject of the Emigration of Indians*, 1: 156–57.
22. William Armstrong to Gibson, September 17, 1832, in *Correspondence on the Subject of the Emigration of the Indians*, 1: 381–82; F. W. to Gibson, September 17, 1832, *Correspondence on the Subject of the Emigration of the Indians*, 1: 379–80; F. W. to Gibson, October 28, 1832, in *Correspondence on the Subject of the Emigration of the Indians*, 1: 391.
23. DeRosier, *Choctaw Removal*, 158.

24. William Armstrong to Gibson, September 1,1832, in *Indian Removal to the West, 1832–1840: Files of the Office of the Commissary General of Subsistence* (microfilm, 19 reels; Bethesda, MD, 2007), reel 2, frames 548–50.
25. F. W. Armstrong to Brown, October 4, 1832, *Indian Removal to the West*, reel 2, frames 616–21.
26. F. W. Armstrong to Gibson, October 21, 1832, in *Correspondence on the Subject of the Emigration of Indians*, 1: 388–89, quotes on 389.
27. William Armstrong to Gibson, October 23, 1832, in *Correspondence on the Subject of the Emigration of Indians*, 1: 389.
28. F. W. Armstrong to Gibson, October 28, 1832, in *Correspondence on the Subject of the Emigration of Indians*, 1: 391.
29. J. A. Phillips to Gibson, October 31, 1832, in *Correspondence on the Subject of the Emigration of Indians*, 1: 787.
30. William Armstrong to Gibson, November 3, 1832, in *Correspondence on the Subject of the Emigration of Indians*, 1: 394–95.
31. William Armstrong to Gibson, November 10, 1832, in *Correspondence on the Subject of the Emigration of Indians*, 1: 398 (emphasis in original).
32. William Armstrong to Gibson, November 3, 1832, in *Correspondence on the Subject of the Emigration of Indians*, 1: 394–95; William Armstrong to Gibson, November 10, 1832, in *Correspondence on the Subject of the Emigration of Indians*, 1: 398.
33. A. S. Langham to Gibson, November 8, 1832, in *Correspondence on the Subject of the Emigration of Indians*, 1: 737.
34. William Armstrong to Gibson, November 10, 1832, in *Correspondence on the Subject of the Emigration of Indians*, 1: 398.
35. William Armstrong to Gibson, November 10, 1832, in *Correspondence on the Subject of the Emigration of Indians*, 1: 398.
36. Entry for November 24, 1832, Journal of J. P. Simonton, Nov. 16, 1832, to Dec. 19, 1832, Records Relating to Indian Removal, Records of the Commissary General of Subsistence, Letters Received, 1830–1836, entry 201, Box 6, Choctaw, 1833, RG 75, NARA. The author wishes to thank Claudio Saunt for sharing his digitized copy of this source.
37. F. W. Armstrong to Gibson, December 2, 1832, in *Correspondence on the Subject of the Emigration of Indians*, 1: 410.
38. W. R. Montgomery to Gibson, October 29, 1832, in *Correspondence on the Subject of the Emigration of Indians*, 1: 770.
39. F. W. Armstrong to Gibson October 31, 1832, in *Correspondence on the Subject of the Emigration of Indians*, 1: 395 (emphasis in the original).
40. W. R. Montgomery to Gibson, January 5, 1833, in *Correspondence on the Subject of the Emigration of Indians*, 1: 772.
41. William S. Colquhoun and J. P. Simonton to Gibson, October 25, 1832, in *Correspondence on the Subject of the Emigration of Indians*, 1: 628.
42. J. P. Simonton to Gibson, April 8, 1833, in *Correspondence on the Subject of the Emigration of Indians*, 1: 886.

43. Entry for November 2, 1832, in Journal of Assistant Agent William Colquhoun During the Choctaw Removal, Letters Received Commissary General of Subsistence, RG 75, NARA, https://catalog.archives.gov/id/38995523.
44. F. W. Armstrong to Gibson, November 21, 1832, in *Correspondence on the Subject of the Emigration of Indians*, 1: 400.
45. W. R. Montgomery to Gibson, January 5, 1833, in *Correspondence on the Subject of the Emigration of Indians*, 1: 772.
46. F. W. Armstrong to Gibson, November 21, 1832, in *Correspondence on the Subject of the Emigration of Indians*, 1: 400.
47. F. W. Armstrong to Lewis Cass, November 21, 1832, in *Indian Removal to the West*, reel 2, frames 652–55 (emphasis in original).
48. Entry for November 17, 1832, in Journal of Assistant Agent William Colquhoun During the Choctaw Removal, Letters Received Commissary General of Subsistence, RG 75, NARA, https://catalog.archives.gov/id/38995523.
49. J. A. Phillips to Gibson, December 2, 1832, in *Indian Removal to the West*, reel 3, frame 948.
50. J. A. Phillips Journal, November 14, 1832, in *Indian Removal to the West*, reel 3, frame 955.
51. Cross's Journal, November 12–December 11, 1832, Letters Received by the Office of Indian Affairs, 1824–1881, RG 75, NARA, microfilm 234, reel 185.
52. Entry for November 24, 1832, in Journal of Simonton, Records Relating to Indian Removal, Records of the Commissary General of Subsistence, Letters Received, 1830–1836, entry 201, Box 6, Choctaw, 1833, RG 75, NARA.
53. J. A. Phillips to Gibson, December 22, 1832, in *Correspondence on the Subject of the Emigration of Indians*, 1: 789.
54. S. T. Cross to Gibson, January 10, 1833, in *Correspondence on the Subject of the Emigration of Indians*, 1: 633.
55. Entry for December 12, 1832, in Journal of Simonton, Records Relating to Indian Removal, Records of the Commissary General of Subsistence, Letters Received, 1830–1836, entry 201, box 6, Choctaw, 1833, RG 75, NARA.
56. Kingsbury to Greene, January 21, 1833, American Board of Commissioners for Foreign Missions Archives, Series 18.3.4, vol. 5, no. 35, Houghton Library, Harvard University, Cambridge, MA.
57. DeRosier, *The Removal of the Choctaw Indians*, 153, 157–58.
58. Little Rock *Weekly Arkansas Gazette*, November 14, 1832; Little Rock *Arkansas Times and Advocate*, November 14, 1832.
59. Little Rock *Weekly Arkansas Gazette*, November 21, 1832; Little Rock *Arkansas Times and Advocate*, November 21, 1832.
60. Little Rock *Weekly Arkansas Gazette*, November 28, 1832.
61. Little Rock *Weekly Arkansas Gazette*, December 5, 1832.
62. Little Rock *Arkansas Times and Advocate*, December 5, 1832.
63. Andrew Jackson, Fourth Annual Message, December 4, 1832, on American Presidency Project, University of California, Santa Barbara, https://www.presidency.ucsb.edu/documents/fourth-annual-message-3.

64. "Lattimore, Josephine Usray, Interview #8822," 5, Indian Pioneer Papers, University of Oklahoma, Western History Collections, accessed April 22, 2024. http://digital.libraries.ou.edu/cdm/ref/collection/indianpp/id/5086.
65. "Lattimore Josephine Usray, Interview #8822," 6.
66. "Lattimore Josephine Usray, Interview #8822," 6.
67. "Lattimore Josephine Usray, Interview #8822," 7.
68. "Lattimore Josephine Usray, Interview #8822," 8.
69. "Lattimore Josephine Usray, Interview #8822," 9.
70. "Lattimore Josephine Usray, Interview #8822," 10.
71. Andrew Jackson, Fifth Annual Message, December 3, 1833, on American Presidency Project, University of California, Santa Barbara, https://www.presidency.ucsb.edu /documents/fifth-annual-message-2.
72. John Pitchlynn to Peter Pitchlynn, January 30, 1834, Peter Pitchlynn Papers, Box 1, fo. 40, Western History Collections, University of Oklahoma.
73. Lane to Gibson, September 6, 1833, in *Indian Removal to the West*, reel 3, frames 919–20; Lane to Gibson, September 24, 1833, in *Indian Removal to the West*, reel 3, frame 922; William Armstrong to Gibson, October 11, 1833, in *Correspondence on the Subject of the Emigration of Indians*, 1: 415–16.

CHAPTER 11

1. Joshua Rothman, *The Ledger and the Chain: How the Domestic Slave Traders Shaped America* (Basic Books, 2021), 102, 7 (quote), 59. Rothman offers the most in-depth examination of Franklin, Armfield, and Co., but other scholars have put the company into the larger context of the business of enslavement. See Michael Tadman, *Speculators and Slaves: Masters, Traders, and Slaves in the Old South* (University of Wisconsin Press, 1989); Robert Gudmestad, *A Troublesome Commerce: The Transformation of the Interstate Slave Trade* (Louisiana State University Press, 2003); Steven Deyle, *Carry Me Back: The Domestic Slave Trade in American Life* (Oxford University Press, 2005); Edward Baptist, *The Half Has Never Been Told: Slavery and the Making of American Capitalism* (Basic Books, 2014); and Calvin Schermerhorn, *The Business of Slavery and the Rise of American Capitalism, 1815–1860* (Yale University Press, 2015).
2. "Testimony of John Boggs, 1863, Canada," in *Slave Testimony: Two Centuries of Letters, Speeches, Interviews, and Autobiographies*, ed. John W. Blassingame (Louisiana State University Press, 1977), 421–23, quote on 422. On Franklin and his colleagues' sexual assaults and impregnating women, see Rothman, *The Ledger and the Chain*, 151–55, 176, 183, 278–80, and 284–85.
3. "Interview of J. W. Lindsay, 1863, Canada," in *Slave Testimony*, 396–404, quotes on 403–4.
4. William Wells Brown, *Narrative of William W. Brown, a Fugitive Slave. Written by Himself* (The Anti-Slavery Office, 1847), 40–41.
5. Schermerhorn, *Business of Slavery*, 10–11, 13–15, 156.
6. "Lewis Hayden, 1853," in *Slave Testimony*, 695–97.

7. John Armfield to David Burford, July 2, 1832, Burford Papers #0935, Box 2, fo. 12, Special Collections, University of Tennessee-Knoxville Libraries.
8. Jourdan Saunders to David Burford, July 4, 1832, Burford Papers, Box 2, fo. 12, Special Collections, University of Tennessee-Knoxville Libraries.
9. Paul Pascal to Bernard Raux, November 14, 1832, Bernard Raux Slave Trade Papers, MS Am 790, Houghton Library, Harvard University, Cambridge, MA. (The author wishes to thank Leslie Tuttle for translating this document.) Rothman, *The Ledger and the Chain*, 192.
10. Isaac Franklin to Rice Ballard, October 5, 1832, Rice C. Ballard Papers #04850, fo. 8, UNC-SHC.
11. Isaac Franklin to Rice Ballard, December 8, 1832, Ballard Papers, fo. 8, UNC-SHC; Franklin wrote a letter to Ballard dated October 31 from Port Gibson. This letter has not been found in Ballard's papers or other collections, but Ballard referred to receiving it in his letter to Franklin, December 2, 1832, Ballard Papers, fo. 8, UNC-SHC.
12. Entry for October 30, 1832, in Journal of Assistant Agent William Colquhoun During the Choctaw Removal, https://catalog.archives.gov/id/38995523.
13. Isaac Franklin to Rice Ballard, December 8, 1832, Ballard Papers, fo. 8, UNC-SHC.
14. James Franklin to Rice Ballard, November 23, 1832, Ballard Papers, fo. 8, UNC-SHC.
15. Alexandria (VA) *Gazette*, August 1, 1832.
16. Rothman, *The Ledger and the Chain*, 188.
17. Rothman, *The Ledger and the Chain*, 186–87.
18. Baltimore *Republican*, September 5, 1832; Easton (MD) *Eastern-Shore Whig*, September 11, 1832; Alexandria (VA) *Gazette*, September 14, 1832; Washington (DC) *National Intelligencer*, September 28, 1832.
19. Baltimore *Republican*, October 1, 1832.
20. Rothman, *The Ledger and the Chain*, 186.
21. Mary Minor Blackford, "Notes illustrative of the wrongs of slavery," Papers of Lancelot Minor Blackford, Mss. 5088, UVA.
22. Alexandria (VA) *Gazette*, November 1, 1832.
23. Inward Slave Manifest, New Orleans, November 26, 1832 (*Brig Tribune*), NARA, microfilm M1895, reel 6.
24. Vicksburg (MS) *Whig*, November 1, 1832; Natchez (MS) *Courier*, November 2, 1832; New Orleans *Louisiana Courier*, November 5, 1832; Nashville *National Banner*, November 7, 1832; New Orleans *Louisiana Courier*, November 14, 1832; Tallahassee (FL) *Floridian*, December 1, 1832; Rachael O'Connor to David Weeks, November 14, 1832, David Weeks and Family Papers, Box 4, LSU; Isaac Franklin to Rice Ballard, December 8, 1832, Ballard Papers, Box 1, fo. 8, UNC-SHC.
25. William Trowbridge To Roxana Smith, December 23, 1832, Trowbridge Family Papers, Mss. Col. 470, LRCTU.
26. History of Evan Hall Plantation, Plantation Collection, Mss. Col. 531, fo. 13, LRCTU.

27. Mary Austin Holley to Harriette Brand, November 25, 1832, Mary Austin Holley Papers, Box 2R39, Dolph Briscoe Center for American History, University of Texas at Austin.
28. Mary Austin Holley to Harriette Brand, December 23, 1832, Mary Austin Holley Papers, Box 2R39, Dolph Briscoe Center for American History, University of Texas at Austin.
29. Rice Ballard to Isaac Franklin, December 2, 1832, Ballard Papers, fo. 8 (emphases in the original), UNC-SHC.
30. Inward Slave Manifest, New Orleans, November 9, 1832, (*Ajax*), NARA, microfilm M1895, reel 6.
31. Paul Pascal to Bernard Raux, November 14, 1832, Bernard Raux Slave Trade Papers, MS Am 790, Houghton Library, Harvard University, Cambridge, MA.
32. Jourdan Saunders to David Burford, December 8, 1832, Burford Papers, Box 2 fo. 18, Special Collections, University of Tennessee-Knoxville Libraries.
33. Isaac Franklin to Rice Ballard, December 8, 1832, Ballard Papers, fo. 8, UNC-SHC.
34. James Franklin to Jourdan Saunders, January 2, 1833, Burford Papers, Box 2, fo.19, Special Collections, University of Tennessee-Knoxville Libraries.
35. Jourdan Saunders to David Burford, February 13, 1833, Burford Papers, Box 2, fo. 20, Special Collections, University of Tennessee-Knoxville Libraries.
36. Isaac Franklin to Rice Ballard, January 29, 1833, Ballard Papers, fo. 10, UNC-SHC.
37. Richmond (VA) *Compiler*, January 12, 1833, in Alexandria (VA) *Gazette*, January 14, 1833.
38. Rothman, *The Ledger and the Chain*, 199–200.
39. John Armfield to Rice Ballard, December 21, 1832, Ballard Papers, fo. 9, UNC-SHC.
40. Alexandria (VA) *Gazette*, January 15, 1833.
41. Rothman, *The Ledger and the Chain*, 201.
42. Alexandria (VA) *Gazette*, January 22, 1833, January 30, 1832.
43. Rothman, *The Ledger and the Chain*, 201; Alexandria (VA) *Gazette*, February 26, 1832, February 28, 1832.
44. Isaac and James Franklin to Rice Ballard, February 19, 1833, Ballard Papers, fo. 10, UNC-SHC.
45. Alexandria (VA) *Gazette*, April 29, 1833.
46. Not all of the shipping records have survived. Rothman examined all available records and tabulated that eighty-three were on the *Lafayette* and "at least 250" were on the two voyages of the *Tribune* and the voyage of the *Ariel* plus a later voyage of the *Renown* that took place between April 20 and May 24. The manifest of the *Renown* survives and shows that Franklin, Armfield, and Co. shipped 31 enslaved people. If these are subtracted from Rothman's calculations, then a figure of 302 is derived for the total that arrived by April 9. See Rothman, *The Ledger and the Chain*, 201, 431 fn. 115. Inward Slave Manifest, New Orleans, April 20, 1833 (*Sch. Renown*), NARA, M1895, reel 7.

47. Thom Rosenblum, "Driving Out the Slave Traders: The Natchez Uprising of 1833," *Journal of Mississippi History* 67 (March 2005), 56.
48. Isaac and James Franklin to Rice Ballard, March 6, 1833, Ballard Papers, fo. 10, UNC-SHC.
49. Isaac and James Franklin to Rice Ballard, March 24, 1833, Ballard Papers, fo. 10, UNC-SHC.
50. Franklin (LA) *Republican*, January 16, 1833, in Natchez *Mississippi Free Trader*, January 25, 1833; Franklin (LA) *Republican*, March 20, 1833, in Natchez *Mississippi Free Trader*, March 29, 1833.
51. Baltimore *American*, April 6, 1833.
52. Natchez *Mississippi Free Trader*, April 19, 1833.
53. Natchez *Mississippi Free Trader*, April 26, 1833.
54. Natchez *Mississippi Free Trader*, April 26, 1833.
55. Natchez *Courier*, April 26, 1833.
56. Natchez *Courier*, April 26, 1833.
57. Citizens Petition, April 22, 1833, Petitions, 1824–1833, Natchez Municipal Records, MF# 36713, Mississippi Department of Archives and History, Jackson, Mississippi (emphasis in original).
58. Certificates of Negro Traders, April 22, 1833, Natchez Municipal Records, MF #36702, Mississippi Department of Archives and History, Jackson, Mississippi.
59. Samuel Gustain to President and Selectmen of the City of Natchez, n.d, Natchez Municipal Records, Health Officer Reports, MF# 36723, Mississippi Department of Archives and History, Jackson, Mississippi.
60. Natchez *Courier*, April 26, 1833.
61. An Ordinance to Prevent the exhibition of slaves as merchandize within the City of Natchez, April 24, 1833, Natchez Municipal Records, Ordinances, 1829–1854, 1870–1872, MF #36711, Mississippi Department of Archives and History, Jackson, Mississippi.
62. James R. Franklin to Rice Ballard, April 24, 1833, Ballard Papers, fo. 11, UNC-SHC.
63. Natchez *Courier*, May 3, 1833.
64. James R. Franklin to Rice Ballard, May 7, 1833, Ballard Papers, fo. 11, UNC-SHC.
65. Rothman, *The Ledger and the Chain*, 309.
66. R. C. Ballard & Co., Slaves Bought, 1832–1834, Ballard Papers, fo. 421, UNC-SHC.
67. James Franklin identified the man as Phillip Willis. See James Franklin to Jourdan Saunders, January 2, 1832, Burford Papers, Box 2, fo. 19, Special Collections, University of Tennessee-Knoxville Libraries. A name that appears to be Phillip Willis appears on the *Tribune*'s slave manifest. See Inward Slave Manifest, New Orleans, November 26, 1832 (*Brig Tribune*), NARA, microfilm M1895, reel 6.

CHAPTER 12

1. Charleston (SC) *Courier*, February 26, 1833.

2. Louise W. Knight, "Grimké, Thomas Smith," *American National Biography*, accessed July 12, 2024, https://doi-org.proxy.library.stonybrook.edu/10.1093/anb/9780198606697.article.1101229.
3. Thomas Grimké, *Address on the Patriot Character of the Temperance Reformation: Delivered Before the Charleston Temperance Society, and the Young Men's Temperance Society of Charleston, On Tuesday Evening, 26th February, 1833* (Observer Office Press, 1833), 8 (emphases in original).
4. Grimké, *Address on the Patriot Character of the Temperance Reformation*, 9 (emphasis in original).
5. Albany (NY) *The Temperance Recorder* 1, no. 8 (October 2, 1832), 64. The call then was relayed throughout the nation, including the following: Brandon *Vermont Telegraph*, October 16, 1832; Jamestown (NY) *Journal*, October 17, 1832; New York *Evangelist*, October 20, 1832; Boston *Christian Herald*, October 24, 1832; Boston *Courier*, October 25, 1832; Boston *Daily Advertiser*, October 25, 1832; St. Johnsbury (VT) *The Weekly Messenger*, October 30, 1832; Baltimore *American*, October 31, 1832; Boston *Weekly Messenger*, November 1, 1832; Alexandria (VA) *Gazette*, November 2, 1832; Cincinnati *Baptist Weekly Journal*, November 2, 1832; Concord *New Hampshire Statesman*, November 10, 1832; Haverhill (MA) *Gazette*, November 10, 1832; Paris (ME) *Jeffersonian*, November 13, 1832; Cincinnati *Gazette*, November 15, 1832; Hallowell (ME) *American Advocate*, November 16, 1832; Brattleboro (VT) *Messenger*, November 17, 1832; Hudson *Ohio Observer*, November 22, 1832; Lancaster (PA) *Examiner*, November 29, 1832; Worcester *Massachusetts Spy*, December 5, 1832; Boston *Trumpet and Universalist Magazine*, December 15, 1832; Pittsfield (MA) *Sun*, December 20, 1832; Woodstock *Vermont Courier*, December 28, 1832; Woodstock (VT) *Mercury*, December 28, 1832; Bridgeton (NJ) *West Jersey Observer*, January 12, 1833.
6. Alvan Stewart, *An Essay on the Evils of Intemperance: Pronounced in the First Presbyterian Church, in Utica, on the 26th February, 1833, at the Request of the Two Temperance Societies in the County of Oneida* (Gardiner Tracy, 1833), 14.
7. New York *Evangelist*, March 2, 1833.
8. Edwin Hall, *An Address in Behalf of the Temperance Society, Norwalk, Connecticut* (James Reed, Jr., 1833), 5.
9. Reverend Thomas H. Stockton, *Address Delivered in the Methodist Episcopal Church in Easton, Before the Temperance Society of Talbot County, Maryland, on the 26th day of February, 1833* (John J. Harrod, 1833), 11 (emphasis in original).
10. Sag Harbor (NY) *Corrector*, February 11, 1832; New-Bedford (MA) *Courier*, February 14, 1832; Salem (MA) *Gazette*, February 14, 1832; Keene (NH) *Sentinel*, February 17, 1832; Worcester *Massachusetts Spy*, February 22, 1832; Boston *Liberator*, March 3, 1832; Montpelier *Vermont Patriot*, February 27, 1832; Morristown (NJ) *Jerseyman*, March 10, 1832; Haverhill (MA) *Essex Gazette*, March 17, 1832.
11. The following printed the Leipsic piece with the commentary that the Baltimore *Gazette* added: Baltimore *Gazette*, August 1, 1832; Cincinnati *Catholic Telegraph*, August 11, 1832; Washington (DC) *United States Telegraph*, August 14, 1832; Maysville

(KY) *Eagle*, August 16, 1832; Charleston (SC) *Mercury*, August 8, 1832; Nashville *National Banner*, August 13, 1832; Lancaster (PA) *Intelligencer*, August 17, 1832; Salisbury (NC) *Western Carolinian*, September 3, 1832. Papers that printed it with no commentary: Pawtucket (RI) *Chronicle*, August 3, 1832; Boston *Traveller*, August 10, 1832; Dedham (MA) *Patriot*, August 10, 1832; New York (NY) *Christian Intelligencer*, August 18, 1832; Portland (ME) *Eastern Argus*, August 31, 1832; Newark (NJ) *Daily Advertiser*, September 4, 1832.

12. Camden (SC) *Journal*, in Alexandria (VA) *Gazette*, September 1, 1832; New Haven (CT) *Columbian Register*, September 8, 1832; Richmond (VA) *Constitutional Whig*, August 31, 1832; Leesburg (VA) *Genius of Liberty*, September 8, 1832.
13. Washington Irving to Charles King, August 9, 1832, in *The Complete Works of Washington Irving. Miscellaneous Writings, 1803–1859*, 2 vols., ed. Wayne R. Clime (Twayne, 1979), 2: 714.
14. Reprinted in Boston *New England Farmer*, November 14, 1832.
15. K. Ahmad, K. Jahan, and I. Huq, "Decontamination of Drinking Water by Alum for the Preparation of Oral Rehydration Solution," *Food and Nutritional Bulletin* 6, no. 2 (1984): 1–4.
16. Cincinnati *Gazette*, October 18, 1832; also published in Cincinnati *Journal*, October 19, 1832. Little is known about Henry Boyd except brief details that appeared in *Ohio Anti-Slavery Convention. Held at Putnam, on the Twenty-Second, Twenty-Third, and Twenty-Fourth of April, 1835* (Beaumont and Wallace, [1835]), 34.
17. Daniel Drake, "Epidemic Cholera. Miscellaneous Observations—Historical, Statistical, Etiological and Therapeutic, on the Prevailing Epidemic," *Western Journal of the Medical and Physical Sciences* 7, no. 26 (July, August, and September 1833): 161–81 (quote on 165).
18. Kevin Franklin, "A Short Biography of Engineer Benjamin Prescott," *New York Almanac*, June 25, 2015, https://www.newyorkalmanack.com/2015/06/a-short-biography-of-engineer-benjamin-prescott/; Documentary History of American Water-Works, accessed July 12, 2024, http://www.waterworkshistory.us/NY/Albany/; David Stevenson, *Sketch of the Civil Engineering of North America* (John Weale, Architectural Library, 1838), 291.
19. Albany (NY) *Evening Journal*, August 24, 1832.
20. Albany (NY) *Evening Journal*, August 24, 1832.
21. Albany (NY) *Argus*, August 27, 1832.
22. Albany (NY) *Evening Journal*, August 27, 1832. The *Evening Journal* identifies the letter's author by the initials J. P. G. His full name is given in the Poughkeepsie (NY) *Journal*, August 29, 1832.
23. Albany (NY) *Evening Journal*, August 28, 1832.
24. New York *Evening Post*, August 25, 1832; Baltimore *Gazette*, August 27, 1832; Maysville (KY) *Eagle*, September 13, 1832; Philadelphia *Inquirer*, August 27, 1832; Nashville *National Banner*, September 8, 1832.
25. Baltimore *Gazette*, August 27, 1832.
26. Baltimore *Gazette*, October 16, 1832.

27. Nelson Manfred Blake, *Water for the Cities: A History of the Urban Water Supply Problem in the United States* (Syracuse University Press, 1956), 92–93, 131–37, 225–27; Rosenberg, *Cholera Years*, 103 n.6; Kolb, "At the Confluence of Science and Power," 22, 92–96.
28. Montreal *Menervie*, June 22, 1832, in Plattsburg (NY) *Republican*, June 25, 1832; Albany (NY) *Argus*, June 29, 1832; Greenfield (MA) *Recorder*, July 3, 1832.
29. George Duffield, *An Address Delivered in the Presbyterian Church, Before the Young Men's Temperance Society of Carlisle, by Rev. George Duffield, July 4, 1832* (Geo. Fleming Printer, 1832), 9.
30. "An Authentic Record of Deaths in the City of Albany, from the Commencement to the Cessation of the Daily Reports, in the Summer of 1832; Omitting All Under the Age of 16 Years," *Temperance Recorder. Extra*. 1, no. 9 (November 6, 1832).
31. New York *Commercial Advertiser*, November 9, 1832; New York *Spectator*, November 12, 1832; Alexandria (VA) *Gazette*, November 13, 1832; Boston *Recorder*, November 14, 1832; New York *Observer*, November 17, 1832; Hartford *Connecticut Observer*, November 18, 1832; Albany (NY) *Argus*, November 20, 1832; Savannah *Georgian*, November 21, 1832; Northampton (MA) *Gazette*, November 21, 1832; Worcester *Massachusetts Spy*, November 21, 1832; Portland (ME) *Christian Mirror*, November 22, 1832; Keene *New-Hampshire Sentinel*, November 22, 1832; Bellows Falls *Vermont Chronicle*, November 23, 1832; Annapolis *Maryland Republican*, November 24, 1832; Boston *American Traveller*, November 27, 1832; Boston *Christian Herald*, November 28, 1832; Philadelphia *Philadelphian*, November 29, 1832; Salem (MA) *Gazette*, November 29, 1832; Amherst (MA) *Farmer's Cabinet*, November 30, 1832; Haverhill (MA) *Gazette*, December 1, 1832; Boston *Liberator*, December 1, 1832; Portsmouth (NH) *Journal of Literature and Politics*, December 1, 1832; Cincinnati *Baptist Weekly Journal*, December 7, 1832; Troy (OH) *Times*, December 21, 1832.
32. *Temperance Recorder* 1, no. 10 (December 4, 1832): 79. This was picked up and published in New York *Evangelist*, December 15, 1832; Boston *Recorder*, December 12, 1832; Portland (ME) *Christian Mirror*, December 20, 1832; Lowell (MA) *Observer*, December 28, 1832; Boston *Liberator*, December 29, 1832; Portsmouth (NH) *Journal and Rockingham Gazette*, December 29, 1832; Brandon *Vermont Telegraph*, January 8, 1833; Cincinnati *Baptist Weekly Journal*, February 8, 1833.
33. Congressional Temperance Society, *Proceedings and Speeches at a Meeting for the Promotion of the Cause of Temperance in the United States: Held at the Capitol, in Washington City, February 24, 1833* (Way and Gideon, 1833), 29.
34. Bellamy Storer, *An Address Delivered Before the Cincinnati Temperance Society, on the Twenty-Sixth Day of February, 1833* (F. S. Benton, 1833), 6–7.
35. Washington (DC) *National Intelligencer*, August 8, 1833.
36. Reuben H. Walworth, "Address," in *Fourth Annual Report of the New-York State Society for the Promotion of Temperance* (Packard and Van Benthuysen, 1833), 4. His address was also published in the *American Quarterly Temperance Magazine*, 1 (May 1833). References to his speech noted here and below are to the former.

37. Walworth, "Address," 5.
38. Walworth, "Address," 5.
39. Sherrill, *An Essay on Epidemics*, 25 ("liberal doses"), 27 ("fatal cases").
40. Thomas Spencer, *An Essay on the Nature of the Epidemic Usually Called Asiatic Cholera* (Webster and Skinners, 1833), 300, 302.
41. Samuel Jackson, "Personal Observations and Experience of Epidemic or Malignant Cholera in the City of Philadelphia," *American Journal of Medical Sciences* 12 (May 1833): 119. (Jackson published his personal observations in two parts; the first came in the February 1833 issue and the second in the May 1833 issue.)
42. Jackson, "Personal Observations and Experience of Epidemic or Malignant Cholera in the City of Philadelphia," *American Journal of Medical Sciences* 11 (February 1833): 306–7.
43. Jackson, "Personal Observations and Experience of Epidemic or Malignant Cholera in the City of Philadelphia," *American Journal of Medical Sciences* 12 (May 1833): 119.
44. Jackson, "Personal Observations and Experience of Epidemic or Malignant Cholera in the City of Philadelphia," *American Journal of Medical Sciences* 11 (February 1833): 331; Jackson, "Personal Observations and Experience of Epidemic or Malignant Cholera in the City of Philadelphia," *American Journal of Medical Sciences* 12 (May 1833): 120.
45. David Meredith Reese, MD, *A Plain and Practical Treatise on the Epidemic Cholera, as It Prevailed in the City of New York, in the Summer of 1832; Including Its Nature, Causes, Treatment and Prevention. Designed for Popular Instruction. To Which Is Added, by Way of Appendix, A Brief Essay on the Medical Use of Ardent Spirits; Being an Attempt to Show That Alcohol Is as Unnecessary and Mischievous in Sickness as in Health* (Conner & Cooke, 1833), 3–4.
46. The New York *Spectator* gave readers advance notice of its impending publication, telling its readers that they knew the author and vouched for his expertise. See New York *Spectator*, May 23, 1833. Notices of the book's publication and advertisements for it can be found in the following: New York *Evening Post*, June 8, 1833; New York *American*, June 10, 1833; Boston *Courier*, June 12, 1833; Boston *Post*, June 13, 1833; Philadelphia *United States Gazette*, June 15, 1833; again in the New York *Spectator*, June 13, 1833, excerpts from, reiterating common theme of who was vulnerable and why and means of prevention; Philadelphia *National Gazette*, June 14, 1833; Philadelphia *Inquirer*, June 18, 1833: gives it a review (positive) and summary in a column; Portland (ME) *Weekly Advertiser*, June 18, 1833; Washington (DC) *National Intelligencer*, July 2, 1833; Washington (DC) *Globe*, July 2, 1833; Piqua (OH) *Courier and Enquirer*, July 13, 1833; Columbus *Ohio State Journal*, July 20, 1833; New Bedford (MA) *Mercury*, July 26, 1833; Charleston (SC) *Mercury*, June 19, 1833 (reprints an extract from New York *Commercial Advertiser* but does not give book title); Piqua (OH) *Courier and Enquirer*, July 13, 1833 (summary of one fills a whole column); Indianapolis *Indiana Journal*, September 21, 1833; Cincinnati *Daily Republican*, September 27, 1833.

47. Reese, *A Plain and Practical Treatise*, 5.
48. Reese, *A Plain and Practical Treatise*, 33.
49. Reese, *A Plain and Practical Treatise*, 59.
50. Shah, *Pandemic*, 64.
51. Reese, *A Plain and Practical Treatise*, 88 ("villainous pump water"), 86 ("intemperate foreigners"), 87 ("Among the hundreds of thousands...").
52. John S. Haller, Jr., *The People's Doctors: Samuel Thomson and the American Botanical Movement, 1790–1860* (Southern Illinois University Press, 2000).
53. Columbus (OH) *Thomsonian Recorder*, September 15, 1832, 22; October 20, 1832, 8; November 3, 1832, 72; and December 29, 1832, 158, 171, 185–86.
54. Columbus (OH) *Thomsonian Recorder*, December 15, 1832, 132–38, and December 29, 1832, 149–50.
55. Columbus (OH) *Thomsonian Recorder*, September 15, 1832, 15, and November 3, 1832, 62 ("regular habits").
56. Columbus (OH) *Thomsonian Recorder*, December 15, 1832, 139–40 (quote on 139).
57. Columbus (OH) *Thomsonian Recorder*, April 27, 1833, 330.
58. Columbus (OH) *Thomsonian Recorder*, June 15, 1833, 399.
59. Ian R. Tyrrell, *Sobering Up: From Temperance to Prohibition in Antebellum America, 1800–1860* (Greenwood Press, 1979), 87.
60. Kerri K. Greenidge, *The Grimkes: The Legacy of Slavery in an American Family* (Liveright, 2023), 12–36.
61. The finding aid of the Weld-Grimké papers records Bettle's death as cholera, but verification could not be found in available primary sources. See https://findingaids.lib.umich.edu/catalog/umich-wcl-M-400wel (accessed July 16, 2024). His death was first reported in Philadelphia *Poulson's American* on October 11, 1832. The lengthier obituary noting the duration of his illness and risky treatment was published in *Poulson's American* on October 15, 1832.
62. Angelina Grimké Diary, November 17, 1829–May 18, 1833, pp. 62–63, Weld-Grimké Papers, Box 15, WLCL.
63. For background on Angelina Grimké during the years 1832–1833, her relationship with Bettle, and her brother's role in comforting her, see Gerda Lerner, *The Grimké Sisters of South Carolina: Pioneers for Women's Rights and Abolition*, revised and expanded ed., (University of North Carolina Press, 2004), 71–75.
64. Angelina Grimké to Thomas Grimké, June 3, 1833, Weld-Grimké Papers, Box 1, fo. 27, WLCL.

CHAPTER 13

1. Louisville *Herald*, November 24, 1905.
2. Dumesnil Memoir, Dumesnil Family Papers, fo. 3, pp. 6–7, FHS.
3. Dumesnil Memoir, Dumesnil Family Papers, fo. 3, p. 7, FHS.
4. Dumesnil Memoir, Dumesnil Family Papers, fo. 3, p. 7, FHS.

5. [Mary Bryan Harford] to Julia Cumming, New Orleans, June 11, 1833, in *Tokens of Affection: The Letters of a Planter's Daughter in the Old South*, ed. Carol Bleser (University of Georgia Press, 1996), 157–58 (quote on 157).
6. New Orleans *Commercial Bulletin*, June 15, 1833.
7. Natchez *Courier*, June 14, 1833.
8. Carl Kohn to Samuel Kohn, July 7, 1833, Carl Kohn Letter Books, HNOC.
9. Carl Kohn to Samuel Kohn, May 15, 1833, Carl Kohn Letter Book, HNOC; N. and J. Dick to Dr. James M. Morris, June 13, 1833, Richard Morris Papers, Mss. 38–79, Box 2, UVA; Charleston (SC) *Courier*, June 18, 1833; Cary Robinson to Conway Robinson, June 27, 1833, Moncure Robinson Papers, 01/Mss. 65 R56, 77–14, Box 3, fo. 25, WMU.
10. John Starker to Levi Lewis, June 21, 1833, Levi Lewis Archive, Box 2, fo. 93, HNOC.
11. Michel Halphen, *Observations Sur Le Choléra-Morbus Qui a Régné a La Nouvelle-Orléans en 1833 et en 1834 Faisant Suite au Mémoire Sur Le Choléra-Morbus De 1832* (Chez J. B. Baillière, Libraire, 1835), 3. The author wishes to thank Nathan Greenhaw for translating this work.
12. Edward Rawle to [Robert Corbin], July 27, 1833, Francis P. Corbin Papers, Box 1, Duke.
13. Edward Rawle to Francis Corbin, August 11, 1833, Francis P. Corbin Papers, Box 1, Duke.
14. A. Harris to Sarah B. Evans, May 28, 1833, Nathaniel Evans and Family Papers, Box 1, fo. 11, LSU. Another planter in the area rounded down the number of fatalities on the Proctor plantation to eighty. See [Robert Corbin to Francis Corbin], June 18, 1833, Francis Corbin Papers, Box 1, Manuscripts and Archives Division, New York Public Library, New York.
15. H. B. Trist to Nicholas Trist, June 21, 1833, Trist Papers, fo. 65, UNC-SHC; H. B. T. to Nicholas Trist, July 3, 1833, Trist Papers, fo. 66, UNC-SHC; H. B. T. to Nicholas Trist, September [7], 1833, Trist Papers, fo. 67, UNC-SHC; John B. Craighead to Col. Andrew Hynes, July 6, 1833, Gay (Edward and Family) Papers, Box 4, LSU; E. Butler to Thomas Butler, August 19, 1833, Butler Family Papers (1026), Box 3, LSU; Natchez *Courier*, August 23, 1833; Mary Stirling to Mary Louisa Stirling, August 20, 1833, Butler (Thomas and Family) Papers, Box 1a, fo. 4, LSU.
16. Natchez *Courier*, June 21, 1832; see also Caiaphas K. Ham to Sterling C. Robertson, August 28, 1833, in *Papers Concerning Robertson's Colony*, vol. VII: *December 6, 1831, Through October 1833. Those Eleven-League Grants* (University of Texas at Arlington Press, 1980), 512.
17. Baton Rouge (LA) *Gazette*, March 30, 1833 (15 near Franklin, LA); Baltimore *Niles Weekly Register*, June 22, 1833, and Lynchburg (VA), *Virginian*, June 29, 1833 (195 enslaved people on plantations around Franklin); Fayette *Missouri Intelligencer and Boon's Lick Advertiser*, September 14, 1833 (60 in St. Martinsville, LA), and Philadelphia *Inquirer*, September 14, 1833 (12 in St. Martinsville, LA, after previous report); Fayette *Missouri Intelligencer*, September 14, 1833 (26 in Opelousas, LA); Philadelphia *Inquirer*, September 7, 1833 (35 at "The Pointe" near St. Martinsville, LA).

18. Natchez *Mississippi Journal and Natchez Advertiser*, July 19, 1833.
19. New York *American*, August 9, 1833. These figures first appeared in the *American* and then were republished in numerous papers throughout the United States.
20. Rothman, *The Ledger and the Chain*, 217–18.
21. On the activities of Franklin, Armfield, and Co. during the third wave, see the following in the Ballard Papers, UNC-SHC: James Franklin to Rice Ballard, November 14, 1833, fo. 12; [James Franklin] to Rice Ballard, December 9, 1833, fo. 12; James Franklin to Rice Ballard, December 13, 1833, fo. 12; Isaac Franklin to Rice Ballard, December 25, 1833, fo. 12; Isaac Franklin to Rice Ballard, March 30, 1834, fo. 13.
22. Sexton reports published in Natchez (MS) *Courier*, April 26, 1833–July 5, 1833. Totals reflect deaths attributed to "cholera" and "cholera asphyxia" but not "cholera infantum."
23. Natchez (MS) *Courier*, June 21, 1833, June 28, 1833.
24. Port Gibson (MS) *Herald and Correspondent*, June 1, 1833; Vicksburg (MS) *Whig*, May 29, 1833; Natchez (MS) *Courier*, June 21, 1833; Natchez *Mississippi Free Trader*, June 28, 1833.
25. Jackson (MS) *State Rights Banner*, June 13, 1833.
26. Natchez *Mississippi Journal and Natchez Advertiser*, July 19, 1833.
27. Little Rock *Arkansas Gazette*, July 3, 1833.
28. Little Rock *Arkansas Gazette*, July 17, 1833, August 14, 1833.
29. Charles E. Wilson to Isaac McCoy, August 15, 1833, McCoy Papers, microfilm reel 8, fr. 322–24, KHS; John Campbell to Elbert Herring, September 4, 1833, in *Correspondence on the Subject of the Emigration of Indians*, 4: 541.
30. G. J. Rains to George Gibson, November 4, 1833, in *Correspondence on the Subject of the Emigration of Indians*, 1: 851.
31. Nashville *National Banner*, June 17, 1833.
32. Jackson (TN) *Southern Statesman*, July 6, 1833.
33. Original report in the Jackson (MO) *Eagle*, June 8, 1833, in Washington (DC) *National Intelligencer*, June 28, 1833.
34. Jackson (MO) *Eagle*, in Washington (DC) *National Intelligencer*, July 6, 1833.
35. St. Louis *Missouri Republican*, August 27, 1833, in Boston *Spirit of the Age and Journal of Humanity*, September 12, 1833.
36. New Bern (NC) *Sentinel*, June 7, 1833.
37. St. Louis *Missouri Republican*, July 12, 1833, in Nashville *National Banner*, July 25, 1833; Fayette *Missouri Intelligencer*, August 17, 1833.
38. Jefferson City (MO) *Jeffersonian Republican*, August 17, 1833.
39. Fayette *Missouri Intelligencer*, August 10, 1833.
40. Hiram Martin Chittenden, *History of Early Steamboat Navigation on the Missouri River*, 2 vols, (Francis P. Harper, 1903) 1: 32–36; New York *Evening Post*, July 31, 1833.
41. Isaac McCoy to Rev. Dr. Bolles, July 22, 1833, McCoy Papers, microfilm reel 8, fr. 287–89, KHS.
42. E. A. Ellsworth, Talk with the Kickapoos, September 2, 1833, in *Correspondence on the Subject of the Emigration of Indians*, 4: 643.

43. Maximilian Wied, *Maximilian, Prince of Wied's Travels in the Interior of North America, Part III*, vol. 24 of *Early Western Travels, 1748–1846*, ed. Reuben Gold Thwaites (Arthur H. Clark Company, 1906), 14, 108.
44. Ninian Wirt Edwards, *History of Illinois, from 1778–1833; and Life and Times of Ninian Edwards* (The Illinois State Journal Company, 1870), 250. Obituary in St. Louis *Missouri Republican*, July 23, 1833, in Nashville *National Banner*, August 3, 1833.
45. Olson, "Plague on the Prairie," 7.
46. Jacob Wyeth to Charles Wyeth, June 27 [or 29?], 1833, Wyeth Family Papers, Box 1, Beinecke Rare Book and Manuscript Library, Yale.
47. Vandalia *Whig and Illinois Intelligencer*, July 24, 1833.
48. St. Louis *Times* in Jefferson City (MO) *Jeffersonian Republican*, June 22, 1833.
49. Palmyra (MO) *Courier*, in Fayette *Missouri Intelligencer*, July 6, 1833. Palymra's tragedy received notice in many newspapers, which reported varying death tolls that are in parentheses that follow these citations: New Orleans *Commercial Bulletin*, July 22, 1833 (105); Alton (IL) *Spectator*, June 25, 1833 (180); Nashville *National Banner*, July 2, 1833 (120) and July 9, 1833 (106); Vandalia *Whig and Illinois Intelligencer*, July 17, 1833 (120).
50. Nashville *National Banner*, April 24, 1833.
51. Nashville *National Banner*, April 23, 1833, May 3, 1833.
52. Nashville *National Banner*, May 29, 1833.
53. Nashville *National Banner*, June 3, 1833, reported thirty deaths during this time period, but in the June 4, 1833, issue, one more was added to the number.
54. Nashville *National Banner*, June 1, 1833.
55. Nashville *National Banner*, June 3, 1833.
56. Andrew Hynes to John B. Craighead, June 5, 1833, Gay (Edward and Family) Papers, Box 4, LSU.
57. Nashville *National Banner*, June 22, 1833.
58. Nashville *National Banner*, June 22, 1833.
59. Nashville *National Banner*, June 17, 1833; J. R. Killick, "Yeatman, Thomas," American National Biography, 2000, https://doi.org/10.1093/anb/9780198606697.article.1002178.
60. Nashville *National Banner*, June 19, 1833, July 8, 1833.
61. Knoxville *Republican*, July 10, 1833.
62. Nashville *National Banner*, July 8, 1833.
63. Nashville *National Banner*, July 22, 1833.
64. Columbia (TN) *Herald and Mail*, June 14, 1901.
65. R. S. Wheatly to Adam Beatty, June 12, 1833, Beatty-Quisenberry Papers, fo. 10, FHS; Lynchburg *Virginian*, July 11, 1833, August 8, 1833; Sarah Trebell Galt Browne and Mary Browne to Elizabeth J. Galt, July 15, 1833, Galt Papers (I), Mss. 78 G13,

Box 2, fo. 22, WMU; [Mary Browne?] to Elizabeth J. Galt, August 5, 1833, Galt Papers (I), Mss. 78 G13, Box 2, fo. 22, WMU.

66. Cincinnati *Gazette*, July 25, 1833, August 1, 1833.
67. Daniel Drake, "Epidemic Cholera. Miscellaneous Observations—Historical, Statistical, Etiological and Therapeutic, on the Prevailing Epidemic," *Western Journal of the Medical and Physical Sciences* 7, no. 26 (July, August, and September 1833): 173.
68. Maysville (KY) *Eagle*, May 25, 1833, in Nashville *National Banner*, June 1, 1833.
69. Frankfort (KY) *The Commonwealth*, June 4, 1833.
70. Charles Morgan to A. Falconer June 8, 1833, Morgan-Falconer Family Papers, Box 1, fo. 34, HNOC; Maysville (KY) *Eagle*, May 31, 1833, in Lynchburg *Virginian*, June 13, 1833.
71. Forrest L. Marion, "Perspective: 'The Dreaded Cholera' in Kentucky, 1832–1833," March 27, 2020, https://theaquilareport.com/perspective-the-dreaded-cholera-in-kentucky-1832-1833/.
72. Maysville (KY) *Eagle*, June 17, 1833, in Washington (DC) *National Intelligencer*, June 27, 1833.
73. Lynchburg *Virginian*, July 15, 1833.
74. John Cabell, M.D. to Richard K. Cralle, July 7, 1833, Cabell Family Papers, Brock Collection, Box 48, Huntington Library, San Marino, California.
75. James Lewis to Henry Massie, July 16, 1833, Massie Family Papers, Mss1 M3811, c307–26, Sec. 7, VHS.
76. Washington (DC) *National Intelligencer*, June 1, 1833.
77. Lynchburg *Virginian*, June 13, 1833.
78. Lynchburg *Virginian*, July 11, 1833.
79. Lynchburg *Virginian*, June 20, 1833.
80. Pittsburgh (PA) *Weekly Gazette*, August 5, 1832.
81. "Our History," Pittsburgh Water, accessed December 19, 2024, https://www.pgh2o.com/about-us/mission-vision-and-core-values/our-history#:~:text=The%20first%20documented%20effort%20to,with%20pumps%2C%20on%20Market%20Street.
82. Thomas F. Purcell to the President of C&O [John H. Eaton], June 24, [1833], COCCP, Box 6, NARA, CPM; Lynchburg *Virginian*, July 15, 1833.
83. The population of Lexington in the 1830 census was 6,026. The city did not grow much during the decade, in part because of the 1833 outbreak. Its population in the 1840 census was 6,997. See Gibson, "Population of the 100 Largest Cities and Other Urban Places in the United States."
84. Baird, "Asiatic Cholera's First Visit to Kentucky," 229.
85. Lunsford Yandell, "An Account of Spasmodic Cholera, as it appeared in the City of Lexington, in June 1833," *Transylvania Journal of Medicine* 6, no. 2 (April, May, and June 1833), 197–99.

86. Sara Kathryn Dawson, "The 1833 Cholera Epidemic in Lexington: A Study of Devastation and Recovery," MA Thesis, University of Kentucky, 1994, 18, 32; J. S. Chambers, *The Conquest of Cholera* (Macmillan Company, 1838), 175.
87. Philadelphia *National Gazette*, June 26, 1833.
88. Sarah A. Bell to Mary Offutt, June 13, 1833, Moxley-Offutt Papers, fo. 1., FHS.
89. Lexington *Kentucky Gazette*, June 22, 1833.
90. Maysville (KY) *Monitor*, July 4, 1833, in Pittsburgh (PA) *Weekly Gazette*, August 15, 1833.
91. Autobiography, vol. 1 (transcription), in the John Rogers Papers #2659-z, UNC-SHC.
92. Frankfort (KY) *Commonwealth*, July 2, 1833.
93. Frankfort (KY) *Commonwealth*, July 9, 1833.
94. Frankfort (KY) *Commonwealth*, July 2, 1833.
95. Frankfort (KY) *Argus*, July 31, 1833; Snyder, *Great Crossings*, 147–48.
96. Frankfort (KY) *Commonwealth*, July 3, 1833; Thomas Burford to Sidney P. Clay, [June 27, 1833], Sidney Payne Clay Papers, FHS.
97. Otis Ammidon to John Corlis, July 25, 1832, Corlis-Respess Papers, fo. 69, FHS.
98. John Corlis to Otis Ammidon, October 19, 1833, Corlis-Respess Papers, fo. 72, FHS.
99. Otis Ammidon to John Corlis, October 29, 1833, Corlis-Respess Papers, fo. 72, FHS.
100. Joseph Huber to Sidney P. Clay, June 26, 1833, Sidney Clay Papers, FHS.
101. Joseph Huber to Sidney P. Clay, July 20, 1833, Sidney Clay Papers, FHS.
102. Frankfort (KY) *Commonwealth*, July 9, 1833.
103. Frankfort (KY) *Commonwealth*, July 16, 1833; James A. Ramage, *Kentucky Rising: Democracy, Slavery, and Culture from the Early Republic to the Civil War* (University of Kentucky Press, 2011), 55.
104. Frankfort (KY) *Commonwealth*, July 2, 1833.
105. Henry Clay to Julia Prather Clay, June 23, 1833, in *The Papers of Henry Clay*, vol. 8, 654.
106. Frankfort (KY) *Commonwealth*, July 16, 1833.
107. Ramage, *Kentucky Rising*, 225.
108. Frankfort (KY) *Commonwealth*, June 25, 1833.
109. Lexington (KY) *Western Luminary*, July 24, 1833.
110. Frankfort (KY) *Commonwealth*, July 10, 1833.
111. Hector Green to Ellen Green, July 7, 1833, Green Family Papers, fo. 9, FHS.
112. Lexington (KY) *Western Luminary*, July 24, 1833.
113. William M. Awl, "A Brief History of the Epidemic Cholera as It Appeared in the Town of Columbus, and the Penitentiary of Ohio, in the Summer of 1833," *Western Journal of the Medical and Physical Sciences* 1, no. 3 (October, November, and December 1833): 343.
114. George Green to William Dickinson, October 7, 1833, Morton and Dickinson Family Correspondence, MSS 9755, Box 5, UVA.
115. Columbus (OH) *Thomsonian Recorder*, August 3, 1833, 484 (population of one thousand); Cincinnati *Gazette*, July 21, 1833 (population of eight hundred).

116. Rice McCoy to Isaac McCoy, January 1, 1834, McCoy Papers, microfilm reel 8, fr. 434–36, KHS.
117. Josephine Chandler, T. Tenny Chandler, and Charles Chandler, "Dr. Charles Chandler: His Place in the American Scene," *Journal of the Illinois State Historical Society* 24, no. 3 (October 1931): 426–29.
118. Quotes in Olson, "Plague on the Prairie," 8.
119. Vandalia *Whig and Illinois Intelligencer*, August 14, 1833, August 21, 1833.
120. Quotes in Olson, "Plague on the Prairie," 8.
121. Washington (DC) *Globe*, July 1, 1833; Baltimore *Gazette*, July 1, 1833; Philadelphia *Inquirer*, July 3, 1833; Philadelphia *Daily Chronicle*, July 3, 1833; Gettysburg (PA) *Adams Sentinel*, July 8, 1833; Gettysburg (PA) *Compiler*, July 9, 1833; Savannah *Georgian*, July 13, 1833; Dover (NH) *Gazette & Strafford Advertiser*, July 16, 1833; Harrisburg *Pennsylvania Telegraph*, July 17, 1833; Milledgeville (GA) *Southern Recorder*, July 24, 1833.
122. Yandell, "An Account of Spasmodic Cholera," 202.
123. Yandell, "An Account of Spasmodic Cholera," 204.
124. Yandell, "An Account of Spasmodic Cholera," 202.
125. Susan Yandell to David Wendel, June 11, 1833, Yandell Family Papers, fo. 12, FHS.
126. Susan Yandell to David Wendel, June 12, 1833, Yandell Family Papers, fo. 12, FHS.
127. Susan Yandell to Sarah Wendel, July 28, 1833, Yandell Family Papers, fo. 13, FHS.
128. Susan Yandell to David Wendel, June 24, 1833, Yandell Family Papers, fo. 12, FHS.
129. Charles Wilkins Short to William Short, June 16, 1833, Short Papers, fo. 18, FHS.
130. Charles Wilkins Short to William Short, June 23, 1833, Short Papers, fo. 18, FHS.
131. The full list was published in Lexington (KY) *Observer and Reporter*, August 22, 1833, and is transcribed and available online. There were calculation errors that I accounted for as well as deaths denoted as having a cause as other than cholera, which I excluded. See https://sites.rootsweb.com/~kyfayett/1833_deaths_reporter.htm (accessed August 14, 2024).
132. C. W. Short, "A Brief Historical Sketch of the Origin and Progress of Cholera Asphyxia," *Transylvania Journal of Medicine and Associate Sciences* 11, no. 1 (January, February, and March 1838): 20.
133. Dumesnil Memoir, Dumesnil Family Papers, fo. 3, pp. 6–7, FHS.
134. Dumesnil Memoir, Dumesnil Family Papers, fo. 3, p. 2, FHS.
135. Dumesnil Memoir, Dumesnil Family Papers, fo. 3, p. 34, FHS.

CHAPTER 14

1. The Erodelphian Society, Miami University, to Thomas S. Grimké, February 15, 1834, Lowcountry Digital Library, College of Charleston Libraries, https://lcdl.library.cofc.edu/lcdl/catalog/lcdl:80642?tify={%22pages%22:[3],%22panX%22:0.447,%22panY%22:0.917,%22view%22:%22info%22,%22zoom%22:0.835}.

2. Thomas S. Grimké, *The Temperance Reformation the Cause of Christian Morals. An Address Delivered Before the Charleston Temperance Society and the Young Men's Temperance Society of Charleston, On Tuesday Evening, February 25, 1834* (Observer Office Press, 1834), 21.
3. Daniel Drake to Sarah Daniel Drayton Grimké, October 25, 1834, Lowcountry Digital Library, College of Charleston Libraries, 1834-10-25. https://lcdl.library.cofc.edu/lcdl/catalog/lcdl:78618?tify={%22view%22:%22info%22}.
4. Halphen, *Observations Sur Le Choléra-Morbus Qui A Régné A La Nouvelle-Orléans En 1833 Et En 1834*, 172–73; Charles Town *Virginia Free Press*, March 20, 1834; Frederick [illegible last name] to Sarah [McGehee?], April 5, 1834, Burruss (John C. and Family) Papers, Box 1, LSU; New Orleans *Commercial Bulletin*, April 26, 1834; New Orleans *Courier*, May 1, 1834; Little Rock *Arkansas Advocate*, May 2, 1834; New Orleans *Bee*, April 24, 1834; Little Rock *Arkansas Gazette*, April 29, 1834; Indianapolis *Indiana Journal*, May 10, 1834; Philadelphia *Inquirer*, May 9, 1834; Rufus Williams to Lewis Alderson, June 12, 1834, Lewis Alderson Papers, KHS.
5. Manchester (now Yazoo City), Mississippi: Vicksburg *Mississippian*, June 27, 1834. Randolph, Tennessee: Nashville *Republican*, August 26, 1834; Little Rock *Arkansas Times and Advocate*, September 5, 1834; Clinton (MS) *Gazette*, September 13, 1834; New York *Evening Post*, October 2, 1834; Nashville *National Banner*, September 1, 1834; Frankfort (KY) *Commonwealth*, October 4, 1834; Columbia, Tennessee: Nashville *National Banner*, August 18, 1834; Nashville *National Banner*, September 6, 1834; J. P. Spindle to Daniel Gold, September 5, 1834, Daniel Lewis Gold Papers, Section A, Box 53, Duke; J. P. Spindle to Daniel Gold, October 4, 1834, Daniel Lewis Gold Papers, Section A, Box 53, Duke; Allen Brown to Hamilton Brown, December 7, 1834, Hamilton Brown Papers, Box 1, fo. 5, UNC-SHC. Princeton, Kentucky: Fayette *Missouri Intelligencer*, July 19, 1834; Murfreesboro (TN) *Weekly Monitor*, July 19, 1834; Princeton (KY) *Record of the Times*, July 11, 1834, in Frankfort (KY) *Commonwealth*, July 22, 1834; Fayette *Missouri Intelligencer*, August 2, 1834, and August 9, 1834; Frankfort (KY) *Argus*, July 23, 1834. Springfield, Illinois: Springfield (IL) *Sangamo Journal*, September 6, 1834, September 13, 1834, September 20, 1834, and September 27, 1834. Rushville, Illinois: "Cholera of 1834," Schuyler County, Illinois Genealogy and History, accessed December 19, 2024, https://genealogytrails.com/ill/schuyler/1834CholeraEpidemic.html. Pekin, Illinois: Springfield (IL) *Sangamo Journal*, July 12, 1834, and July 19, 1834; Jared Olar, "Pekin in the Time of Cholera: The 'Blue Death' Comes to Pekin," Pekin Public Library website, November 2, 2023, https://pekinpubliclibrary.org/pekin-in-the-time-of-cholera-the-blue-death-comes-to-pekin/.
6. "Journal of Lieutenant Harris," in *The River Trail: A Saga of the Cherokee Removal*, ed. Jane B. Noble (Cross Cultural Education Center, n.d.), 143. At Cadron Creek, near Conway, Arkansas, the Conway Chamber of Commerce and Faulkner County Historical Society, in Cooperation with the US Army Corps of Engineers, erected a

historical marker in 1989 noting the nearby burials of fifty individuals from Harris's contingent. These are named on a plaque. The author wishes to express his thanks to Vaughn Scriber for providing this information.

7. "Journal of Lieutenant Harris," 143.
8. New Echota (Cherokee Nation) *Cherokee Phoenix*, May 31, 1834.
9. Benjamin Curry to Lewis Cass, September 15, 1834, Letters Received by the Office of Indian Affairs, 1824–1881, RG 75, NARA, microfilm 234, reel 76.
10. Joseph Smith to William W. Phelps, July 31, 1832, and Joseph Smith to Noah C. Saxton, January 4, 1833, both letters in Joseph Smith Papers: The Authoritative Source for the Writings, Teachings, and Records of Joseph Smith, online https://www.josephsmithpapers.org/.
11. Independence (MO) *Evening and Morning Star*, June 1833.
12. Matthew B. Lund, "A Society of Like-Minded Men: American Localism and the Mormon Expulsion from Jackson County," *Journal of Mormon History* 40 (Summer 2014): 170.
13. Isaac McCoy Letter of November 28, 1833, in St. Louis *Daily Missouri Republican*, December 20, 1833.
14. Charles Rich Daybook, Beinecke Rare Book and Manuscript Library, Yale.
15. Quoted in Andrea G. Radke, "We Also Marched: the Women and Children of Zion's Camp, 1834," *BYU Studies Quarterly* 39, no. 1 (2000), 155.
16. Radke, "We Also Marched," 156.
17. Quoted in Matthew C. Godfrey, "'We Believe the Hand of the Lord Is in It': Memories of Divine Intervention in the Zion's Camp Expedition," *BYU Studies Quarterly* 56, no.4 (2017): 116.
18. Godfrey, "'We Believe the Hand of the Lord Is in It,'" 131.
19. Steve Fidel, "Zion's Camp Monument Recalls 15 Members Who Died of Cholera," *Deseret News*, August 30, 1997, online https://www.deseret.com/1997/8/30/19331274/zion-s-camp-monument-recalls-15-members-who-died-of-cholera/.
20. "Osages," *Missionary Herald* 30, no. 1 (January 1834): 23; Tai Edwards, *Osage Women and Empire: Gender and Power* (University of Kansas Press, 2018).
21. Nathaniel B. Dodge to Greene, September 4, 1834, American Board of Commissioners for Foreign Missions Archives, Series 18.4.4, vol. 1, Houghton Library, Harvard.
22. Harriet Montgomery to "Dear Brother and Sister," August 25, 1834, Harriet Wooley Letterbook, Beinecke Rare Book and Manuscript Library, Yale; Abraham Redfield to Greene, August 25, 1834, American Board of Commissioners for Foreign Missions Archives, Series 18.4.4, vol. 1, Houghton Library, Harvard.
23. Abraham Redfield to Greene, September 18, 1834, American Board of Commissioners for Foreign Missions Archives, Series 18.4.4, vol. 1, Houghton Library, Harvard.
24. "Mission to the Osage," *Missionary Herald* 32, no. 1 (January 1836): 24.

25. Willard Hughes Rollins, *Unaffected by the Gospel: Osage Resistance to the Christian Invasion (1673–1906): A Cultural History* (University of New Mexico Press, 2004), 109–13.
26. The town was in Beaver County, where a total of nineteen fatalities were recorded up to August 15, 1834. See Philadelphia *Inquirer*, August 23, 1834, and Canton *Ohio Repository*, August 22, 1834.
27. New York *Evening Post*, September 29, 1834; Albany (NY) *Argus*, September 23, 1834.
28. Elizabeth T. Baird, "Reminiscences of Life in Territorial Wisconsin," *Collections of the State Historical Society of Wisconsin*, vol. 15 (State Historical Society of Wisconsin, 1900), 238.
29. Sister Mary Alphonsa Corry, *The Story of Father Van den Broek, O.P.; a Study of Holland and the Story of the Early Settlement of Wisconsin* (Ainsworth & Company, 1907), 50–51.
30. Towns known to have significant fatalities that newspapers enumerated are listed in table 14.1. Some other towns made the news but without enumeration. The following papers gave mortality figures for Huron, Sandusky, and Lower Sandusky and reference Venice, Norwalk, Perrysburg, and Tiffin as sustaining losses but offering no numbers: Norwalk (OH) *Huron Reflector*, August 19, 1834, August 26, 1834; Cleveland *Whig* August 20, 1834; Hudson *Ohio Observer*, August 21, 1833. Cincinnati's board of health began making weekly reports in mid-July and ceased by the end of August. These can be found here: Cincinnati *Daily Republican*, July 22, 1834, July 30, 1834, August 7, 1834, August 14, 1834, August 21, 1834. Butler County's figures are in Cyrus Falconer, "XV.—Epidemic Cholera in Butler County, Ohio," *Western Journal of Medical and Physical Sciences* 2, no. 2 (July, August, and September 1834): 326–28; Fulton's death toll was reported in Cincinnati *Western Christian Advocate*, July 25, 1834; New Carlisle's total deaths were reported in Philadelphia *Inquirer*, September 13, 1834; Chester's, Massillon's, and Newark's can be found in Columbus (OH), *The Ohio State Journal*, August 30, 1834; Cleveland's in Cleveland *Whig*, September 10, 1834.
31. Donald A. Hutslar, "'God's Scourge': The Cholera Years in Ohio," *Ohio History Journal* 105 (Summer-Autumn 1996): 174.
32. Detroit *Free Press*, July 30, 1834; New York *American*, August 26, 1834.
33. New York *Commercial Advertiser*, August 23, 1834.
34. Detroit *Free Press*, August 20, 1834.
35. Aaron Hulin to Samuel Hunter, September 20, 1834, Aaron Hulin Letters to Samuel Hunter, Beinecke Rare Book and Manuscript Library, Yale.
36. Susan Farley to Mother, September 7, 1834, Farley Family Papers, Box 1, fo. 38, WLCL. Farley relays the "official" count of 350 to her mother and gives a population figure of 5,000. The press relayed the official toll. Population figures that editors chose to contextualize the mortality with vary. New York, *Commercial Advertiser*, August 30, 1834, indicated only 2,500 in Detroit, while the same paper on September 8, 1834, indicated that with its "suburbs" the population numbered 7,000.

37. New Bedford, MA: New Bedford (MA) *Gazette*, September 8, 1834. New York: Charles Lee, "Medical Statistics of New York," *The American Journal of Medical Sciences* 19 (November 1836): 27, 30, 33 (Lee tabulates 971 deaths from the board of health reports of 1834 but gives a total of 1021, without explaining where the extra 50 came from. Since most deaths tolls were undercounts, I am using the higher figure.) Albany: Albany (NY) *Argus*, September 5, 1834. Poughkeepsie: New York *American*, August 13, 1834. Philadelphia: "Statement of Deaths, with the Diseases and Ages, in the City and Liberties of Philadelphia, During the Year 1834," *American Journal of Medical Sciences* 17 (November 1835): 264; Philadelphia *Inquirer*, November 6, 1834, and November 10, 1834. Petersburg, VA: Philadelphia *Inquirer*, November 8, 1834. Baltimore: Philadelphia *Inquirer*, November 8, 1834. An outbreak also occurred in Washington, NC, but mortality statistics could not be found. See Raleigh *North-Carolina Star*, October 16, 1834; Tarboro (NC) *Press*, October 31, 1834.
38. New York *Commercial Advertiser*, July 30, 1834.
39. New York *Commercial Advertiser*, August 18, 1834.
40. William Dunham to William Gibbons, September 9, 1834, William Gibbons Papers, fo. 8, WLCL; Savannah, *Republican*, September 1, 1834.
41. Charleston (SC) *Courier*, September 10, 1834; S. Dulles to J.H.D. October 4, 1834, Cheves Papers, 12/95/1, SCHS [typescript]; M.E. Cheves to Ann Lovell, September 20, 1834, Ann (Heatly) Reid Lovell Papers, Section A, Box 85, Duke; Alicia [Alice Izard?] to Ewerette B. Middleton, October 4, 1834, Middleton Family Papers, 12/158/7, SCHS; James Louis Petigru to Hugh S. Legaré, September 16, 1834, in James P. Carson, ed., *Life, Letters and Speeches of James Louis Petigru: the Union Man of South Carolina* (Washington, DC: W. H. Lowdermilk & Co, 1920), 161; "The Life and Times of James Hamilton of South Carolina by S. P. Hamilton, His Son," 46, unpublished manuscript, James Hamilton Papers, UNC- SHC; William Dunham to William Gibbons, September 15, 1834, William Gibbons Papers, fo. 8, WLCL
42. Charleston (SC) *Courier*, September 8, 1834, September 9, 1834, September 12, 1834.
43. Charleston (SC) *Mercury*, September 12, 1834.
44. Charleston (SC) *Courier*, September 15, 1834.
45. Charleston (SC) *Courier*, September 20, 1834.
46. Richard Arnold to Thomas Spalding, September 14, 1834, in *Letters of Richard D. Arnold, M.D. 1808–1876*, ed. Richard H. Shyrock (AMS Press, 1929), 11 (emphasis in the original).
47. Richard Arnold to Thomas Spalding, September 24, 1834, in *Letters of Richard D. Arnold*, 12–13.
48. Charleston (SC) *Courier*, September 15, 1834.
49. Charleston (SC) *Courier*, September 24, 1834.
50. Charleston (SC) *Courier*, October 2, 1834.
51. Savannah (GA) *Georgian*, September 29, 1834.

52. Charleston (SC) *Mercury*, September 26, 1834.
53. Philadelphia *Inquirer*, November 7, 1834.
54. James Louis Petigru to Hugh S. Legaré, October 26, 1834, in Carson, *Life, Letters and Speeches of James Louis Petigru*, 164.
55. New Orleans *Bee*, May 9, 1835, in New York *Evening Post*, May 28, 1835.
56. Nashville *National Banner*, April 29, 1835.
57. Several towns listed in table 14.4 are not discussed in this chapter and are herein cited. Alton, IL: New York *Evening Post*, June 26, 1835; Philadelphia *Inquirer*, June 29, 1835. Beardstown, IL: Springfield (IL) *Sangamo Journal*, June 27, 1835; Madison, IN: Madison (IN) *Banner*, July 16, 1835; Red Lion, OH: Lebanon (OH) *Western Star*, June 26, 1835. Bucyrus, OH: Bucyrus (OH) *Journal*, April 25, 1879; Nashville: Nashville *Republican*, June 20, 1835, June 29, 1835 (sexton records indicated thirty-six fatalities); Nashville, *Republican*, August 11, 1835 (twenty-four deaths in the penitentiary). Lebanon, TN: Nashville *National Banner*, July 1, 1835. Murfreesboro, TN: Nashville *National Banner*, July 8, 1835. Clarksville, TN: Nashville *Republican*, July 16, 1835. Franklin, TN: Nashville *National Banner*, July 10, 1835. Beech Grove, TN: Nashville *Republican*, July 21, 1835. Williamsport, TN: Windsor (VT) *Aurora of the Valley*, September 12, 1835; Newnan (GA) *Palladium*, September 26, 1835. Maysville, KY: Frankfort (KY) *Commonwealth*, July 4, 1835. Sharpsburg, KY: Mt. Sterling (KY) *Herald*, June 27, 1835, in Frankfort (KY) *Commonwealth*, July 11, 1835. Millersburg, KY: Frankfort (KY) *Commonwealth*, July 4, 1836; Washington (DC) *United States Telegraph*, July 15, 1835.
58. Jefferson City (MO) *Jeffersonian Republican*, July 4, 1835.
59. Nashville *National Banner*, July 31, 1835.
60. Lexington *Kentucky Gazette*, August 8, 1835.
61. Rebecca Smith Washington to Jane Washington Walker, August 10, 1835, typescript PDF downloaded from Folklife Archives, Manuscripts &, "Washington, Rebecca (Smith), 1776–1861 (SC 1254)" (2014). *Manuscript Collection Finding Aids.* Paper 3363. https://digitalcommons.wku.edu/dlsc_mss_fin_aid/3363. This letter was discussed in a contemporary news outlet, which says the writer lived in Gordonville, which is less than ten miles west of Russellville. See Evelyn Richardson, "Cholera Epidemic Hits Logan County in 1835," Franklin Favorite, accessed January 4, 2025, https://www.franklinfavorite.com/article_1021f63c-7b61-50c1-bb04-bb99bb06965c.html.
62. Rebecca Smith Washington to Jane Washington Walker, August 10, 1835.
63. "A List of Those Attacked with Cholera in Russellville, July & August 1835," David Morton Papers, FHS.
64. Nashville *Republican*, August 8, 1835.
65. Nashville *Republican*, August 8, 1835.
66. Rebecca Smith Washington to Jane Washington Walker, August 10, 1835.
67. Russellville *Messenger*, August 28, 1835, in Lexington *Kentucky Gazette*, September 5, 1835. What appears to be the manuscript version of this list is in the David

Morton Papers, Filson Historical Society, Louisville, Kentucky. The editors added a few names before publishing.

68. Nancy Baird, "Asiatic Cholera in Kentucky 1832 to 1873," Ohio County, Kentucky, accessed January 4, 2025, https://ohiocountykentuckyhistory.blogspot.com/2020/12/cholera.html.
69. Lexington *Kentucky Gazette*, August 22, 1835.
70. Nashville *Republican*, August 25, 1835.
71. Richmond (IN) *Palladium*, August 29, 1835; Frankfort (KY) *The Commonwealth*, August 22, 1835.
72. Frankfort (KY) *The Commonwealth*, August 22, 1835.
73. St. Louis (MO) *Daily Evening Herald*, September 14, 1835.
74. Fayette *Missouri Intelligencer*, July 11, 1835; St. Louis (MO) *Daily Evening Herald*, July 15, 1835.
75. Newark (NJ) *Daily Advertiser*, December 2, 1835; New York *Evening Post*, December 4, 1835. Cholera's visit to the Omahas, Otoes, and Pawnees during any years of the 1830s pandemic cannot be corroborated in government records. See Upper Missouri Agency Records, Letters Received by the Office of Indian Affairs, 1824–1881, RG 75, NARA, microfilm 234, reel 883 and reel 884. John Dougherty, the federal agent who oversaw relations with these nations, and Joshua Pilcher, however, had been in St. Louis during the late summer and early fall of 1835 and would not have witnessed outbreaks at that time. See John Dougherty to Elbert Herring, September 11, 1835, and Joshua Pilcher to Major J. B. Brant, October 6, 1835, both on reel 884.
76. Quoted in Portland (ME) *Daily Advertiser*, June 3, 1836; Philadelphia *Public Ledger*, June 4, 1836; Newburyport (MA) *Herald*, June 7, 1836; New London *Connecticut Gazette*, June 8, 1836; Newport *Rhode-Island Republican*, June 8, 1836; Schenectady (NY) *Cabinet*, June 8, 1836; Pittsburgh (PA) *Post-Gazette*, June 8, 1836; Bennington (VT) *Gazette*, June 14, 1836; Burlington (VT) *Sentinel and Democrat*, June 17, 1836; Wilkes-Barre (PA) *Republican Farmer, and Democratic Journal*, June 22, 1836.
77. Alexandria (VA) *Gazette*, May 25, 1836, reprinted or referred to in Charleston (SC) *Courier*, May 31, 1836; Chambersburg (PA) *Franklin Repository*, June 7, 1836; Black Rock (NY) *Advocate*, June 2, 1836; Buffalo (NY) *Patriot and Commercial Advertiser*, June 8, 1836; St. Louis (MO) *Daily Commercial Bulletin*, June 15, 1836; Dubuque (IA) *Visitor*, June 29, 1836.
78. Rain reported on Sunday, August 29, in Charleston (SC) *Courier*, September 6, 1836.
79. The rancid nature of Charleston's water came up during a discussion of finding alternatives in 1829. The report of that time was later republished in Charleston (SC) *Courier*, November 3, 1836.
80. Charleston (SC) *Mercury*, August 30, 1836.
81. Charleston (SC) *Courier*, September 10, 1836; Charleston (SC) *Mercury*, September 10, 1836.

82. Charleston (SC) *Courier*, September 28, 1836.
83. On Elliot's business dealings, see advertisements in Charleston (SC) *Mercury*, January 5, 1836, February 15, 1836, June 8, 1836, September 23, 1836; Charleston (SC) *Courier*, April 6, 1836, June 15, 1836, July 8, 1836.
84. Charleston (SC) *Mercury*, September 13, 1836.
85. Charleston (SC) *Mercury*, September 27, 1836.
86. Charleston (SC) *Courier*, November 4, 1836.
87. W. Mazyck Porcher to Robert Marion Deveaux, September 15 [1836], William Mazyck Porcher Papers, South Caroliniana Library, Columbia, South Carolina.
88. Charleston (SC) *Courier*, September 26, 1836.
89. Charleston (SC) *Courier*, November 4, 1836.
90. Charleston (SC) *Courier*, September 26, 1832. Funeral notice: Charleston (SC) *Courier*, September 11, 1836. Obituary: Charleston (SC) *Courier*, October 4, 1836 (quote).
91. Jacob Frederic Schirmer, "The Schirmer Diary (continued)," *The South Carolina Historical Magazine* 69, no. 1 (January 1968): 65.
92. A[rthur] M[iddleton] to Mrs. Thomas Middleton, September 27, 1836, Middleton Family Papers, 12/158/8, SCHS.
93. A[rthur] M[iddleton] to Mrs. Thomas Middleton, September 27, 1836, Middleton Family Papers, 12/158/8, SCHS.
94. Charleston (SC) *Courier*, September 26, 1836; Charleston (SC) *Mercury*, September 26, 1836; Charleston (SC) *Southern Patriot*, September 28, 1836.
95. Charleston (SC) *Courier*, September 27, 1836.
96. Schirmer, "The Schirmer Diary (continued)," 65.
97. Charleston (SC) *Courier*, November 4, 1836.
98. Charleston (SC) *Courier*, October 20, 1836; Richard Bacot to Robert Dewar Bacot, October 8, 1836, Bacot Family Papers, 1004: 11/48/9, SCHS.
99. Charleston (SC) *Courier*, October 5, 1836.
100. Charleston (SC) *Courier*, October 13, 1836.
101. Charleston (SC) *Courier*, October 31, 1836.
102. [T. Fayssoux?] to "My Dear Dewar" [Richard Dewar Bacot], November 1, 1836, Bacot Family Papers, 1004:11/48/9, SCHS.
103. Richard [Hartman?] Bacot to Robert Dewar Bacot, November 3, 1836, Bacot Family Papers, 1004: 11/48/9, SCHS.
104. Charleston (SC) *Courier*, November 4, 1836. The newspaper had printed a chart of deaths on November 2 that included an error in addition and listed the total number of deaths at 408. Two days later, the *Courier* corrected the error and provided the total of 380 fatalities.
105. Charleston (SC) *Courier*, September 20, 1836; Alexandria (VA) *Gazette*, October 21, 1836.
106. Memoranda to Daniel Ravenel, Esq. Executor of the Est. of John Emperor Farr, October 26, 1836, D. E. H. Smith Papers, 1101: 11/389/22, SCHS.

107. Thomas M. Logan to General J. Hamilton, October 9, 1836, Pinckney Family Papers, SCHS.
108. Charleston (SC) *Courier*, October 28, 1836.
109. Charleston (SC) *Courier*, November 4, 1836.
110. Philadelphia *United States Gazette*, September 3, 1834.
111. Pittsburgh (PA) *Post-Gazette*, September 11, 1834.
112. Frederick Grimké to Henry Grimké, October 12, 1834, Grimké Family Papers, 11/172/38, SCHS.
113. Charleston (SC) *Courier*, November 5, 1834.
114. Frederick Grimké to Henry Grimké, October 12, 1834, Grimké Family Papers, 11/172/38, SCHS.
115. Charleston (SC) *Courier*, October 24, 1834.
116. Daniel Drake to Sarah Daniel Drayton, October 25, 1834, Lowcountry Digital Library, College of Charleston Libraries, 1834-10-25. https://lcdl.library.cofc.edu/lcdl/catalog/lcdl:78618?tify={%22view%22:%22info%22}.
117. Sarah Drayton Grimké to Angelina Grimké, December 8, 1834, Weld-Grimké Papers, Box 1, WLCL.
118. "Lines addressed to my dear Mother on the death of her precious & beloved son, T.S. Grimké, December 29, 1834," Weld-Grimké Papers, Box 1, WLCL.

CONCLUSION

1. Rosenberg, *The Cholera Years*, 101–72.
2. New York *Evangelist*, January 18, 1834; Fredonia (NY) *Censor*, February 19, 1834; Newport (RI) *Herald of the Times*, February 27, 1834; George Duffield, *The Immorality of the Traffic in Ardent Spirit. A Discourse Delivered in the Presbyterian Church in Carlisle, on the 25th of February, 1834* (George Fleming, 1834); New York *General Refuge*, November 1, 1834; Boston *Liberator*, December 6, 1834; Concord (NH) *New-England Baptist Register*, February 26, 1835; Bangor (ME) *Daily Commercial Advertiser*, December 4, 1835; Pennsylvania State Temperance Society, *Pennsylvania and New-Jersey Temperance Almanac for 1835* (Temperance Depository, 1835).
3. Washington (DC) *National Intelligencer*, July 23, 1834.
4. Reuben Dimond Mussey and Harvey Lindsly, *Temperance Prize Essays* (Duff Green, 1835), 34.
5. Mussey and Lindsly, *Temperance Prize Essays*, 35.
6. Mussey and Lindsly, *Temperance Prize Essays*, 36.
7. Mussey and Lindsly, *Temperance Prize Essays*, 36, 43.
8. New York *Observer*, October 3, 1835.
9. W. G., "Medical Use of Alcohol," *The Moral Reformer and Teacher on the Human Constitution* 1 (October 1835): 319 (emphasis in the original).
10. American Temperance Society, *The Temperance Manual, of the American Temperance Society for the Young Men of the United States* (Seth Bliss, 1836), 6.

11. [Lucius M. Sargent], *Letters to John H. Hopkins, D. D. Bishop of the Protestant Episcopal Church for the Diocese of Vermont: Occasioned by His Lecture in Opposition to the Temperance Society. By an Episcopalian* (Chronicle Press, 1836), 137.
12. "Eighth Annual Report of the American Temperance Society 1835," in *Permanent Documents of the American Temperance Society*, vol. 1 (Seth Bliss, 1835), 458 (quote is on page 4 of the report).
13. William E. Channing, *An Address on Temperance* (Weeks, Jordan & Company, 1837), 32.
14. Channing, *An Address on Temperance,* 68.
15. Pennsylvania State Temperance Society, *Memorial of the Board of Managers of the Pennsylvania State Temperance Society, to the Convention for Revising the Constitution of the State of Pennsylvania* (Brown & Sinquet, Printers, 1837), 22.
16. "Ohio. Western Reserve Temperance Convention," *Journal of the American Temperance Union* 2, no. 9 (September 1838): 141.
17. Executive Committee of the New York Temperance Society, "Address," *Journal of the American Temperance Union* 2, no. 10 (October 1838): 151.
18. Short, "A Brief Historical Sketch," 11.
19. Short, "A Brief Historical Sketch," 16.
20. Short, "A Brief Historical Sketch," 20.
21. Short, "A Brief Historical Sketch," 20.
22. Short, "A Brief Historical Sketch," 21.
23. Short, "A Brief Historical Sketch," 21.
24. Springfield (IL) *Sangamo Journal*, July 12, 1834 (eleven deaths before July 8); Philadelphia *Inquirer*, August 18, 1834 (seven hundred fled the town).
25. Scripps's account of the Rushville cholera outbreak was published in two parts in Rushville *Schuyler Citizen*, August 18, 1858, and August 25, 1858. (Rushville is in Schuyler County.) These issues are available digitally, although the legibility of the second part is difficult, through Community History Archive: https://rushvilleil.advantage-preservation.com/. Transcriptions of both parts of the account can be found on Schuyler County, Illinois Genealogy and History website: https://genealogytrails.com/ill/schuyler/1834CholeraEpidemic.html.
26. In 2007, the town of Rushville erected a tombstone at the old graveyard with the names of the twenty-seven victims engraved. Rushville (IL) *Times*, October 31, 2007, 1, 10A.

Bibliography

MANUSCRIPT COLLECTIONS

Albert and Shirley Small Special Collections Library, University of Virginia, Charlottesville

Ambler Family Papers
Burton Randall Papers
Cocke Family Papers
Ellen Wayles Randolph Coolidge Correspondence
Grinnan Family Papers
James Maury Papers
Joseph C. Cabell and Cabell Family Papers
Lancelot Minor Blackford Papers
Michael Wallace Papers
Morton and Dickinson Family Correspondence
Palmore Family Papers
Preston Bowker Papers
Richard Morris Papers
Thomas Law Papers
Webb-Prentis Papers
William H. Kennon Papers

Beinecke Rare Book and Manuscript Library, Yale University, New Haven, Connecticut

Aaron Hulin Letters
Charles Rich Daybook
Edward Blackmore Shepheard Journal
Harriet Wooley Letterbook
Wyeth Family Papers

Carl A. Kroch Library, Cornell University, Ithaca, New York

Abell Family Papers
Gould Family Papers

Joseph Fellows Papers
Kernan Family Papers
Lyman Stuart Collection
Chester County Historical Society, West Chester, Pennsylvania
Diary of Deborah Bowman
David Rubenstein Rare Book & Manuscript Library, Duke University, Durham, North Carolina
Ann (Heatly) Reid Lovell Papers
Asa Rogers Papers
Charles Watts Letters
Daniel Lewis Gold Papers
Francis P. Corbin Papers
Frank A. Harris Papers
James M. Willcox Papers
Jarratt-Puryear Papers
Joseph Starke Sims Papers
Knight Family Papers
Samuel Smith Downey Papers
Thomas Bradford Papers
William Patterson Smith Papers
William T. Bishop Papers
William Weaver Papers
Dolph Briscoe Center for American History, University of Texas at Austin
Mary Austin Holley Papers
Filson Historical Society, Louisville, Kentucky
Adam McKee Letter
A. P. Thompson Letter
Beall-Boothe Papers
Beatty-Quisenberry Papers
Bodley Papers
Buckner Family Papers
Charles Wilkins Short Papers
Cholera, Mss.
Clay Family Papers
Clay Green Papers
Corlis Family Papers
Corlis-Respess Family Papers
David Morton Papers
Dumesnil Family Papers
Edmund Halsey Collection
Edward Thurman Collection
Garnett Family Correspondence

Green Family Papers
Henry Bacon Family Papers
John Wesley Hunt Papers
Matthew Monroe Campbell Letters
Moxley-Offutt Papers
Sanders Family Papers
Sidney Payne Clay Papers
Taylor-Hay Family Papers
Thomas Crittenden Autobiography
William Clark Letters
Yandell Family Papers
Firestone Library Special Collections, Princeton University, Princeton, New Jersey
Samuel L. Southard Papers
General Theological Seminary, New York
Samuel Roosevelt Johnson papers
Harvey Cushing/John Hay Whitney Medical Library, Yale University, New Haven, Connecticut
Benjamin Lincoln papers
Helmerich Center for American Research, Thomas Gilcrease Museum, Tulsa, Oklahoma
Peter Pitchylnn Collection
Hill Memorial Library Special Collections, Louisiana State University, Baton Rouge
Alexander Porter Letter
Alonzo Snyder Papers
Andrew Kleinpeter Papers
Bass-Farrar Family Papers
Butler Family Papers (Mss. 1026)
Cartwright Cholera Prescription, MISC:C
David Weeks and Family Papers
Edward Gay and Family Papers
Hennen-Jennings Papers
Henry S. Leverich Correspondence
James P. Bowman Family Papers
John C. Burruss and Family Papers
John Close Papers
Lucius Duncan Letters
Marshall Furman Family Papers
Nathaniel Evans and Family Papers
Palfrey Family Papers
Thomas Affleck Papers
Thomas Butler and Family Papers (Mss. 2850)
William S. Hamilton Papers

Historical Society of Pennsylvania, Philadelphia
Claude W. Unger Collection, (Collection 1860A)
Colt Collection
Edwin Shippen Burd Papers
Gratz Collection
John and Henry Nixon Papers
Joseph Turner Chew Papers
Logan Family Papers (Collection 379)
Maria Dickinson Logan Collection
Vaux Family Papers
Wister and Butler Family Papers
Wister Family Papers
Historical Society of Princeton, New Jersey
Delaware and Raritan Canal Files
Stockton Family Papers
Historic New Orleans Collection, New Orleans
Carl Kohn Letter Books
Levi Lewis Archive
Morgan-Falconer Family Papers
Ste-Gême Family Papers
Hodges Library, Special Collections, University of Tennessee-Knoxville
David Burford Papers
Houghton Library, Harvard University, Cambridge, Massachusetts
American Board of Commissioners for Foreign Missions Archives
Bernard Raux Slave Trade Papers
Huntington Library, San Marino, California
Brock Collection
Edmund Kirby Papers
Henry Waller Collection
James Crocker Letter
John Arnold Rockwell Papers
J. B. Cain Archives of Mississippi Methodism, Millsaps College, Jackson.
William Winans Manuscript Papers
Kansas Historical Society, Topeka
Isaac McCoy Papers (microfilm)
Lewis Alderson Papers
Kislak Center for Special Collections, University of Pennsylvania, Philadelphia
Thomas Knights's Writing Book, 1829–1832
Louisiana Research Collection, Howard-Tilton Library, Tulane University, New Orleans
Fanny Leverich Eshleman Craig Collection
Harrison-Hoffman Papers
John McDonogh Papers

Joseph S. Copes Papers
Ker and Texada Families Papers
Morse and Wederstrandt Family Papers
Plantation Collection
Semple Family Papers
Trowbridge Family Papers
William Edwards Clement Collection
Manuscripts and Archives Division, New York Public Library, New York
Asher B. Durand Papers
Francis Corbin Papers
George Batterbury Journal
Jeremiah Briggs Letters
Samuel Tilden Papers
Maryland Historical Society, Baltimore
James Hawkins Letters
Prevost Family Papers
T. J. Wilson, Reminiscences
Th. H. W. Monroe, Record of Cholera Epidemic in Baltimore, 1832
Mississippi Department of Archives and History, Jackson
Natchez Municipal Records
National Archives and Records Administration, College Park, Maryland
Chesapeake and Ohio Canal Company Records
National Archives and Records Administration, Washington, DC
Letters Received by the Office of Indian Affairs, 1824–1881. Record Group 75. M234 (microfilm)
Slave Manifests of Coastwise Vessels Filed at New Orleans, 1807–1860. Record Group 36. M1895 (microfilm)
New Jersey Historical Society, Newark
Canfield-Dickerson family papers
New Orleans Public Library
Conseil de Ville Records (English translations microfilm)
Oberlin College Archives, Oberlin, Ohio
Finney Papers
Oneida County History Center, Utica, New York
Uticana Collection
Patricia D. Klingenstein Library, New York Historical Society, New York
Albany Diary 1831 November 23–1832 December 22
Amos H. Hosmer letter
Anicartha Miller letters
Benjamin Van Zandt Letter to Angelo Ames
Caroline A. Cleveland Letters
Jacob Schiefflen Letters

James Riker, Jr., Diary and Reminiscences, 1836–1868
John Pintard Papers
John W. Taylor Papers
Lyon Family Papers
Ravaud Kearney Letters
Richard Henry Staats Memorandum Book
Samuel Hunter Papers
Thomas Fuller Letter to George W. Wright
Van Ness-Philip Family Papers
Villers Hatton Collection
Winfield Scott Papers
Rose Memorial Library, Drew University, Madison, New Jersey
Gibbons Family Papers
South Carolina Historical Society Archives, College of Charleston
Bacot Family Papers
Baker Family Papers
Barbot Family Papers
Langdon Cheves Papers
D. E. H. Smith Papers
Harriot Horry Ravenel Papers
Haynsworth Family papers
Hering Family Papers
Grimké Family Papers
James Butler Campbell Papers
John B. Adger Papers
Middleton Family Papers
Peter Manigault Collection
Pinckney Family Papers
Pringle Family Papers
Ravenel Family Papers
Read Family Papers
Vander Horst Papers
Yates Family Papers
South Caroliniana Library, University of South Carolina, Columbia
Charles Heyward Journal
William Mazyck Porcher Papers
William Rogers Hart and Sarah Grimball Clark Hart Papers
Southern History Collections, Wilson Library, University of North Carolina at Chapel Hill
Brashear and Lawrence Family Papers
Charles Wilkins Short Papers
Hamilton Brown Papers
Hughes Family Papers

Isaac Jarrett Papers
James Hamilton Papers
John Berkley Grimball Diaries
John Rogers Papers
Mary Hunter Kennedy Papers
Nicholas Philip Trist Papers
Rice C. Ballard Papers

Special Collections, Alexander Library, Rutgers University, New Brunswick, New Jersey
John Hopper Papers
Roswell L. Colt Family Papers

Special Collections Research Center, William & Mary University, Williamsburg, Virginia
Alexander Hamilton, Jr., Papers
Archibald Woods Papers
Blair, Banister, Braxton, Horner, and Whiting Papers
Brown, Coalter, and Tucker Papers
Conway Whittle Papers
Francis P. Lee Papers
Galt Papers
James Barron Papers
Jerdone Family Papers
Maury Family Papers
Moncure Robinson Papers
Southall Papers

Sterling Library Manuscripts and Archives, Yale University, New Haven, Connecticut
Alexander Bryan Johnson Papers
Bernhard Knollegnberg Collection
Jay Family Papers

Virginia Historical Society, Richmond
Blow Family Papers
Carrington Family Papers
Crutchfield Family Papers
Edgar A. MacDonald Papers
Edmundson Family Papers
Elcan Family Papers
Louthan Family Papers
Marshall Papers
Massie Family Papers
Nathaniel Burwell and J. Ambler Johnson Papers
Peter Hoffman Cruse Papers

Western History Collections Library, University of Oklahoma
Peter Pitchlynn Papers

William L. Clements Library, University of Michigan, Ann Arbor
- Almon Underwood Journal
- American Science and Medicine Collection
- Amos Beebe Eaton Collection
- Anna Price Gibson Paschall Diary
- Ann M. Van Wart Journals, 1832–1837
- Dennis Delany Collection, Small Collections
- Farley Family Papers
- Francis W. Edmonds Papers
- George S. Brown Papers
- Hannah and Evi Smith Correspondence
- John W. and Maria Eliza Cutler Family Collection
- Joseph Shipley, Jr., Collection
- Lewis Cass Papers
- Lincoln Family Papers
- Masters-Taylor-Wilbur Papers
- Nathaniel Stacy Papers
- Phelps-Lyon Family Papers
- Suckley Family Papers
- Thomas Bradford Papers
- Warder-Haines Papers
- Weld-Grimké Papers
- William Gibbons Papers
- William Philander and Seth Comstock Correspondence
- Wilson Family Papers
- Young Papers

Wright Library, Princeton Theological Seminary, Princeton, New Jersey
- William Swan Plumer Collection

DIGITAL AND OTHER MANUSCRIPT COLLECTIONS

American Presidency Project, University of California—Santa Barbara. https://www.presidency.ucsb.edu/.

Documenting Ireland: Parliament, People and Migration. https://www.dippam.ac.uk/.

Indian-Pioneer Papers. University of Oklahoma, Western History Collections. https://repository.ou.edu/content/western-history-collections.

Indian Removal to the West, 1832–1840: Files of the Office of the Commissary General of Subsistence. Microfilm. University Publications of America/LexisNexis, Bethesda, MD 2007.

John Pendleton Kennedy Papers. Microfilm. Scholarly Resources, Inc. Wilmington, DE. 1972.

Joseph Smith Papers. https://www.josephsmithpapers.org/.
Journal of Assistant Agent William Colquhoun During the Choctaw Removal. National Archives and Records Administration. https://catalog.archives.gov/id/38995523.
Lowcountry Digital Library. College of Charleston Libraries. https://lcdl.library.cofc.edu/.
Volunteer Voices Digital Collections. University of Tennessee Libraries. https://digital.lib.utk.edu/collections/volvoicescollection.

NEWSPAPERS, 1831–1836

America's Historical Newspapers by Readix
(New York Public Library Institutional Subscription)

Albany (NY) *Argus*
Alexandria (VA) *Gazette*
Amherst (NH) *Farmer's Cabinet*
Baltimore *American and Commercial Daily Advertiser*
Baltimore *Gazette and Daily Advertiser*
Baltimore *Republican and Commercial Advertiser*
Belfast *Maine Working Men's Advocate*
Bennington (VT) *Gazette*
Boston *American Traveller*
Boston *Columbian Centinel*
Boston *Christian Herald*
Boston *Christian Watchman*
Boston *Commercial Gazette*
Boston *Courier*
Boston *Daily Advertiser*
Boston *Investigator*
Boston *Liberator*
Boston *New England Artisan, and Farmer's Mechanic's and Laboring-man's Repository*
Boston *Recorder*
Boston *Statesman*
Boston *Trumpet and Universalist Magazine*
Boston *Weekly Messenger*
Brattleboro (VT) *Messenger*
Bridgeport (CT) *Spirit of the Times*
Bridgeton (NJ) *West Jersey Observer*
Charleston (SC) *Courier*
Charleston (SC) *Mercury*
Charleston (SC) *Southern Patriot*
Charlotte (NC) *Miners' and Farmers' Journal*

Chelsea *Vermont Advocate*
Cincinnati *Baptist Weekly Journal of the Mississippi Valley*
Cincinnati *Catholic Telegraph*
Cincinnati *Journal*
Cincinnati *Liberty Hall and Gazette*
Cincinnati *National Republican and Daily Mercantile Advertiser*
Cincinnati *Western Christian Advocate*
Columbus *Ohio Monitor*
Columbus *Ohio State Journal*
Concord (NH) *New-England Baptist Register*
Concord *New-Hampshire Statesmen*
Dedham (MA) *Patriot, and Farmers', Mechanics' and Manufacturers' Advocate*
Dover (NH) *Enquirer*
Easton (MD) *Gazette*
Eastport (ME) *Sentinel*
Frankfort (KY) *Argus*
Gardiner (ME) *Christian Intelligencer and Eastern Chronicle*
Gloucester (MA) *Telegraph*
Hagerstown (MD) *Torch Light and Public Advertiser*
Hallowell (ME) *American Advocate*
Hartford (CT) *American Mercury*
Hartford *Connecticut Courant*
Hartford *Connecticut Mirror*
Hartford *Connecticut Observer*
Hartford (CT) *Times*
Haverhill (NH) *Essex Gazette*
Jamestown (NY) *Journal*
Keene (NH) *Farmer's Museum*
Keene *New-Hampshire Sentinel*
Litchfield (CT) *Enquirer*
Little Rock *Arkansas Times and Advocate*
Little Rock *Weekly Arkansas Gazette*
Lowell (MA) *Mercury*
Lowell (MA) *Observer*
Lynchburg *Virginian*
Macon (GA) *Telegraph*
Maysville (KY) *Eagle*
Montpelier *Vermont Watchman and State Gazette*
Morristown (NJ) *Jerseyman*
Nantucket (MA) *Inquirer*
Newark (NJ) *Daily Advertiser*
New Bedford (MA) *Courier*

New Bedford (MA) *Gazette*
New Bedford (MA) *Mercury*
Newburyport (MA) *Herald*
New Echota (Cherokee Nation) *Cherokee Phoenix*
New Haven (CT) *Columbian Register*
New Haven *Connecticut Journal*
New London *Connecticut Gazette*
Newport (RI) *Mercury*
Newport *Rhode-Island Republican*
New York *Advertiser*
New York *American*
New York *Christian Intelligencer*
New York *Commercial Advertiser*
New York *Evangelist*
New York *Evening Post*
New York *Mercury*
New York *Observer*
New York *Spectator*
Northampton (MA) *Hampshire Gazette*
Norwich (CT) *Courier*
Paris (ME) *Jeffersonian*
Pawtucket (RI) *Chronicle and Manufacturers' and Artizans' Advocate*
Philadelphia *Daily Chronicle*
Philadelphia *Inquirer*
Philadelphia *National Gazette*
Philadelphia *Philadelphian*
Philadelphia *Poulson's American Daily Advertiser*
Philadelphia *United States Gazette for the Country*
Pittsfield (MA) *Sun*
Portland (ME) *Advertiser*
Portland (ME) *Christian Mirror*
Portland (ME) *Eastern Argus*
Portsmouth (ME) *Journal and Rockingham Gazette*
Portsmouth *New-Hampshire Gazette*
Poughkeepsie (NY) *Independence*
Providence (RI) *Manufacturers' & Farmers' Journal*
Providence (RI) *Microcosm*
Providence (RI) *Patriot*
Providence *Rhode Island American and Gazette*
Rochester (NY) *Union and Advertiser*
Salem (MA) *Gazette*
Saratoga Springs (NY) *Sentinel*

Savannah *Georgian*
Somersworth (NH) *Great Falls Journal*
Washington (DC) *Daily National Journal*
Washington (DC) *Globe*
Washington (DC) *National Intelligencer*
Washington (DC) *United States Telegraph*
Washington (PA) *Review and Examiner*
Windsor *Vermont Republican and Journal*
Woodstock (VT) *Observer*
Woodstock *Vermont Courier and Farmer's, Manufacturer's, and Mechanic's Advocate*
Worcester *Massachusetts Spy*
Worcester (MA) *National Aegis*

Archived Issues
New York *Morning Courier and Enquirer* (New York Society Library, New York)
Rahway *New Jersey Advocate and Middlesex and Essex County Advertiser* (New Jersey State Library, Trenton)
West Chester (PA) *Chester County Democrat* (Historical Society of Pennsylvania, Philadelphia)

Library of Virginia (Open Access: virginiachronicle.com)
Fredericksburg (VA) *Political Arena*
Leesburg (VA) *Genius of Liberty*
Norfolk (VA) *American Beacon*
Richmond (VA) *Constitutional Whig*
Richmond (VA) *Enquirer*
Richmond (VA) *Southern Religious Telegraph*
Richmond (VA) *Whig and Commercial Journal*
Staunton (VA) *Spectator*

Microfilm
Albany (NY) *Evening Journal*
New Orleans *Bee*
New York *Journal of Commerce*
Pottsville (PA) *Miners' Journal*
Trenton (NJ) *Emporium and True American*
Trenton *New Jersey State Gazette*
Utica (NY) *Sentinel and Gazette*
Utica (NY) *Western Recorder*
West Chester (PA) *Village Record and General Advertiser*

Newspaperarchive.com by Storied (Author Subscription)
Annapolis *Maryland Republican*
Augusta (GA) *Constitutionalist*

Canton *Ohio Repository*
Charles Town *Virginia Free Press*
Cincinnati *Daily Republican and Commercial Register*
Easton (MD) *Eastern-Shore Whig and Peoples Advocate*
Gettysburg (PA) *Adams Sentinel*
Gettysburg (PA) *Republican Banner*
Hagerstown (MD) *Mail*
Madison (IN) *Banner*
Madison (IN) *Republican*
Newnan (GA) *Palladium*
Sag Harbor (NY) *Corrector*
Sandusky (OH) *Clarion*
Savannah (GA) *Republican*
Springfield (IL) *Sangamo Journal*
St. Louis (MO) *Daily Evening Herald*
Tuscaloosa *Alabama State Intelligencer*
Woodville (MS) *Southern Planter*
Newspapers.com by Ancestry (Author Subscription)
Alton (IL) *Spectator*
Annapolis *Maryland Gazette*
Baltimore *Niles Weekly Register*
Baton Rouge (LA) *Gazette*
Bellows Falls *Vermont Chronicle*
Black Rock (NY) *Advocate*
Boston *New England Farmer*
Boston *Post*
Brandon *Vermont Telegraph*
Buffalo (NY) *Patriot and Commercial Advertiser*
Burlington (VT) *Sentinel and Democrat*
Burlington (VT) *Weekly Free Press*
Chambersburg (PA) *Franklin Repository*
Danville (VT) *North Star*
Detroit *Free Press*
Dubuque (IA) *Visitor*
Fayette *Missouri Intelligencer and Boon's Lick Advertiser*
Fayetteville (NC) *Observer*
Frankfort (KY) *Commonwealth*
Frederick (MD) *Herald*
Gettysburg (PA) *Compiler*
Greenfield (MA) *Recorder*
Halifax (NC) *Roanoke Advocate*
Jackson (MS) *State Rights Banner*

Jackson (TN) *Southern Statesman*
Jefferson City (MO) *Jeffersonian Republican*
Knoxville (TN) *Republican*
Lancaster (PA) *Examiner*
Lancaster (PA) *Intelligencer*
Lawrenceburg (IN) *Western Statesman*
Lexington *Kentucky Gazette*
Liverpool (UK) *Mercury*
London (UK) *Morning Chronicle*
Middlebury (VT) *Register and Addison County Journal*
Milledgeville (GA) *Southern Recorder*
Montpelier *Vermont Patriot and State Gazette*
Murfreesboro (TN) *Weekly Monitor*
Nashville *National Banner*
Nashville *Republican*
Natchez (MS) *Courier and Adams, Jefferson, and Franklin Advertiser*
Natchez *Mississippi Free Trader*
New Bern (NC) *Sentinel*
Newport (RI) *Herald of the Times*
Norwalk (OH) *Huron Reflector*
Oxford (UK) *Jackson's Oxford Journal*
Piqua (OH) *Courier and Enquirer*
Pittsburgh (PA) *Post-Gazette*
Pittsburgh (PA) *Weekly Gazette*
Port Gibson (MS) *Herald and Correspondent*
Poughkeepsie (NY) *Journal*
Preston (UK) *Preston Chronicle and Lancashire Advertiser*
Raleigh *North-Carolina Star*
Richmond (IN) *Palladium*
Rutland (VT) *Weekly Herald*
Salisbury (NC) *Western Carolinian*
Sheffield (UK) *Sheffield and Rotherham Independent*
Springfield (MA) *Weekly Republican*
St. Johnsbury (VT) *Weekly Messenger and Connecticut and Passumpsic River Valley Advertiser*
Tarboro (NC) *Press*
Troy (OH) *Times*
Tuscaloosa (AL) *Spirit of the Age*
Vandalia *Whig and Illinois Intelligencer*
Vicksburg *Mississippian*
Vicksburg (MS) *Whig*
Wilkes-Barre (PA) *Republican Farmer, and Democratic Journal*

Wilkes-Barre (PA) *Wyoming Republican and Herald*
Windsor (VT) *Aurora of the Valley*
Woodstock (VT) *Mercury*
York (PA) *Gazette*
NYS Historic Newspapers (Open Access: nyshistoricnewspapers.org)
Auburn (NY) *Free Press*
Binghamton (NY) *Broome Republican*
Delhi (NY) *Delaware Gazette*
Fredonia (NY) *Censor*
Geneva (NY) *Courier*
Geneva (NY) *Gazette and Mercantile Advertiser*
Lansingburgh (NY) *Gazette*
Plattsburgh (NY) *Republican*
Schenectady (NY) *Cabinet*
Various
Albany (NY) *Temperance Recorder* (hathitrust.org)
Baltimore *Patriot and Mercantile Advertiser* (genealogybank.com)
Boston *Jesuit: Catholic Sentinel* (https://newspapers.bc.edu)
Boston *Spirit of the Age and Journal of Humanity* (archive.org)
Boston *US Catholic Intelligencer* (https://newspapers.bc.edu)
Boston *Youth's Companion & Weekly Family Visitor* (archive.org)
Columbus (OH) *Thomsonian Recorder* (hathitrust.org)
Dover (NH) *Gazette & Strafford Advertiser* (Gale: 19th Century US Newspapers)
Hudson *Ohio Observer* (Gale: 19th Century US Newspapers)
Independence (MO) *Evening and Morning Star* (https://lib.byu.edu/collections/digital/)
Lebanon (OH) *Western Star* (https://ohiomemory.org/digital/collection/p16007coll84)
Lexington (KY) *Western Luminary* (American Periodical Series by ProQuest)
New Orleans *Commercial Bulletin* (Gale: 19th Century US Newspapers)
New Orleans *Louisiana Courier* (genealogybank.com)
New York *Cholera Bulletin* (compiled and reprinted by Arno Press, 1972)
New York *General Refuge* (American Antiquarian Society Historical Periodical Collection: Series 2)
Philadelphia *Cholera Gazette* (https://curiosity.lib.harvard.edu/contagion)

PUBLISHED PRIMARY MATERIAL

Alexander, James W. *Forty Years, Familiar Letters of James W. Alexander: Constituting, with Notes, a Memoir of His Life*. Scribner, 1870.

American Temperance Society. *Fifth Report of the American Temperance, Presented at the Meeting in Boston, May 1832*. Aaron Russell, 1832.

American Temperance Society. *Permanent Documents of the American Temperance Society*. Vol. 1. Seth Bliss, 1835.

American Temperance Society. *The Temperance Manual, of the American Temperance Society for the Young Men of the United States*. Seth Bliss, 1836.

Atkins, Dudley, ed. *Reports of Hospital Physicians and Other Documents in Relation to the Epidemic Cholera of 1832*. G.&C.&H. Carvill, 1832.

Awl, William M. "A Brief History of the Epidemic Cholera as It Appeared in the Town of Columbus, and the Penitentiary of Ohio, in the Summer of 1833." *Western Journal of the Medical and Physical Sciences* 1, no. 3 (October, November, and December 1833): 341–49.

Baird, Elizabeth T. "Reminiscences of Life in Territorial Wisconsin." In *Collections of the State Historical Society of Wisconsin*. Vol. 15. State Historical Society of Wisconsin, 1900. 205–63.

Barber, John W., and Henry Howe. *Historical Collections of the State of New Jersey*. S. Tuttle, 1846.

Barry, D. "On the Statistics of Epidemic Cholera." *Transactions of the Statistical Society of London*, 1, no. 1 (1837): 83–96.

Beck, Lewis. "Report on Cholera, Made to his Excellency Gov. Throop, August 1832." In *Transactions of the Medical Society of the State of New York. Vol. 1: 1832–1833*. Webster and Skinners, 1833.

Beecher, Lyman "An Appeal on the Subject of Cholera." *Christian Advocate* 10 (August 1832): 356–61.

Beecher, Lyman. *Six Sermons on the Nature, Occasions, Signs, Evils, and Remedy of Intemperance*. American Tract Society, 1827.

Bell, Theodore. "Remarks on Spasmodic Cholera, as It Appeared in Louisville in October 1832." *Transylvania Journal of Medical and Associate Sciences* 5 (October, November, and December 1832): 534–49.

Blassingame, John W., ed. *Slave Testimony: Two Centuries of Letters, Speeches, Interviews, and Autobiographies*. Louisiana State University Press, 1977.

Bleser, Carol, ed. *Tokens of Affection: The Letters of a Planter's Daughter in the Old South*. University of Georgia Press, 1996.

Brown, Henry Box. *Narrative of Henry Box Brown, Who Escaped from Slavery Enclosed in a Box 3 Feet Long and 2 Wide. Written from a Statement of Facts Made by Himself by Charles Stearns*. Brown & Stearns, 1849.

Brown, William Wells. *Narrative of William W. Brown, a Fugitive Slave. Written by Himself*. The Anti-Slavery Office, 1847.

Burden, Jessie Reading. "Report on Arch Street Prison." In *Report of the Committee Appointed to Visit the Eastern Penitentiary and Report on the Condition and Discipline Thereof, with a View to Introduce, as Far as Expedient and Practicable, a Similar Arrangement in That of the West and Also, to Visit the Public Institutions in*

Which the Spasmodic Cholera Prevailed in a Malignant Form, and Report Thereon. Henry Welsh, 1833.

Carson, James P., ed. *Life, Letters and Speeches of James Louis Petigru: The Union Man of South Carolina.* W. H. Lowdermilk & Co, 1920.

"Causes of the Epidemic Cholera." *Journal of Health* 3, no. 2 (September 21, 1831): 27–30.

Channing, William E. *An Address on Temperance.* Weeks, Jordan & Company, 1837.

"Cholera in the Ship Brutus." *The Medico-Chirurgical Review, and Journal of Practical Medicine* 17, no. 33 (July 1, 1832): 285.

"The Cholera Not Contagious." *Journal of Health* 3, no. 10 (January 25, 1832): 147–62.

Clapp, Theodore. *Autobiographical Sketches and Recollections During a Thirty-Five Years' Residence in New Orleans.* 1st ed. Phillips, Sampson & Company, 1857.

Commissary General of Subsistence. *Correspondence on the Subject of the Emigration of Indians, Between the 30th November 1831 and 27th December 1833.* 5 vols. Duff Green, 1834–1835.

Congressional Temperance Society. *Proceedings and Speeches at a Meeting for the Promotion of the Cause of Temperance in the United States: Held at the Capitol, in Washington City, February 24, 1833.* Way and Gideon, 1833.

Corson, Hiram. *Reminiscences of the Cholera Epidemic of 1832: And Notes on the Treatment of the Disease at That Time [Reprinted from the Philadelphia Medical Times for Aug. 9 and Sept. 6, 1884].* n.p., n.d.

Delany, Martin Robison. *The Condition, Elevation, Emigration, and Destiny of the Colored People of the United States.* Published by the Author, 1852.

Douglass, Frederick. *Life and Times of Frederick Douglass, Written by Himself.* DeWolf & Fiske Company, 1892.

Drake, Daniel. *An Account of the Epidemic Cholera, as It Appeared in Cincinnati.* Cincinnati: Chronicle Office, 1832.

Drake, Daniel. *A Discourse on Intemperance: Delivered at Cincinnati, March 1, 1828, Before the Agricultural Society of Hamilton County and Subsequently Pronounced, by Request to a Popular Audience.* Looker & Reynolds, 1828.

Drake, Daniel. "Epidemic Cholera in Cincinnati." *Western Journal of Medical and Physical Sciences* 6 (October, November, and December 1832): 321–64.

Drake, Daniel. "Epidemic Cholera. Miscellaneous Observations—Historical, Statistical, Etiological and Therapeutic, on the Prevailing Epidemic." *Western Journal of the Medical and Physical Sciences* 7, no. 26 (July, August, and September 1833): 161–81.

Duffield, George. *An Address Delivered in the Presbyterian Church, Before the Young Men's Temperance Society of Carlisle, by Rev. George Duffield, July 4, 1832.* Geo. Fleming Printer, 1832.

Duffield, George. *The Immorality of the Traffic in Ardent Spirit. A Discourse Delivered in the Presbyterian Church in Carlisle, on the 25th of February 1834.* George Fleming, 1834.

Dunn, Taylor, ed. "'Cincinnati Is a Delightful Place': Letters of a Law Clerk [Isaac Jewett], 1831–1834." *Bulletin of the Historical and Philosophical Society of Ohio* 10, no. 4 (October 1952): 257–77.

Executive Committee of the New York Temperance Society. "Address." *Journal of the American Temperance Union* 2, no. 10 (October 1838): 150–51.

Falconer, Cyrus. "XV.—Epidemic Cholera in Butler County, Ohio." *Western Journal of Medical and Physical Sciences* 2, no. 2 (July, August, and September 1834): 326–28.

Feller, Daniel, Thomas Coens, and Laura-Eve Moss, eds. *The Papers of Andrew Jackson, Volume 10, 1832*. University of Tennessee Press, 2016.

Finney, Charles G. *Memoirs of Rev. Charles G. Finney. Written by Himself.* A. S. Barnes & Company, 1876.

Finney, Charles G. "Sermon," *Oberlin Evangelist*, May 9, 1849.

Fulton, Ambrose Cowperthwaite. *A Life's Voyage: A Diary of a Sailor and Land, Jotted Down During a Seventy-Years' Voyage*. Published by the Author, 1898.

"Further Quarantine Regulations." *Boston Medical and Surgical Journal* 6, no. 6 (March 28, 1832): 111.

G., W. "Medical Use of Alcohol." *The Moral Reformer and Teacher on the Human Constitution* 1 (October 1835): 319.

Gayle, Sarah Haynesworth. *The Journal of Sarah Haynsworth Gayle, 1827–1835*. Edited by Sarah Woolfolk Wiggins and Ruth Smith Truss. University of Alabama Press, 2013.

General Synod Reformed Church in America. *The Acts and Proceedings of the General Synod of the Reformed Dutch Church in North America at New York, in June, and Albany, October 1832*. General Synod, 1832.

Grimké, Thomas. *Address on the Patriot Character of the Temperance Reformation: Delivered Before the Charleston Temperance Society, and the Young Men's Temperance Society of Charleston, on Tuesday Evening, 26th February 1833*. Observer Office Press, 1833.

Grimké, Thomas S. *The Temperance Reformation the Cause of Christian Morals. An Address Delivered Before the Charleston Temperance Society and the Young Men's Temperance Society of Charleston, on Tuesday Evening, February 25, 1834*. Observer Office Press, 1834.

Hall, Edwin. *An Address in Behalf of the Temperance Society, Norwalk, Connecticut.* James Reed, Jr., 1833.

Halphen, Michel. *Mémoire sur le Cholera-Morbus, compliqué d'une Epidémie de Fièvre Jaune, qui a régné simultanément a la Nouvelle Orléans en 1832*. Chez J. B. Baillière, Libraire 1833.

Halphen, Michel. *Observations Sur Le Choléra-Morbus Qui a Régné a La Nouvelle-Orléans en 1833 et en 1834 Faisant Suite au Mémoire Sur Le Choléra-Morbus De 1832*. Chez J. B. Baillière, Libraire, 1835.

Henry, John. "A Letter on the Cholera as It Occurred in Cincinnati, Ohio, in the Month of October 1832." *Transylvania Journal of Medical and the Associate Sciences* 5, no. 4 (October, November, and December 1832): 507–33.

Herr, Benjamin. "Journal, 1830." *German American Annals* 1 (January 1903): 8–31.

Hoffman, A. K. "Communication from A. K. Hoffman, M.D. Physician of the Sing Sing State Prison, December 25, 1832." In *Transactions of the Medical Society of the State of New York*. Vol. 2. E. W. and C. Skinner, 1835.

Hone, Philip. *Diary of Philip Hone, 1828–1851*. Edited by Bayard Tuckerman. Dodd, Mead, and Company, 1889.

Irving, Washington. *The Complete Works of Washington Irving. Miscellaneous Writings, 1803–1859*. Vol. 2. Edited by Wayne R. Clime. Twayne, 1979.

Jackson, Samuel. "Personal Observations and Experiences of Epidemic or Malignant Cholera in the City of Philadelphia." *American Journal of the Medical Sciences* 11 (February 1833): 289–346.

Jackson, Samuel. "Personal Observations and Experiences of Epidemic or Malignant Cholera in the City of Philadelphia." *American Journal of the Medical Sciences* 12 (May 1833): 76–121.

Jameson, Horatio G. "Consulting Physicians Report, December 31, 1832." In *The Ordinances of the Mayor and City Council of Baltimore, Passed at the Extra Sessions in 1832, and at the January Session, 1833. To Which Is Annexed Sundry Acts of Assembly; Passed at December Session, 1832; A List of the Officers of the Corporation, The Summary of the Register, and the Annual Reports and Returns of the Officers of the Corporation*. Sands & Neilson, 1833.

Jameson, Horatio G. "An Epitome of the More Important Circumstances Connected with the Epidemic Cholera." *Maryland Medical Recorder* 3, no. 1 (1832): 193–229.

Jameson, Horatio. *A Treatise on Epidemic Cholera*. Lindsay and Blakiston, 1855.

Latrobe, John H. B. *Picture of Baltimore, Containing a Description of All Objects of Interest in the City; and Embellished with Views of the Principal Public Buildings*. F. Lucas, Jr., 1832.

Latrobe, John H. B. *Southern Travels: Journal of John H. B. Latrobe*. Edited by Samuel Wilson. Historic New Orleans Collection, 1986.

Lee, Charles. "Medical Statistics of New York." *The American Journal of Medical Sciences* 19 (November 1836): 25–52.

Manley, James R. *Letters Addressed to the Board of Health, and to Richard Riker, Recorder of the City of New-York*. Peter Van Pelt, 1832.

McLean, Malcolm, ed. *Papers Concerning Robertson's Colony. Vol. 7: December 6, 1831, Through October 1833. Those Eleven-League Grants*. University of Texas at Arlington Press, 1980.

Mercer, Charles F. *Memorial of the Chesapeake and Ohio Canal Company to the General Assembly of Maryland, December 31, 1832*. Gales and Seaton, 1832.

"Mission to the Osage." *Missionary Herald* 32, no. 1 (January 1836): 24–25.

Mussey, Reuben Dimond, and Harvey Lindsly. *Temperance Prize Essays*. Duff Green, 1835.

New York Board of Health. *Report of the Commissioners Employed to Investigate the Origin and Nature of Epidemic Cholera in Canada*. Peter Van Pelt, 1832.

"No Great Loss Without Some Small Gain." *Christian Magazine: Conducted Under the Supervision of the Associate Reformed Synod of New-York* 1, no. 5 (May 1832): 159.

"Ohio. Western Reserve Temperance Convention." *Journal of the American Temperance Union* 2, no. 9 (September 1838): 141.

"On the Apartment for Criminals and Untried Prisoners, in the Arch Street Jail." *Hazard's Register of Pennsylvania* 11, no. 12 (March 23, 1833): 177–84.

"Osages." *Missionary Herald* 30, no. 1 (January 1834): 22–24.

Pennington, Samuel H. "Report for the Eastern District." In *The Rise, Minutes, and Proceedings, of the New Jersey Medical Society, Established July 23d, 1766*. Jennings & Hardham, 1875.

Pennsylvania General Assembly. *Report of the Committee Appointed to Investigate the Local Causes of Cholera in the Arch Street Prison*. Henry Welsh, 1833.

Pennsylvania State Temperance Society. *Memorial of the Board of Managers of the Pennsylvania State Temperance Society, to the Convention for Revising the Constitution of the State of Pennsylvania*. Brown & Sinquet, Printers, 1837.

Pennsylvania State Temperance Society. *Pennsylvania and New-Jersey Temperance Almanac for 1835*. Temperance Depository, 1835.

Pintard, John. *Letters from John Pintard to His Daughter, Eliza Noel Pintard Davidson, 1816–1833*. New York Historical Society, 1911.

Prucha, Francis Paul, ed. *Cherokee Removal: The "William Penn" Essays and Other Writings by Jeremiah Evarts*. University of Tennessee Press, 1981.

Reese, David Meredith. *A Plain and Practical Treatise on the Epidemic Cholera, as It Prevailed in the City of New York, in the Summer of 1832; Including Its Nature, Causes, Treatment and Prevention. Designed for Popular Instruction. To Which Is Added, by Way of Appendix, A Brief Essay on the Medical Use of Ardent Spirits; Being an Attempt to Show That Alcohol Is as Unnecessary and Mischievous in Sickness as in Health*. Conner & Cooke, 1833.

Report of the Committee Appointed to Investigate the Local Causes of Cholera in the Arch Street Prison, in the City of Philadelphia. Henry Welsh, 1833.

"Resolution for the Relief of William B. Mitchell." In *Compilation of the Laws of Pennsylvania, Relative to the Internal Improvements: Together with the Canal and Railway Regulations, as Established by the Board of Canal Commissioners*. Barrett and Parke, 1840.

"Sanitary Cordon." *Journal of Health* 3, no. 5 (November 9, 1831): 75–76.

[Sargent, Lucius M.] *Letters to John H. Hopkins, D. D. Bishop of the Protestant Episcopal Church for the Diocese of Vermont: Occasioned by His Lecture in Opposition to the Temperance Society. By An Episcopalian*. Chronicle Press, 1836.

Schirmer, Jacob Frederic. "The Schirmer Diary (continued)." *The South Carolina Historical Magazine* 69, no. 1 (January 1968): 59–65.

Scoutetten, Henri. *A Medical and Topographical History of the Cholera Morbus: Including the Mode of Prevention and Treatment*. Translated by A. S. Doane. Carter and Hendee, 1832.

Seager, Robert and Melba Porter Hay, eds. *The Papers of Henry Clay. Vol. 8: Candidate, Compromiser, Whig, March 5, 1829–December 31, 1836*. University of Kentucky Press, 1984.

Shattuck, Lemuel. *Report of the Sanitary Commission of Massachusetts, 1850*. Harvard University Press, 1948.

Sherrill, Hunting. *An Essay on Epidemics: as They Appeared in Dutchess County, from 1809 to 1824 . . . with an Appendix, Containing an Account of the Epidemic Cholera, as It Appeared in Poughkeepsie in 1832*. Booth & Smith, 1832.

Sherrill, Hunting. *On the Pathology of Epidemic Cholera*. S. Wood and Sons, 1835.

Short, Charles Wilkins. "A Brief Historical Sketch of the Origin and Progress of Cholera Asphyxia." *Transylvania Journal of Medicine and Associate Sciences* 11, no. 1 (January, February, and March 1838): 11–21.

Shyrock, Richard H., ed. *Letters of Richard D. Arnold, M.D. 1808–1876*. AMS Press, 1929.

Smith, Margaret Bayard. *The First Forty Years of Washington Society: Portrayed by the Family Letters of Mrs. Samuel Harrison Smith from the Collection of Her Grandson*. Scribner, 1906.

Smith, Mather J. *A Discourse on the Epidemic Cholera Morbus of Europe and Asia*. J. Seymour, 1831.

Southard, Samuel Lewis. *An Eulogium upon the Hon. Charles Ewing: Late Chief Justice of New Jersey*. D. Fenton, 1832.

Spencer, Thomas. *An Essay on the Nature of the Epidemic Usually Called Asiatic Cholera*. Webster and Skinners, 1833.

"Statement of Deaths, with the Diseases and Ages, in the City and Liberties of Philadelphia, During the Year 1834." *American Journal of Medical Sciences* 17 (November 1835): 261–264.

Stewart, Alvan. *An Essay on the Evils of Intemperance: Pronounced in the First Presbyterian Church, in Utica, on the 26th February 1833, at the Request of the Two Temperance Societies in the County of Oneida*. Gardiner Tracy, 1833.

Stockton, Rev. Thomas H. *Address Delivered in the Methodist Episcopal Church in Easton, Before the Temperance Society of Talbot County, Maryland, on the 26th day of February 1833*. John J. Harrod, 1833.

Storer, Bellamy. *An Address Delivered Before the Cincinnati Temperance Society, on the Twenty-Sixth Day of February 1833*. F. S. Benton, 1833.

Tanner, Henry Schenk. *Geographical and Statistical Account of the Epidemic Cholera*. Published by the Author, 1832.

"Treaty with the Choctaw, 1830." In *Indian Affairs: Laws and Treaties*. Vol. 2, edited by Charles Kappler. Government Printing Office, 1904.

US Census Office. *Abstract of the Returns of the Fifth Census*. Duff Green, 1832.

US Census Office. *Compendium of the Enumeration of the Inhabitants and Statistics of the United States, as Obtained at the Department of State, from the Returns of the Sixth Census*. Thomas Allen, 1841.

US Congress. Cholera Morbus, 22d Cong., 1st sess., January 20, 1832, House Report 226.

US Congress. *Register of Debates in Congress*. 22nd Cong., 1st sess., Vol. 8, pt. 1. Gales and Seaton, 1833.

Walworth, Reuben H. "Address." In *Fourth Annual Report of the New-York State Society for the Promotion of Temperance*. Packard and Van Benthuysen, 1833.

Watson, John, and Willis Hazard, eds. *Annals of Philadelphia, and Pennsylvania, in the Olden Time: Being a Collection of Memoirs, Anecdotes, and Incidents of the City and Its Inhabitants and of the Earliest Settlements of the Inland Part of Pennsylvania*. Vol. 3. E. S. Stuart, 1891.

"What Shall We Do?" *Journal of Health* 3, no. 23 (August 8, 1832): 355–58.

Wied, Maximilian. *Maximilian, Prince of Wied's Travels in the Interior of North America, Part III. Vol. 24: Early Western Travels, 1748–1846*, edited by Reuben Gold Thwaites. Arthur H. Clark Company, 1906.

Williams, James. *Narrative of James Williams, an American Slave, Who Was for Several Years a Driver on a Cotton Plantation in Alabama*. American Anti-Slavery Society; Isaac Knapp, 1838.

Yandell, Lunsford. "An Account of Spasmodic Cholera, as It Appeared in the City of Lexington, in June 1833." *Transylvania Journal of Medicine* 6, no. 2 (April, May, and June 1833): 197–222.

Yates, Christopher C. *Observations on the Epidemic Now Prevailing in the City of New-York; Called the Asiatic or Spasmodic Cholera; with Advice to the Planters of the South, for the Medical Treatment of Their Slaves*. George P. Scott and Co., 1832.

SELECTED SECONDARY MATERIAL

Books

Adler, Richard. *Cholera in Detroit: A History*. McFarland, 2013.

Akers, Donna L. *Living in the Land of Death: The Choctaw Nation, 1830–1860*. Michigan State University Press, 2004.

Archer, Randolph Edwin. *The Life of Rev. John Jasper, Pastor of Sixth Mt. Zion Baptist Church, Richmond, Va., from His Birth to the Present Time, with His Theory on the Rotation of the Sun*. R. T. Hill & Co., Publishers, 1884.

Baldasty, Gerald. *The Commercialization of News in the Nineteenth Century*. University of Wisconsin Press, 1992.

Baptist, Edward. *The Half Has Never Been Told: Slavery and the Making of American Capitalism*. Basic Books, 2014.

Bilson, Geoffrey. *A Darkened House: Cholera in Nineteenth-Century Canada*. University of Toronto Press, 1989.

Blake, Nelson Manfred. *Water for the Cities: A History of the Urban Water Supply Problem in the United States*. Syracuse University Press, 1956.

Bragg, George F. "Lewis G. Wells, M.D." In *Men of Maryland*. Church Advocate Press, 1914.

Bristow, Nancy. *American Pandemic: The Lost Worlds of the 1918 Influenza Pandemic*. Oxford University Press, 2012.

Brockman, R. John. *Commodore Robert F. Stockton, 1795–1866: Protean Man for a Protean Nation*. Cambria Press, 2009.

Campbell, Stephen W. *The Bank War and the Partisan Press: Newspapers, Financial Institutions, and the Post Office in Jacksonian America*. University of Kansas Press, 2019.

Chambers, J. S. *The Conquest of Cholera*. Macmillan Company, 1838.

Chittenden, Hiram Martin. *History of Early Steamboat Navigation on the Missouri River*. Vol 1. Francis P. Harper, 1903.

Cincinnati (Ohio) Board of Administration. *The Cincinnati Waterworks: A Paper Submitted by the Board of Administration for the Consideration of the Members of Hamilton County Delegation to the LXXII. General Assembly of Ohio*. Cincinnati Board of Administration, 1896.

Cohn, Samuel K., Jr. *Epidemics: Hate and Compassion from the Plague of Athens to AIDS*. Oxford University Press, 2018.

Corry, Sister Mary Alphonsa. *The Story of Father Van den Broek, O. P.; A Study of Holland and the Story of the Early Settlement of Wisconsin*. Ainsworth & Company, 1907.

Delaporte, François. *Disease and Civilisation, the Cholera in Paris, 1832*. Translated by A. Goldhammer. Harvard University Press, 1986.

DeRosier, Arthur. *The Removal of the Choctaw Indians*. University of Tennessee Press, 1981.

Deyle, Steven. *Carry Me Back: The Domestic Slave Trade in American Life*. Oxford University Press, 2005.

Durey, Michael. *The Return of the Plague: British Society and the Cholera, 1831–1832*. Gill and Macmillan, 1979.

Edwards, Ninian Wirt. *History of Illinois, from 1778–1833; and Life and Times of Ninian Edwards*. The Illinois State Journal Company, 1870.

Edwards, Tai. *Osage Women and Empire: Gender and Power*. University of Kansas Press, 2018.

Evans, Richard J. *Death in Hamburg: Society and Politics in the Cholera Years, 1830–1910*. Oxford University Press, 1987.

Fenn, Elizabeth. *Pox Americana: The Great Smallpox Epidemic of 1775–82*. Farrar, Straus and Giroux, 2001.

Foreman, Grant. *Indian Removal: The Emigration of the Five Civilized Tribes of Indians*. University of Oklahoma Press, 1972.

Freehling, Alison Goodyear. *Drift Toward Dissolution: The Virginia Slavery Debate of 1831–1832*. Louisiana State University Press, 1982.

Greenidge, Kerri K. *The Grimkes: The Legacy of Slavery in an American Family*. Liveright, 2023.

Gudmestad, Robert. *A Troublesome Commerce: The Transformation of the Interstate Slave Trade*. Louisiana State University Press, 2003.

Haller, John S., Jr. *The People's Doctors: Samuel Thomson and the American Botanical Movement, 1790–1860*. Southern Illinois University Press, 2000.

Hamlin, Christopher. *Cholera: The Biography*. Oxford University Press, 2009.

Handy, Rt. Rev. James A. *Scraps of African Methodist Episcopal History*. A. M. E. Book Concern, [1902].

Harper, Kyle. *Plagues upon the Earth: Disease and the Course of Human History*. Princeton University Press, 2021.

Hirota, Hidetaka. *Expelling the Poor: Atlantic Seaboard States and the Nineteenth-Century Origins of American Immigration Policy*. Oxford University Press, 2017.

Horine, Emmet Field. *Daniel Drake: Pioneer Physician of the Midwest*. University of Pennsylvania Press, 1961.

Howe, David Walker. *What God Hath Wrought! The Transformation of America, 1815–1848*. Oxford University Press, 2007.

Jacobson, Matthew Frye. *Whiteness of a Different Color: European Immigrants and the Alchemy of Race*. Harvard University Press, 1998.

Jung, Patrick J. *The Black Hawk War of 1832*. University of Oklahoma Press, 2007.

Kelton, Paul. *Cherokee Medicine Colonial Germs: An Indigenous Nation's Fight Against Smallpox, 1518–1824*. University of Oklahoma Press, 2015.

Kenny, Kevin. *The American Irish: A History*. Longman, 2000.

Lawrence, Charles. *History of the Philadelphia Almshouses and Hospitals from the Beginning of the Eighteenth to the Ending of the Nineteenth Centuries, Covering a Period of Nearly Two Hundred Years, Showing the Mode of Distributing Public Relief Through the Management of the Boards of Overseers of the Poor, Guardians of the Poor and the Directors of the Department of Charities and Correction*. n.p., 1905.

Lerner, Gerda. *The Grimké Sisters of South Carolina: Pioneers for Women's Rights and Abolition*. Rev. ed. University of North Carolina Press, 2004.

McCracken, Henry Noble. *Blithe Dutchess: The Flowering of an American County from 1812*. Hastings House, 1958.

McGrew, Roderick. *Russia and the Cholera, 1823–1832*. University of Wisconsin Press, 1965.

Melosi, Martin. *The Sanitary City: Environmental Services in Urban America from Colonial Times to the Present*. University of Pittsburgh Press, 2008.

Mifflin, Benjamin C. *Charles Mifflin, M.D., with an Account of his Ancestors and Ancestral Connections*. Riverside Press, 1876.

Miller, Kerby A. *Emigrants and Exiles: Ireland and the Irish Exodus to North America*. Oxford University Press, 1985.

Morris, R. J. *Cholera, 1832: The Social Response to an Epidemic*. Holmes & Meier, 1976.

Mould, Tom. *Choctaw Tales*. University of Mississippi Press, 2004.

Muser, Janet. *Rocky Hill, Kingston, and Griggstown*. Arcadia Publishing, 1998.

Noble, Jane B., ed. *The River Trail: A Saga of the Cherokee Removal*. Cross Cultural Education Center, n.d.

O'Brassill-Kulfan, Kristin. *Vagrants and Vagabonds: Poverty and Mobility in the Early American Republic*. New York University Press, 2019.

Olivarius, Kathryn. *Necropolis: Disease, Power, and Capitalism in the Cotton Kingdom*. Harvard University Press, 2022.

Osborn, Matthew Warner. *Rum Maniacs: Alcoholic Insanity in the Early American Republic*. University of Chicago Press, 2014.

Oshinsky, David. *Bellevue: Three Centuries of Medicine and Mayhem at America's Most Storied Hospital*. Doubleday, 2016.

Pelling, Margaret. *Cholera, Fever, and English Medicine, 1825–1865*. Oxford University Press, 1978.

Porter, Roy. *The Greatest Benefit to Mankind: A Medical History of Humanity*. Norton, 1999.

Ramage, James A. *Kentucky Rising: Democracy, Slavery, and Culture from the Early Republic to the Civil War*. University of Kentucky Press, 2011.

Rhodes, Richard. *John James Audubon: The Making of an American*. Knopf, 2004.

Richmond (VA) Department of Public Utilities. *Watering the City of Richmond*. William Byrd Press, 1930.

Rollins, Willard Hughes. *Unaffected by the Gospel: Osage Resistance to the Christian Invasion (1673–1906): A Cultural History*. University of New Mexico Press, 2004.

Rothman, Joshua. *The Ledger and the Chain: How Domestic Slave Traders Shaped America*. Basic Books, 2021.

Rohrbaugh, W. J. *The Alcoholic Republic: An American Tradition*. Oxford University Press, 1981.

Rosenberg, Charles. *The Cholera Years: The United States in 1832, 1849, and 1866*. University of Chicago Press, 1962.

Saunt, Claudio. *Unworthy Republic: The Dispossession of Native Americans and the Road to Indian Territory*. W. W. Norton, 2020.

Schermerhorn, Calvin. *The Business of Slavery and the Rise of American Capitalism, 1815–1860*. Yale University Press, 2015.

Shah, Sonia. *Pandemic: Tracking Contagions, From Cholera to Ebola and Beyond*. Sarah Crichton Books/Farrar, Straus and Giroux, 2016.

Snowden, Frank. *Naples in the Time of Cholera, 1884–1911*. Cambridge University Press, 1995.

Snowden, Frank. *Epidemics and Society from the Black Death to the Present*. Yale University Press, 2019.

Snyder, Christina. *Great Crossings: Indians, Settlers, and Slaves in the Age of Jackson*. Oxford University Press, 2017.

Starr, Paul. *The Social Transformation of American Medicine*. 2nd ed. Basic Books, 2017.

Stevenson, David. *Sketch of the Civil Engineering of North America*. John Weale, Architectural Library, 1838.

Tadman, Michael. *Speculators and Slaves: Masters, Traders, and Slaves in the Old South*. University of Wisconsin Press, 1989.

Tomes, Nancy. *The Gospel of Germs: Men, Women, and the Microbe in American Life*. Harvard University Press, 1998.

Tyrell, Ian R. *Sobering Up: From Temperance to Prohibition in Antebellum America, 1800–1860*. Greenwood Press, 1979.

Valenčius, Conevery Bolton. *The Health of the Country: How American Settlers Understood Themselves and Their Land*. Basic Books, 2002.

Watson, William E., and J. Francis Watson. *Massacre at Duffy's Cut: Tragedy & Conspiracy on the Pennsylvania Railroad*. The History Press, 2018.

Way, Peter. *Common Labour: Workers and the Digging of North American Canals, 1780–1860*. Cambridge University Press, 1993.

Wilentz, Sean. *The Rise of American Democracy: Jefferson to Lincoln*. Norton, 2005.

Woodworth, John M. *The Cholera Epidemic of 1873 in the United States*. Government Printing Office, 1875.

Articles

Ahmad, K., K. Jahan, and I. Huq. "Decontamination of Drinking Water by Alum for the Preparation of Oral Rehydration Solution." *Food and Nutritional Bulletin* 6, no. 2 (1984): 1–4.

Anderson, Warwick. "Excremental Colonialism: Public Health and the Poetics of Pollution." *Critical Inquiry* 21, (1995): 640–69.

Arnold, David. "Cholera and Colonialism in British India." *Past & Present* 113 (1986): 118–51.

Baird, Nancy D. "Asiatic Cholera's First Visit to Kentucky: A Study in Panic and Fear." *Filson Club Historical Quarterly* 48, no. 3 (1974): 228–40.

Barabanova, Kseniya. "The First Cholera Epidemic in St. Petersburg." *Arcadia* 6 (2014). Rachel Carson Center for Environment and Society. https://doi.org/10.5282/rcc/5385.

Barr, Marleen. "Deborah Norris Logan, Feminist Criticism, and Identity Theory: Interpreting a Woman's Diary Without the Danger of Separatism." *Biography* 8, no. 1 (1985): 12–24.

Berdan, Marshall S. "The Pestilence That Walketh in Darkness: The Cholera Epidemic of 1832." *Virginia Cavalcade* 43, no. 1 (1993): 14–23.

Bordelon, Christine. "New Park Celebrates Irish Contributions to New Orleans." *Clarion Herald: Official Newspaper of the Archdiocese of New Orleans*. https://clarionherald.org/news/new-park-celebrates-irish-contributions-to-new-orleans.

Carter, Ruth C. "Cincinnatians and Cholera: Attitudes Toward the Epidemics of 1832 and 1849." *Queen City Heritage* 50, no. 3 (1992): 32–48.

Chandler, Josephine, T. Tenny Chandler, and Charles Chandler. "Dr. Charles Chandler: His Place in the American Scene." *Journal of the Illinois State Historical Society* 24, no. 3 (October 1931): 369–552.

Chari, S., S. Teyssen, and M. V. Singer. "Alcohol and Gastric Acid Secretion in Humans." *Gut* 34, no. 6 (1993): 843–47.

"Cholera Epidemic of 1832." *Encyclopedia of Cleveland History*. 2025. https://case.edu/ech/articles/c/cholera-epidemic-1832

"The Colored People. A Day's Account of What They Are Doing and Saying. An Address by Frederick Douglass." *Baltimore Sun*, September 7, 1891.

"Death Ends Long Career of Optimism and Charity." *Louisville Herald*, November 24, 1905.

Donaldson, Gary A. "Bringing Water to the Crescent City: Benjamin Latrobe and the New Orleans Waterworks System." *Louisiana History: The Journal of the Louisiana Historical Association* 28 (Autumn 1987): 381–96.

"'Duffy's Cut Part Two' as Team Uncovers Fresh Mass Burial Site." *Derry Journal*, June 5, 2020. https://www.derryjournal.com/news/people/duffys-cut-part-two-as-teamuncovers-fresh-mass-burial-site-2875720.

Edwards, Tai, and Paul Kelton. "Germs, Genocides, and America's Indigenous Peoples." *Journal of American History* 107, no. 1 (June 2020): 52–76.

Espinosa, Mariola. "The Question of Racial Immunity to Yellow Fever in History and Historiography." *Social Science History* 38 (Winter 2014): 437–52.

Evans, Richard J. "Epidemics and Revolutions: Cholera in Nineteenth-Century Europe." *Past & Present* 120 (August 1988): 123–46.

Fidel, Steve. "Zion's Camp Monument Recalls 15 Members Who Died of Cholera." *Deseret News*, August 30, 1997. https://www.deseret.com/1997/8/30/19331274/zion-s-camp-monument-recalls-15-members-who-died-of-cholera/.

Foreman, Carolyn Thomas. "The Armstrongs of Indian Territory." *Chronicles of Oklahoma* 30 (Autumn 1952): 292–307.

Francis, Samuel W. "Biographical Sketches of Distinguished Living New York Physicians, X. Isaac Wood, M.D." *The Medical and Surgical Reporter* 15 (July–December 1866): 454–58.

Frost, Meigs O. "Filling Recalls Death of 10,000 in Digging Canal." *The Times-Picayune New Orleans States*, July 18, 1937.

Galishoff, Stuart. "Cholera in Newark, New Jersey." *Journal of the History of Medicine and Allied Sciences* 25 (October 1970): 438–48.

Godfrey, Matthew C. "'We Believe the Hand of the Lord Is in It': Memories of Divine Intervention in the Zion's Camp Expedition." *BYU Studies Quarterly* 56, no. 4 (2017): 99–132.

Greenberg, Zoe. "Evidence Suggesting a Second Mass Grave of Irish Railroad Workers is Unearthed in Downington." *Philadelphia Inquirer*, July 15, 2025.

Halley, R. A. "Paul Fitzsimons Eve, A.M., M.D., LL.D." *The American Historical Magazine and Tennessee Historical Quarterly* 9, no. 4 (October 1904): 281–342.

Harrison, Mark. "A Dreadful Scourge: Cholera in Early Nineteenth-Century India." *Modern Asian Studies* 54, no. 2 (2020): 502–33.

Harvey, Katherine A. "Practicing Medicine at the Baltimore Almshouse, 1828–1850." *Maryland Historical Magazine* 74, no. 3 (September 1979): 223–37.

Hutslar, Donald. "'God's Scourge': The Cholera Years in Ohio." *Ohio History* 105 (Summer/Autumn 1996): 174–91.

Jortner, Adam. "Cholera, Christ, and Jackson: The Epidemic of 1832 and the Origins of Christian Politics in Antebellum America." *Journal of the Early Republic* 27 (Summer 2007): 233–64.

Kanungo, Suman, Andrew S. Azman, Thandavarayan Ramamurthy, Jaqueline Deen, Shanta Dutta. "Cholera." *The Lancet* 399 (April 2022): 1429–40.

Kelton, Paul. "Pandemic Injustice: Irish Immigrant, Enslaved African American, and Choctaw Experiences with Cholera in 1832." *Journal of Southern History* 88, no. 1 (February 2022): 73–110.

Killick, J.R. "Yeatman, Thomas (1787–1833), Merchant and Banker." *American National Biography* (February 2000). https://doi.org/10.1093/anb/9780198606697.article.1002178.

Knight, Louise W. "Grimké, Thomas Smith," *American National Biography* (October 2015). https://doi.org/10.1093/anb/9780198606697.article.1101229.

Lauck, George. "Early History of the Lutheran Sunday School." Bucyrus (OH) *Journal*, April 25, 1879.

Lund, Matthew B. "A Society of Like-Minded Men: American Localism and the Mormon Expulsion from Jackson County." *Journal of Mormon History* 40 (Summer 2014): 169–200.

McCabe, Louise B. "Cholera, Germantown, 1832: Suspicion and Science." *Germantown Crier* 64 (Spring 2014): 21–25.

O'Brassill-Kulfan, Kristin, "'People First': Interpreting and Commemorating Houselessness and Poverty." *The Public Historian* 45 (February 2023): 25–50.

Olson, Greg. "Plague on the Prairie: The Cholera Epidemic of 1833 and Its Impact on One Illinois Town." *Illinois Heritage* 5 (January 2002): 6–9.

Osborne, John B. "Preparing for the Pandemic: City Boards of Health and the Arrival of Cholera in Montreal, New York, and Philadelphia in 1832." *Urban History Review* 36 (Spring 2008): 29–42.

Osborne, John B. "Cholera." *Encyclopedia of Greater Philadelphia*. 2010. https://philadelphiaencyclopedia.org/archive/cholera/.

Pan, Jiaqi, Li Cen, Weixing Chen, Chaohui Yu, Youming Li, and Zhe Shen. "Alcohol Consumption and the Risk of Gastroesophageal Reflux Disease: A Systematic Review and Meta-Analysis." *Alcohol and Alcoholism* 54, no. 1 (January 2019): 62–69.

Petriello, David. "'A People So Well Fed and So Clean': The 1832 Cholera Pandemic in New Jersey." *NJS: An Interdisciplinary Journal* (Winter 2020): 91–115.

Prashad, Viyah. "Native Dirt/Imperial Ordure: The Cholera of 1832 and the Morbid Resolutions of Modernity." *Journal of Historical Sociology* 7, no. 3 (1994): 243–60.

Radke, Andrea G. "We Also Marched: The Women and Children of Zion's Camp, 1834." *BYU Studies Quarterly* 39, no. 1 (2000): 147–65.

"Recollections of an Old Citizen." *New Orleans Times-Democrat*, September 10, 1893.

Rosenberg, Charles. "Cholera in Nineteenth-Century Europe: A Tool for Social and Economic Analysis." *Comparative Studies in Society and History* 8 (July 1966): 452–63.

Rosenblum, Thom. "Driving Out the Slave Traders: The Natchez Uprising of 1833." *Journal of Mississippi History* 67 (March 2005): 45–67.

Rowley, William E. "The Albany Microscope: Gadfly for Jacksonian Democracy." *New York History* 71, no. 2 (April 1990): 172–206.

Schuetze, Sarah. "Mapping a Demon Malady: Cholera Maps and Affect in 1832." *Common-Place: The Interactive Journal of Early American Life* 17, no. 1 (Fall 2016). https://commonplace.online/article/mapping-a-demon-malady/.

Schwartz, James Z. "'A Melancholy and Trying Season': Cholera and the Conflict over Cultural Boundaries in Early Michigan." *Journal of the Early Republic* 26 (Spring 2006): 95–116.

Singer, M. V., and C. Leffmann. "Alcohol and Gastric Acid Secretion in Humans: A Short Review." *Scandinavian Journal of Gastroenterology*. Supplement 146. (1988): 11–21.

Tuite, Ashleigh R., Christina H. Chan, and David N. Fisman. "Cholera, Canals, and Contagion: Rediscovering Dr. Beck's Report." *Journal of Public Health Policy* 32, (August 2011): 320–33.

Warring, Joseph. "Asiatic Cholera in South Carolina." *Bulletin of the History of Medicine* 40, (September 1966): 459–66.

Wilford, John Noble. "How Epidemics Helped Shape the Modern Metropolis." *New York Times*, April 15, 2008.

DISSERTATIONS, THESES, AND REPORTS

Dawson, Sara Kathryn. "The 1833 Cholera Epidemic in Lexington: A Study of Devastation and Recovery." MA Thesis, University of Kentucky, 1994.

Hawn, Virginia. "Baltimore's Reaction to the Cholera Epidemic, Summer, 1832, as Reflected by the City's Newspapers." Typed Report, Goucher College, 1962, in possession of Maryland Historical Society.

Kolb, Carolyn Goldsby. "At the Confluence of Science and Power: Water Struggles of New Orleans in the Nineteenth Century." PhD Dissertation, University of New Orleans, 2006.

WEBSITES

Baird, Nancy. "Asiatic Cholera in Kentucky 1832 to 1873." Ohio County, Kentucky, History (blog). December 9, 2020. https://ohiocountykentuckyhistory.blogspot.com/2020/12/cholera.html.

Brinegar, Pam. "List of Deaths—1833." RootsWeb. 2006. https://sites.rootsweb.com/~kyfayett/1833_deaths_reporter.htm.

Campanella, Richard. "Managing Streets, Utilities, and Municipal Services in Historic New Orleans." Preservation Resource Center of New Orleans. December 1, 2012. https://prcno.org/managing-streets-utilities-municipal-services-historic-new-orleans/.

Chance, Lil. "Stenton's Cultural Landscape, Part 1: 1730–1900." Stenton: A House of Learning, Past and Present. 2015. https://www.stenton.org/cultural-landscape-1.

City of Norfolk. "City of Norfolk Utilities." 2025. https://www.norfolk.gov/DocumentCenter/View/74743/Utilities-Pamphlet.

Delaware and Raritan Canal Commission. "A Brief History of the Delaware and Raritan Canal." Official Site of the State of New Jersey. 1996–2020. https://www.nj.gov/dep/drcc/about-canal/history/.

Drinkaware. "Is Alcohol Harming Your Stomach?" October 22, 2025. https://www.drinkaware.co.uk/facts/health-effects-of-alcohol/general-health-effects/is-alcohol-harming-your-stomach.

Ewing Township Historic Preservation Society. "Biography of Charles Ewing." Ewing Township. https://www.ewingnj.org/charlesewing.

Francis, Gerald A. "The Philadelphia & Columbia Railway." The Lower Merion Historical Society. 2025. https://collections.lowermerionhistory.org/home/full-text/contents/columbia-railway/.

Franklin, Kevin. "A Short Biography of Engineer Benjamin Prescott." New York Almanack. June 25, 2015. https://www.newyorkalmanack.com/2015/06/a-short-biography-of-engineer-benjamin-prescott/.

Gibson, Campbell. "Population of the 100 Largest Cities and Other Urban Places in the United States: 1790–1990." Working Paper POP-WOP0327. United States Census Bureau. https://www.census.gov/library/working-papers/1998/demo/POP-twps0027.html.

Investing in Native Communities. "First Choctaw Forced Removal Causes Death of Thousands." 2025. https://nativephilanthropy.candid.org/events/first-choctaw-forced-removal-causes-death-of-thousands/.

IrishCentral. "Inspiring Emigrant Letters Home to Ireland from America in the Famine Era." October 31, 2024. https://www.irishcentral.com/roots/history/letters-ireland-america-famine.

Le Canada: A People's History/Une Histoire Populaire. "Rising Population and Immigration." 2001. https://www.cbc.ca/history/EPCONTENTSE1EP7CH1PA2LE.html.

Marion, Forrest L. "Perspective: 'The Dreaded Cholera' in Kentucky, 1832–1833." Aquila Report. 2020. https://www.baruch.cuny.edu/nycdata/disasters/cholera-1832.html.

Olar, Jared. "Pekin in the Time of Cholera: The 'Blue Death' Comes to Pekin." Pekin (IL) Public Library. November 2, 2023. https://pekinpubliclibrary.org/pekin-in-the-time-of-cholera-the-blue-death-comes-to-pekin/.

Pierce, Morris A. *Documentary History of American Waterworks*. http://www.waterworkshistory.us/.

Pittsburgh Water. "Our History." 2025. https://www.pgh2o.com/about-us/mission-vision-and-core-values/our-history.

Richardson, Evelyn. "Cholera Epidemic Hits Logan County in 1835." Franklin Favorite. December 23, 2020. https://www.franklinfavorite.com/article_1021f63c-7b61-50c1-bb04-bb99bb06965c.html.

Schuyler County, Illinois, Genealogy and History. "News of Epidemics." 2025. https://genealogytrails.com/ill/schuyler/1834CholeraEpidemic.html.

Starr, S. Frederick, and Jack Stewart, "The Rise and Fall of the New Orleans Cistern." Preservation Resource Center of New Orleans. March 14, 2018. https://prcno.org/rise-fall-new-orleans-cistern/.

State of New Jersey Department of Environmental Protection. "Honoring the Irish Who Built the D&R Canal." News release, March 17, 2003. https://dep.nj.gov/newsrel/03_0030/.

University of Cincinnati, College of Medicine. "About Daniel Drake." 2025. https://med.uc.edu/about/daniel-drake-medal/daniel-drake.

World Health Organization, Eastern Mediterranean Region. "WHO Regional Director's Statement on Cholera Outbreaks." November 2, 2022. https://www.emro.who.int/media/news/who-regional-director-for-the-eastern-mediterraneans-statement-on-cholera-outbreaks.html.

Index

For the benefit of digital users, indexed terms that span two pages (e.g., 52–53) may, on occasion, appear on only one of those pages.